Clinical Topics in Teaching Psychiatry

Clinical Topics in Teaching Psychiatry

A Guide for Clinicians

Edited by

Sarah Huline-Dickens
Peninsula Deanery

Patricia Casey
Hermitage Medical Clinic, Dublin

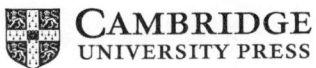

CAMBRIDGE
UNIVERSITY PRESS

University Printing House, Cambridge CB2 8BS, United Kingdom

One Liberty Plaza, 20th Floor, New York, NY 10006, USA

477 Williamstown Road, Port Melbourne, VIC 3207, Australia

314–321, 3rd Floor, Plot 3, Splendor Forum, Jasola District Centre,
New Delhi – 110025, India

103 Penang Road, #05–06/07, Visioncrest Commercial, Singapore 238467

Cambridge University Press is part of the University of Cambridge.

It furthers the University's mission by disseminating knowledge in the pursuit of
education, learning, and research at the highest international levels of excellence.

www.cambridge.org
Information on this title: www.cambridge.org/9781009054690
DOI: 10.1017/9781009053938

© Royal College of Psychiatrists 2023

First published 2023

A catalogue record for this publication is available from the British Library.

ISBN 978-1-009-05469-0 Paperback

....

With sincere gratitude to Professor Peter Tyrer, my longstanding educational and professional mentor
Patricia Casey

To Michael Carter
Sarah Huline-Dickens

Contents

Contributors

Elizabeth Anderson is a professor of interprofessional education at the University of Leicester Medical School, UK.

Oliver Batham is a specialty trainee in child and adolescent psychiatry at South London and Maudsley NHS Foundation Trust, UK.

Joshua Bellevue de Sylva is a higher trainee working in Cheshire and Wirral Partnership NHS Foundation Trust, UK. Formerly CPD Lead for The Royal College of Psychiatrists

Dinesh Bhugra is an emeritus professor of mental health and diversity at the Institute of Psychiatry at King's College London, UK and an honorary consultant psychiatrist at the South London and Maudsley NHS Foundation Trust, UK.

Guy Brookes is a consultant general adult psychiatrist at the Leeds and York Partnerships Foundation Trust, UK. Formerly CPD Lead for The Royal College of Psychiatrists

Nick Brown is a retired consultant psychiatrist and senior assessment adviser for the National Clinical Assessment Service. Formerly, he was Associate Dean at the Royal College of Psychiatrists.

Andrea Cipriani is a professor of psychiatry at the Department of Psychiatry, University of Oxford, UK and an honorary consultant psychiatrist at Oxford Health NHS Foundation Trust, UK.

Patricia Casey is Consultant in Liaison Psychiatry at the Hermitage Medical Clinic, Dublin, Professor Emeritus of Psychiatry at University College, Dublin, Republic of Ireland and is the editor of *BJPsych Advances*, Royal College of Psychiatrists, London, UK.

Christopher C. S. Cheok is chief and senior consultant psychiatrist at the Department of Forensic Psychiatry, Institute of Mental Health, Singapore.

Victor Cohn is an ST6 specialty trainee in general adult psychiatry at Camden and Islington NHS Foundation Trust, UK.

David Cottrell is an emeritus professor of child and adolescent psychiatry at the University of Leeds, UK.

Arthita Das is a consultant psychiatrist in Rotherham, Doncaster and South Humber Trust, UK and a specialist advisor to the Royal College of Psychiatrists on foundation training.

Subodh Dave is a consultant psychiatrist and Deputy Director of Undergraduate Medical Education at Derbyshire Healthcare NHS Foundation Trust, UK, a professor of psychiatry at the University of Bolton, UK and Dean of the Royal College of Psychiatrists.

Riccardo De Giorgi is a Wellcome Trust doctoral training fellow at the Department of Psychiatry, University of Oxford, and an honorary clinical fellow at Oxford Health NHS Foundation Trust, UK.

Monica Doshi is a semi-retired consultant psychiatrist. Formerly, she was an honorary associate professor in medical education at the Warwick Medical School, UK.

Eleanor Dryhurst is a consultant child and adolescent psychiatrist and Medical Lead for RISE Children's Services in Coventry and Warwickshire Partnership Trust, UK. and Training Programme Director for the Birmingham MRCPsych Course.

John R. Geddes is WA Handley Professor of Psychiatry, University of Oxford and director of the National Institute for Health Research Oxford Health Biomedical Research Centre, Oxford Health NHS Foundation Trust, UK.

Jayne Greening is the head of West Midlands Post-Graduate School of Psychiatry and a consultant in adult psychiatry in Burton on Trent, UK.

Allys Guérandel is a consultant psychiatrist in the Department of Psychiatry and Mental Health Research, St Vincent's University Hospital, Dublin, and a clinical professor in the School of Medicine and Medical Science, University College Dublin, Republic of Ireland.

Cyrus S. H. Ho is a consultant psychiatrist at the National University Hospital, Singapore and also an assistant professor in the Department of Psychological Medicine, Yong Loo Lin School of Medicine, National University of Singapore.

Roger C. M. Ho is a professor and senior consultant psychiatrist at the National University of Singapore.

Gareth Holsgrove is a retired head of postgraduate educational services at the Royal College of Psychiatrists and former head of the academic unit of medical and dental education at St Bartholomew's and the Royal London Hospital Medical School, UK.

Sarah Huline-Dickens is a consultant in child and adolescent psychiatry at Livewell Southwest and Associate Dean for Peninsula Deanery, UK.

Thomas Hewson is an academic clinical fellow at the University of Manchester, UK and a core training level 3 clinical trainee at the Health Education North West School of Psychiatry, UK.

Antonina Ingrassia is a consultant child and adolescent psychiatrist and lead clinician at South London and Maudsley NHS Foundation Trust, and an honorary senior lecturer at King's College London, UK.

Radhika Kanessan is a community consultant psychiatrist at Sutherland Centre, Stoke on Trent, North Staffordshire Combined Healthcare NHS Trust and the MRCPSych course lead for Keele University–University Hospitals of North Midlands NHS Trust, UK.

Brendan D. Kelly is a professor of psychiatry at Trinity College Dublin and a consultant psychiatrist at Tallaght University Hospital, Dublin, Republic of Ireland.

Daniel Kinnair is a consultant general adult psychiatrist at the Leicester Partnership NSH Trust and an honorary associate professor at the University of Leicester, UK.

Anna Ludvigsen is the simulation-based-learning lead at Nottinghamshire Healthcare NHS Foundation Trust, Nottingham, UK.

Amit Malik has worked in mental health globally as a senior clinical psychiatrist and professional leader.

Fiona McMaster has been a public health and behavioral science academic, an innovation consultant and now runs the training and research company, Eskal Ltd, UK.

Andrew Northern is a teacher of academic STEMM research communication at the Centre for Academic English, Imperial College London, UK and a senior fellow of the Higher Education Academy.

Brían Ó Ruairc is a medical graduate from the National University of Ireland, Galway, and a graduate in history and political science at Trinity College Dublin, Republic of Ireland and currently working as an intern in the University College Dublin intern network,

Gareth Rees is a consultant in general adult psychiatry in Birmingham Women's and Children's NHS Foundation Trust, and honorary clinical lecturer at the University of Birmingham, UK.

Kris Roberts is a core training level 3 doctor in psychiatry at the Leicestershire Partnership NHS Trust, UK.

S. Neil Sarkar is a Consultant Psychiatrist in Women's Psychiatric Intensive Care at Camden and Islington NHS Foundation Trust, Honorary Clinical Senior Teaching Fellow at University College London, and Fellow of the Higher Education Academy, UK.

Sridevi Sira Mahalingappa is a consultant psychiatrist at Western Sydney Local Health District, Australia, an honorary assistant professor at the University of Nottingham, UK, and honorary clinical teaching fellow at Derbyshire Healthcare NHS Foundation Trust, UK.

Holly Smith is a higher trainee in Rotherham, Doncaster and South Humber Trust, UK.

Katharine A. Smith is an Honorary Consultant Psychiatrist at the Department of Psychiatry, University of Oxford, UK and Oxford Health NHS Foundation Trust, Warneford Hospital, Oxford, UK.

Katherine E. Stevens was the research administrator of the Oxford Precision Psychiatry Laboratory at the National Institute for Health Research Biomedical Research Centre, Oxford, UK.

Geraldine Swift is a consultant in liaison psychiatry and Director of Medical Education in Cheshire and Wirral Partnership NHS Foundation Trust, UK.

Hiberet Tessema Belay is a consultant general adult psychiatrist in the Department of Psychiatry, Connolly Hospital Blanchardstown, Dublin, Republic of Ireland.

Erin Turner is a consultant psychiatrist at the Solihull Early Intervention for Psychosis Service, Birmingham and Solihull Mental Health NHS Foundation Trust (BSMHFT) and head of the BSMHFT Clinical Teaching Academy, UK.

Peter Tyrer is an emeritus professor of community psychiatry at Imperial College, London and a consultant in transformation psychiatry in Lincolnshire Partnership NHS Foundation Trust, UK.

Guy Undrill was an acute psychiatrist and Director of Medical Education at Gloucestershire Health and Care NHS Foundation Trust, UK.

Caroline Winkle is a consultant in old age psychiatry at Midlands Partnership NHS Foundation Trust, and Undergraduate Support Tutor at Keele Medical School, UK.

Anne Worrall-Davies is Senior Psychiatrist Lead (Children and Young People) for the Learning Disability and Autism Programme, NHS England and NHS Improvement, UK.

Melvyn W. B. Zhang is a consultant psychiatrist at the National Addictions Management Service, Institute of Mental Health, Singapore Institute of Mental Health, Singapore.

A Note on the Cover

Sarah Huline-Dickens and Patricia Casey

There are few well known images in medical education. This one, *Une leçon clinique à la Salpêtrière* (A clinical lesson at the Salpêtrière) by Brouillet, 1887, is supposed to show a group portrait of the famous neurologist Charcot (1825–1893) giving a demonstration of clinical signs in a female patient to postgraduate students.

Charcot has been the subject of much critique culturally and scientifically; but his teaching courses on hysteria and hypnotism were much celebrated in the 1870s, and he was an important influence on Freud at the start of his academic career. The picture captures the sense of drama of the event: students with rapt attention clearly spellbound by what they are seeing or have just seen. Maybe a few are sceptical. The light from the obscured windows softly illuminates their fascinated faces. Whatever one's thoughts about Charcot and what he was doing to the woman at the centre of the picture - and the male gaze upon her half-covered torso - this image was perhaps intended to show the shedding of light on unexplained phenomena, the progress of scientific investigation, and that feeling of wonder which can happen when a group of learners meet to witness something extraordinary.

Introduction

Sarah Huline-Dickens and Patricia Casey

Drawing on case studies, updated papers from *BJPsych Advances* and specially commissioned new chapters, this book takes a scholarly approach to the whole range of teaching and learning as applied to psychiatry. This covers direct teaching of the speciality of psychiatry through to educational management, coaching and mentoring. It provides essential information on topics not often covered, and it will provide guidance for busy clinicians who are acting as trainers, and for those who teach and train medical students in university departments

Many of the chapters are written by figures of significant educational status within clinical psychiatry. These include a new chapter on literature searching; chapters on technological aspects of teaching such as webinars and virtual placements (the importance of which has been brought into focus by the recent effects of the pandemic on how training is organized); and writing for learning and publication.

Teaching teachers how to teach is a neglected topic in medicine generally and this book aim to fill this vacuum with accessible and clearly written material on basics such as how to deliver a 'good' lecture, how to run a webinar, how to make 'Powerpoint' interesting and how to gain access to up-to-date information without feeling overwhelmed

Before and after COVID-19

This book was conceived before the coronavirus (COVID-19) pandemic which has so dramatically transformed the clinical and training lives of so many doctors. Before this event there were already many concerns about the welfare of trainees (not just psychiatrists) in clinical environments. This theme is addressed in this book in a way that may be helpful: no longer should it be seen as stigmatizing to admit that you are struggling in your working environment. The new chapters on coaching and mentoring and how best to support trainees in difficulty remind us of the importance of the human connection between trainers and trainees.

Virtual clinics and virtual conferences and meetings are good examples of some of the developments that trainers and trainees were obliged to adopt when the pandemic struck in 2020. How reassuring it was at that time to watch the webinars rapidly produced by the Royal College of Psychiatrists. We are yet to see how many of the changes made to accommodate remote teaching and learning will remain (probably quite a few). Professor Subodh Dave, now Dean of the College, along with colleagues, was also instrumental in helping many of us come to terms with virtual teaching, very soon after the start of the pandemic, through informative webinars suggesting imaginative strategies broadcast from the Association of University Teachers of Psychiatry (AUTP). A new landscape of technical terms of engagement has emerged including being 'on mute'; how to raise your virtual hand and remembering to lower it again; and those comments about 'it's in the chat'. And what to do about 'lurkers' (i.e., those who seem to be at the meeting but make no contributions). Other ways of harnessing technology have been demonstrated by the use of smartphones and portfolio-based learning and e learning.

However, for psychiatrists who are always attentive to the non-verbal cues in the consultation and mindful of what is going on off camera, the exclusive use of telephone calls and video clinics, common modes of consultation during the pandemic, are always going to limit the possibilities of human interaction in the here and now.

All of these developments highlight the importance of continuous professional development (CPD) for the trainer and many of the chapters in this book return us to sound principles on how to deliver a good lecture, involve patients in teaching, consider assessment, supervision, feedback, small- and large-group learning, critical reflection and the use of journal clubs and workshops. This was the staple of learning for many of us as we matured into competent clinicians, teachers, trainers and academics.

Topical Developments in Medical Education and Psychiatry

Two immediate and two more remote topics deserve particular mention here. The two immediate ones are the expansion of the foundation programme in psychiatry and differential attainment.

The foundation programme in psychiatry has been a topic of much interest in the College and has also been the focus of national reviews. In Chapter 15 of this volume, Das and colleagues bring up us to date with the developments and inform us of the recommendations that have been made for foundation trainees and also for those trainers supervizing them. The ambitious plans for the expansion of psychiatry posts in the foundation programme will have a large impact on the number of doctors who will have had some grounding in the specialty and, we hope, a more favourable attitude towards it. They also of course have an impact on supervisors: often keen to train but always struggling to find extra time to support trainees.

Whilst not the subject of a dedicated chapter, differential attainment is described in Chapter 2 by Greening et al. on the Membership of the Royal College of Psychiatrists (MRCPsych) courses and also Chapter 22 by Huline-Dickens on trainees in difficulty. It is still the case that some supervisors are unfamiliar with the term and literature on this important subject, in spite of the fact that so many of our trainees are international medical graduates who may miss out on opportunities and often need more support with some aspects of their training.

The two slightly more remote topics are the introduction of the new UK Medical Licensing Assessment and the increasing emphasis on patient safety. Although not a focus of this book it will be relevant to many trainers to know that, from 2024, there will be a requirement for international medical graduates who would have sat the Professional and Linguistic Assessments Board test (PLAB), as well as all UK medical students, to sit a licensing exam, the UK Medical Licensing Assessment (UKMLA). This will consist of an applied knowledge test (AKT) and clinical and professional skills assessment (CPSA).

Educating for patient safety is another topical area, and simulation is a good way to teach this. The World Health Organization (WHO) have produced a curriculum guide, *Patient Safety Curriculum Guide* (WHO 2011), and many other resources are available to support teaching and training with patient safety in mind such as the Institute for Healthcare Improvement or the National Collaborative For Improving the Clinical Learning Environment (NCICLE).

Psychiatrists are uniquely placed to understand systems, apply human factors approaches, engage patients and families and use knowledge of team dynamics to this end.

The Teaching and Training Roles of the Psychiatrist

As psychiatrists we have many roles within training and in the arena of the scholarship of teaching and learning. Many colleagues will have been introduced to teaching or training when asked to supervise trainees or medical students early in their career, and have been confronted with the need to master the material they teach and also communicate it in a way that is engaging. Seeking feedback, reflecting on this and adapting resources and refining the goals for the session, and the methods of presenting these, are activities that quickly follow and form the basis of scholarly teaching.

Over the careers of the two editors of this book, the roles and activities of academically inclined psychiatrists have changed dramatically: where once we had clinicians who were doing teaching merely as an additional activity, some more expertly than others, academically minded doctors now have the possibility of pursuing teaching as a portfolio career available to them. Teaching has become professionalized and time needs to be included in job plans to do it.

The Professionalization of Teaching and Training

Many colleagues will have been aware of the increasing trend towards professionalization of teaching, and this is mentioned in Chapter 17 by Ingrassia and Batham. In this context too it is interesting to reflect on the work of Boyer (1990) and his work *Scholarship Reconsidered: Priorities for the Professoriate*. In this, he distinguished four categories of scholarship: application, discovery, integration and teaching. Not everyone will wish to engage with all levels, but institutions would do well to support individuals who do. Scholarship thought of broadly is the ability to think, communicate and learn.

Colleagues interested in teaching should bear in mind the helpful distinction drawn by Cleland et al. (2021). These authors distinguish *scholarly teaching* from the *scholarship of teaching and learning*. Within this document, the guide produced by Association for Medical Education in Europe (AMEE), 'Redefining scholarship for health professions education: AMEE Guide No. 142', they describe the importance of the scope of influence one can have as an experienced clinician and educator spanning different institutions.

According to these authors, scholarly teaching uses the work produced by others (the literature) to inform and guide one's practice. Scholarly teaching involves reflection and observation of one's teaching, curriculum design, development and maintenance, and evaluation of practice and has a pragmatic focus. The scholarship of teaching and learning, on the other hand, is the systematic inquiry into student learning which advances the practice of teaching and is likely to involve research and dissemination, and to advance the profession of teaching itself. Cleland et al. believe that every teacher should work towards becoming a scholarly teacher, but every scholarly teacher need not engage in the scholarship of teaching and learning.

For those new to either category, learning on the job is available through courses and conferences offered, among others, by the Association for the Study of Medical Education (ASME) and Association for Medical Education in Europe (AMEE). These international organizations are communities of practice (a term coined by Lave and Wenger 1991) and offer activities and resources for members supporting scholarship. Colleagues can also study education through Certificate, Diploma and Masters' programmes.

We believe this textbook will fill a vacuum for teachers of psychiatry, whether they are clinicians using their experience to enhance the knowledge of medical students, or trainees in psychiatry. Teaching and imparting knowledge is also an excellent way of learning and of continuing one's own personal and professional development. So here's to a long life of learning. In the words of Michelangelo (aged 87), 'I am still learning'.

References

Boyer EL (1990) *Scholarship Reconsidered: Priorities for the Professoriate.* Carnegie Foundation for the Advancement of Teaching.

Cleland JA, Jamieson S, Kusurkar RA, et al. (2021) Redefining scholarship for health professions education: AMEE Guide No. 142. *Medical Teacher,* 43: 824–38.

Lave J, Wenger E (1991) *Situated Learning: Legitimate Peripheral Participation.* Cambridge University Press.

WHO (2011) *Patient Safety Curriculum Guide.* World Health Organization.

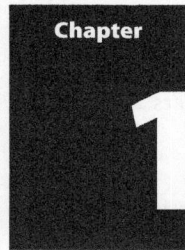

Chapter

1

Improving Patient Care through Continuing Professional Development

Guy Brookes

Introduction

Medicine is a rapidly developing field. Much of what many of us learned in medical school is now obsolete, and an expanding knowledge base has led to increasingly specialized services. If you add to this the fact that many doctors – by choice or as the result of service changes – change their areas of clinical practice, the need to continue learning and developing after completion of formal training is undeniable.

We learn on a day-to-day basis in our clinical practice. As well as taking the relatively obvious forms of reading a literature review or asking the advice of a colleague, learning will also be through continuous feedback, for example from patients about a particular approach we take or a good clinical outcome. Being open to everyday feedback and thoughtfully working in teams is therefore an important part of remaining a safe and effective practitioner.

Given this essential and unavoidable day-to-day learning, it is reasonable to ask what the additional benefit guidance from the Royal College of Psychiatrists and Academy of Medical Royal Colleges alongside requirements set out by the General Medical Council (GMC) add.

What Is Continuing Professional Development?

The General Medical Council (GMC) has defined continuing professional development (CPD) as follows:

> CPD is any learning outside of undergraduate education or postgraduate training that helps you maintain and improve your performance. It covers the development of your knowledge, skills, attitudes and behaviours across all areas of your professional practice. It includes both formal and informal learning activities (GMC 2012).

This definition acknowledges the continuous learning within clinical practice described above and the importance of this in a doctor's development. It emphasizes that CPD should consider the full scope of a doctor's practice and that, while the majority of psychiatrists are primarily clinicians, other roles such as teaching or research, must not be forgotten.

The College's CPD programme supports a structured and objective approach to learning and seeks to make CPD more effective for the individual. It does not aim to encourage the doctor to record and explicitly consider all learning that they undertake. This would be unrealistic and would not reflect the way in which thoughtful practitioners develop. Key to the College's programme is the development and completion of a personal development plan (PDP) within a CPD peer group that can support the doctor in reflecting on current practice (and therefore areas for development) and the implications of new learning for their practice.

If CPD is intended to help 'maintain and improve your performance', it is reasonable to assume that the outcome of good CPD is improved patient care. This makes intuitive sense but, although it is possible to show evidence of improved outcomes individually, demonstrating that CPD as a whole improves care is far more challenging (Mathers 2012).

What Are the Requirements for CPD?

There are three bodies that provide guidance or requirements for psychiatrists' CPD. This can lead to confusion if their roles are not understood.

1. The General Medical Council

The role of the GMC is set out in the Medical Act 1983. It maintains a register of doctors ensuring appropriate qualifications, sets standards for a 'good' doctor, including undergraduate and postgraduate education, through revalidation ensures that doctors keep up to date with knowledge and skills and, if needed, investigates concerns raised about doctors. Therefore, though it seeks to improve practice, the GMC is there to ensure a minimum and safe standard. In keeping with this, there is a requirement for annual appraisal to ensure that doctors are keeping up to date and in line with the standards set out in Good Medical Practice. There is no minimum amount of CPD required and demonstration that you have met the standard is through annual appraisal and ultimately revalidation.

2. The Academy of Medical Royal Colleges

The Academy of Medical Royal Colleges seeks to ensure standards are consistent across the many specialties in medicine. This is similar to the role of the GMC in that it is essential that the public has equal confidence in a general practitioner as a psychiatrist or a surgeon. The Academy of Medical Royal Colleges is essentially the product of its constituent colleges and so its guidance applies to all colleges but focuses on areas that are universally applicable. As such it has defined seven core principles of CPD:

(1) **Individual responsibility**. In line with the GMC, whatever support is in place (e.g., appraisal, CPD peer groups), doctors, themselves, are ultimately responsible for maintain and improving their practice.

(2) **The importance of reflection**. Learning has no value unless considered against current practice and the opportunity for improvement.

(3) **Scope of work**. All areas of a doctor's role need to be considered. Realistically this cannot (and might not be desired) be completed every year but needs to be covered within the five-year cycle.

(4) **CPD and annual appraisal**. CPD undertaken within the year should be considered within the annual appraisal but identifying development needs should not be limited to this annual event.

(5) **Balance of CPD**. Different learning approaches offer different benefits. It is important to have opportunities for learning outside organizations to broaden experience and learn with colleagues as well as alone.

(6) **Documenting CPD**. It is essential that doctors are able to evidence learning undertaken and the consequences of this.

(7) **Employers' responsibilities**. Doctors need access to funding and time to keep up to date and develop their practice.

3. The Royal College of Psychiatrists

The College is the professional body responsible for supporting psychiatrists throughout their careers and setting and raising standards. It thus promotes our development.

Guidance from the College therefore focuses on improvement and specifically relates to psychiatrists' needs. Our guidance differs somewhat from the Academy of Medical Royal Colleges while adhering to the shared principles. For example, while the Royal College of Psychiatrists has set a minimum of 50 hours of CPD each year approved by the CPD peer group, not all colleges (as with the GMC) do so there is no quantity required by the Academy of Medical Royal Colleges. The range of specialties and different needs across the profession means that it is the CPD peer group rather than educational providers that determines whether any learning has been effective for an individual. As a result, to be in good standing with the College for CPD requires active engagement with the CPD peer group.

Because the College's requirements for being in good standing for CPD differ from those set out by the GMC, being in good standing is not necessary for annual appraisal and thus revalidation.

How to Link CPD to Improved Patient Care

Good CPD can have many potential outcomes – for example, improved confidence, greater job satisfaction, innovation, networking and sharing with peers – but the ultimate outcome should be improved care for patients. How can this be achieved?

Developing a Focused PDP

As doctors, we receive feedback from many sources. Some sources are formal, such as complaints, incident reviews or structured multi-source feedback; others are less formal, such as individual patient outcomes, peer discussion and our own reflections on our practice. Being able to consider this feedback honestly and thoughtfully is essential to understanding our learning needs. When developing a PDP, it is natural to be drawn to our areas of interest or expertise. Of course, to stay up to date, ongoing learning in such areas is necessary but we must also pay attention to areas of our practice that we are less enthusiastic about and have perhaps not focused on previously.

It is the individual doctor's responsibility to identify their needs and consider how they will address them (GMC 2012). However, psychiatrists are helped to do this in two ways: by their CPD peer group and by the appraisal process.

- The peer group will use an informal process to help the doctor to develop a PDP that reflects their needs (rather than interests or wishes).
- At appraisal, information about the full scope of the doctor's practice and performance (e.g., outcome measures, complaints, incident reviews, activity levels) is formally discussed. Using this information as a foundation, the appraiser and doctor will create a PDP. The full scope of practice – both clinical and non-clinical aspects – should be considered.

This can mean that the doctor ends up with two PDPs: one from the peer group and one from appraisal. The PDP developed in the peer group will inform the one developed in appraisal. If the processes resulting in each have been robust, the PDPs should not be too dissimilar. A significant difference in the PDPs should raise concerns that there has not been fair or honest discussion about the psychiatrist's work and needs in one, or both, of the processes.

It is important that CPD reflects the doctor's practice (or intended practice for the future), rather than their own personal interests. Although all doctors, whatever their experience, need to stay up to date with relevant therapeutic developments, it is inevitable that their needs will change over their career. Developing skills that are not going to be used in practice will not benefit patients.

Successfully Addressing Development Needs

To evaluate how successful learning has been, it is necessary to be clear about what is to be achieved. The PDP should be specific and the outcomes must be, to some extent, measurable (Box 1.1).

How to best meet development needs will depend on a variety of factors. We all have preferred ways of learning; some may prefer individual reading, others group discussion or learning through experience. In addition, different objectives will be best achieved in different ways; attending a lecture might help to meet an objective of understanding the evidence base of pharmacological treatments, but would be unlikely to offer a doctor much if their objective was to improve their communication skills, in which case observation and practice with a respected colleague are more likely to be effective. The Academy of Medical Royal Colleges (2012) has created a useful template to help doctors structure their reflections when considering how new information relates to current practice and whether further actions are required (Fig. 1.1). Use of this template is encouraged by the Royal College of Psychiatrists (2015). There are many alternative approaches that can be adjusted as needed, but all tend to cover the same areas: what the activity was, what the learning was and how it will change practice. See Box 1.2 for examples (taken from Borton 1970). Such notes can be used in peer-group discussions, to demonstrate value and justify the allocation of CPD credits, and within the appraisal process, to demonstrate ongoing personal development and quality improvement.

Box 1.1 How to develop a good PDP

1. Gather information about the full scope of your practice (e.g., multi-source feedback, clinical activity, complaints and compliments, incident reports)
2. Make time to reflect on what the information says about your practice -- what should you aim to improve?
3. Discuss it in a supportive and formative environment with others (e.g., a CPD peer group)
4. Agree specific objectives – SMART objectives are good:

   - Specific
   - Measurable (or demonstrable)
   - Achievable (personally and within the service)
   - Relevant to current or proposed practice
   - Time-bound

Title and description of activity

18/09/14: CPD Online Module – The Pharmacological Treatment of Resistant Depression: An Overview

What was the learning need or objective that was addressed?

CPD peer group agreed on an objective to better understand the evidence base behind different pharmacological interventions for treatment-resistant depression , as I had reflected that I had less confidence in poly-pharmacological interventions in this field than other peers.

The modules set out a series of steps to take to assess and then consider options at various stages of 'treatment resistance'. Some evidence was presented in the form of meta-analysis. It was useful to be reminded of the importance of thoroughly assessing past treatments, response, other symptoms (e.g. psychotic or bipolar spectrum) before making any decisions about treatment options.

Potential adverse interactions were usefully summarised. The potential benefits of drugs I rarely use (e.g. MAOIs) were discussed and I need to consider my confidence in prescribing these . Although other interventions (e.g. ECT and CBT) were briefly discussed I would need to consider how, in practice, these would be used alongside changes to medication .

In terms of involving the patient in the decision making process more understanding of potential side effects would be needed.

What was the outcome of the activity?

Key learning points:
1. The importance of key areas to remember to include in the initial assessment – bipolar, psychotic symptoms – was emphasised.

2. I have learned a useful stepped model to consider and manage resistant depression

3. I have a good overview of the evidence base for augmentation therapies.

Changes to practice:
– In future my assessment will include specific areas for exploration .

Practice reinforced:
– Augmentation of antidepressant medication with other antidepressants or atypical antipsychotics is safe and effective.
– Caution when using antidepressants for people with bipolar spectrum disorders and consider non-antidepressant options.

Further learning needs

1. Understand the effectiveness of ECT, particularly earlier on in the process of treatment.

2. Revise prescribing and side effect of MAOIs. How will this activity improve patient care or safety?

Number of CPD hours claimed

1 h (agreed by peer group)

Fig. 1.1 Example of a reflective note using the Academy of Medical Royal Colleges (2012) template.

Box 1.2 Borton's model of reflection

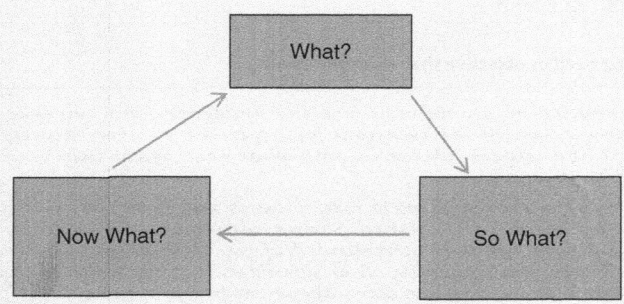

What?

Describe the event. Consider:
* What happened?
* What was the response?
* Who was involved?

So what?

Think about the impact and meaning of the event. Reflect on the event. Consider:
* What happened as a result?
* How did this affect me?
* Why is this important?

Now what?

What are the consequences for you and others? What are you going to do as a result? Consider:
* What would you want to do differently?
* What needs to change?
* How are you going to achieve change?

Klob's learning cycle

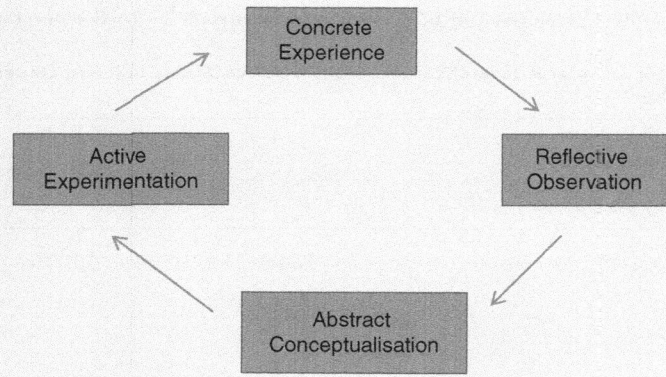

Concrete experience

- Describe what actually happened.
- Who was involved and what was the outcome.

Reflective observation

- What was good, what could have been better?
- Why did the event occur? Why did it happen in that way?

Abstract conceptualization

- How could it have been better?
- What needs to change for a better outcome?
- How could you do better in future?

Active experimentation

- Make the change
- Assess the impact of any changes
- Is further development required?

However, completing the learning event will not in itself improve practice. The knowledge and skills acquired need to be put into practice in the psychiatrist's work.

Modifying Practice after Acquiring New Skills or Knowledge

CPD is only important inasmuch as it improves a doctor's practice; it is not an end in itself. The College's guidance emphasizes this and places the responsibility for ensuring that learning relates to practice on the peer group. The College supports psychiatrists to achieve this through CPD peer groups. The peer group will help you reflect on how the learning has changed or reinforced your practice and from this reflection award CPD credits which will count towards being in good standing with the College for CPD. In a relationship between peers, this requirement might not feel comfortable but it is a professional responsibility.

Collating evidence of improvement can be difficult in some circumstances and will be impossible if the initial objective is not specific. Organizations are now collecting more clinically relevant outcome measures (although this is not yet universal) and clinical audit is a useful tool for measuring performance against predetermined standards. In its guidance on revalidation, the College acknowledges the benefit of clinical audit in both identifying the need for improvement and demonstrating that it has taken place (Royal College of Psychiatrists 2014). Showing that learning has been incorporated into practice need not and should not be onerous. Considering learning in relation to clinical practice through, for example, a case-based discussion, is a useful way to gain feedback where outcome measures are lacking. If honestly and openly approached, such a process could identify further, previously unconsidered learning as needed. The result, therefore, is one of continued learning, reflection and change (Fig. 1.2).

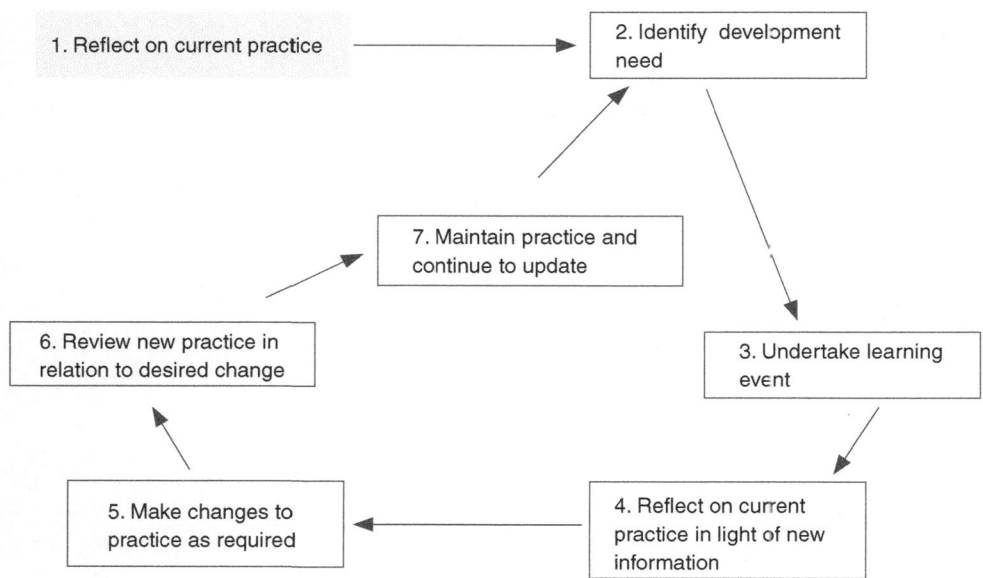

Fig. 1.2 The learning cycle.

Reflection as Part of Effective CPD

In CPD, reflection is the process of thinking about our actions, responses or practice in a conscious, open and considered way in order to learn from them. It encourages us to ask why we do things or make particular decisions and thus whether there are other, better options.

There are two times at which reflection is particularly important in ensuring that CPD improves patient care:

- when identifying development needs – often in response to feedback, we must review our practice and why we came to a particular decision or work in a certain way;
- after a learning event, we should consider the new information in relation to our own practice, and decide whether we need to make changes or whether it supports our current approach.

Reflecting on Current Practice to Identify Development Needs

We need to consider not just what we are doing but why. This often happens after significant events such as a serious incident or a complaint and this is, of course, necessary and good practice. However, if reflection is restricted to such times, consideration of our practice will be limited and probably unfairly critical. We need to evaluate our practice on an ongoing basis, and to do that we need mechanisms to support us.

- Reflective practice groups allow teams to consider how they respond in (often) challenging situations and the feelings that patients and situations can evoke.
- CPD peer groups help the psychiatrist to explore their practice and, from formal or informal feedback, consider which areas could improve through the CPD process.

- Appraisal considers the whole of a doctor's practice and uses both hard and soft data to support discussion about the care they provide and the relationships they form with patients and colleagues.
- Case-based discussion and clinical supervision with peers will explore a relatively small area of practice in detail. Although it is not required by the GMC, the College recommends that psychiatrists undertake at least two case-based discussions each year.
- Review processes should allow doctors and clinical teams to learn from incidents and consider their development needs.
- The cycle of clinical audit requires considering the findings (comparing practice with established or agreed standards) to develop an action plan for improvement.

Alongside these are many less formal discussions that clinicians have with colleagues during day-to-day practice.

If they are committed to improvement and learning, any of the above mechanisms will provide the psychiatrist with a rich view of their practice and therefore suggest what their development needs are.

Reflecting on New Learning to Change Practice

Even if new knowledge has been acquired, without changes to practice patients will not experience any benefit. Reflection is the process that bridges the gap between theory and practice. However, changing practice is not necessarily simple. Most psychiatrists work within teams and interact closely with others. Changing an individual's practice might, therefore, not be possible without changing a wider system. It is thus essential, when setting objectives, that not only the needs of the doctor but the needs of the teams and services in which they work are considered.

As when setting development objectives, considering how new learning will affect practice requires space and honest consideration of our own behaviour. Through regular meetings the peer group will allow space for the doctor to consider both their needs and later, through reflection and appropriate challenge, whether they have met their learning objectives.

Some reflection will need to take place in other arenas (such as incident reviews or clinical audit meetings) or by the doctor alone. Achieving meaningful reflection might require practice. As shown in Fig. 1.1, the Academy of Royal Colleges' template provides a useful framework.

What Is Effective CPD?

Put simply, effective CPD is learning that meets the doctor's developmental needs and leads to improved patient care. Better care does not solely come from improved clinical skills. Teachers and trainers who enhance their educator's skills through CPD indirectly improve the care of all the patients their students go on to treat. Similarly, those who use CPD to develop their leadership skills improve patient care provided by the clinicians working in their service.

There are several factors related to learning that make CPD more likely to improve patient care.

- Learning objectives should be set after honest consideration of the doctor's range of practice and feedback from various sources.
- Learning that relates to the doctor's work is best suited to improving their practice.

> **Box 1.3** Principles of effective CPD
>
> - The doctor feels able to honestly and openly discuss their development needs
> - Information about their practice is accurate and readily available
> - There is a supportive environment in which needs can be considered
> - There is space for new learning to be considered alongside current practice
> - Needs and improvements in the doctor's practice are not considered in isolation from the team/service in which they work
> - Changes to practice are evaluated and further learning identified

- Various forms of education should be considered to acquire the learning. This is an important point, as it is always tempting to look for a taught course rather than considering other forms of learning, such as working alongside a colleague.
- New knowledge should be considered alongside current practice to identify any changes that are needed.
- Time must be available to implement any necessary changes.
- Any change should be evaluated after implementation – has the desired improvement actually been achieved?

Box 1.3 summarizes the principles of effective CPD.

Who and What Is Needed to Make CPD Effective?

The Doctor

The GMC (2012) simply states that 'you are responsible for identifying your CPD needs, planning how these needs should be addressed and undertaking CPD that will support your professional development and practice'. To identify relevant CPD, the doctor needs to consider the available information about their practice and reflect on areas for improvement. This should cover the entirety of practice, both clinical and non-clinical. Without this open and honest reflection, the effect of any subsequent learning will be limited. The doctor is also responsible for reflecting how new learning should be considered alongside current practice and, as far as they are able, for changing practice as appropriate. In both these areas, although the individual doctor is responsible, they should be supported to do this effectively.

To be in good standing with the College for CPD, all clinically active psychiatrists are required to undertake, on average, 30 hours of clinical CPD and thus ensure a high standard of care is experienced uniformly by patients.

The CPD Peer Group

A doctor's peers are a useful asset in identifying development needs and how and when these needs should be met. The College relies on the effective functioning of a peer group when considering whether someone is in good standing for CPD (Box 1.4). The peer group should 'support the individual in developing and completing a relevant PDP that leads to an improvement in that person's skills or competence and therefore an improvement in care

> **Box 1.4** Responsibilities of the CPD peer group
>
> The College relies on the CPD peer group to ensure that learning is relevant and incorporated into practice. Peers should choose their peer group; it should not be allocated by employers. The peer group should:
> - help the psychiatrist to honestly reflect on their practice and identify areas for improvement
> - help convert development needs into achievable goals for a PDP
> - help identify how these goals can be met
> - allow the psychiatrist to reflect on how new learning relates to their current practice
> - consider whether the learning has been relevant to the goal and whether appropriate reflection in relation to practice has been achieved (are there further learning needs?)
> - allocate CPD credits to the learning if it has been relevant to practice and followed by appropriate reflection

provided to patients' (Royal College of Psychiatrists 2015: p. 4). In addition, the peer group is responsible for accrediting learning as CPD activity. A learning activity can only be allocated CPD credits if:

- it is relevant to the psychiatrist's scope of practice (or intended practice);
- it is of sufficient quality;
- learning has been understood and, through reflection, considered alongside current practice.

The peer group is not fulfilling its duty to the psychiatrist if it does not robustly consider these points.

Appraisal

The appraisal process is at the core of revalidation and thus the assurance we give to the public that doctors are safe practitioners. It examines the full scope of the doctor's practice and encourages reflection. CPD is one way in which a doctor can demonstrate that they are up to date in their practice and developing the skills required in their work.

During appraisal, information about the doctor's practice is considered and the doctor is required to reflect on it, with a view to developing a PDP. A good appraiser will support reflection in a way that promotes learning and a formative approach. They will also seek to understand how quality or improvement has been demonstrated.

The following information should be used to develop a PDP within the appraisal:

- information from and reflection on complaints and other forms of patient feedback;
- information from and reflection on incidents relating to the doctor or the service in which they work;
- multi-source feedback;
- clinical activity information;
- clinical outcome information;
- reflections on incidents or feedback relevant to the doctor's practice.

- the PDP as agreed with the CPD peer group.

Good appraisal, therefore, will start the cycle by developing a PDP that reflects the doctor's scope of practice and development needs within it and challenges the doctor to reflect on their development and demonstrate ongoing improvement in practice.

Employers

Employers have a responsibility to ensure that their workforce is up to date and working to appropriate standards. CPD is one mechanism for achieving this. The health service is facing unprecedented financial challenges, but effective CPD does not come without sufficient resources. This is not simply an adequate study leave budget (learning is not necessarily met through taught courses), but also allows doctors the time to reflect on their development needs and the meaning of new knowledge in relation to their own practice, and also to evaluate the impact of any change.

As already mentioned, psychiatrists rarely work in isolation. If the ambition of CPD is to improve patient care, learning in teams is an important option, at least for some people. Therefore, it will be necessary for a whole team, not just a single doctor, to find time for reflection.

Finally, honest and open reflection has been described as a key element to effective CPD. This includes being able to reflect on our actions when things go wrong. Learning from serious incidents is essential to developing safe doctors and safe services and is understandably what the public demands of us. Employers have a major role in providing an environment that is supportive of this approach.

Conclusion

CPD should not be seen as an optional 'add-on' to our everyday work and cannot live in conference halls and lecture theatres. It needs to be an integrated part of our everyday practice, with the aim of continually improving the care we provide to patients and their families. It requires us to reflect on our work and behaviour so that we can identify what improvements to make and then consider whether we have achieved them.

Being in good standing with the Royal College of Psychiatrists for CPD is one way in which we can assure the public that we are maintaining our skills and continuing to develop. It requires the psychiatrist to reflect on their current practice, undertake relevant and effective learning, put that learning into practice and evaluate the outcome. The College relies on the CPD peer group to ensure that learning is relevant and that it is incorporated into practice. To do this requires a constructive, enquiring relationship between peers that can only exist if they are comfortable being open and honest with each other.

References

Academy of Medical Royal Colleges (2012) Academy reflective template for revalidation. Available at: www.aomrc.org.uk/wp-content/uploads/2016/06/Reflective_template_for_revalidation_0312-2.pdf.

Borton T (1970) *Reach, Touch and Teach.* Hutchinson.

GMC (2012) *Continuing Professional Development: Guidance for All Doctors.* General Medical Council.

Mathers N, Mitchell C, Hunn A (2012) Assessing the impact of continuing professional development (CPD) on doctors' performance and patient/service outcomes. GMC. Available at: www .gmc-uk.org/about/research/25022.asp.

Royal College of Psychiatrists (2014) Supporting information for appraisal and revalidation: guidance for psychiatrists (College Report CR194). Royal College of Psychiatrists. Available at: www.rcpsych.ac.uk/docs/default-source/improving-care/better-mh-policy/college-reports/college-report-cr194.pdf?sfvrsn=954f9053_4.

Royal College of Psychiatrists (2015) Continuing professional development: guidance for psychiatrists (Occasional Paper OP98). Royal College of Psychiatrists. Available at: www .rcpsych.ac.uk/docs/default-source/members/cpd/members-cpd-op98.pdf?sfvrsn=1de40c5f_4.

The MRCPsych: Preparing Trainees and Improving Courses

Jayne Greening, Erin Turner, Gareth Rees, Caroline Winkle, Eleanor Dryhurst and Radhika Kanessan

Introduction

Changes to the Member of the Royal College of Psychiatrists (MRCPsych) examination and the current COVID-19 pandemic require adaptation of existing teaching and training for core psychiatry trainees. With the General Medical Council (GMC) also limiting the number of times that a candidate can attempt the MRCPsych examination, there is growing pressure to ensure that course organizers are maximizing trainees' potential to pass. Using our experiences of running MRCPsych courses in Birmingham and Keele we discuss how courses can be developed to best prepare trainees for the MRCPsych written papers and the Clinical Assessment of Skills and Competencies (CASC).

Changes to the MRCPsych Examination

Since April 2015, the MRCPsych examination has consisted of two written papers (Paper A and Paper B) and the CASC.

Written Papers

Unless additional time has been pre-approved by the College, candidates have up to three hours to complete each of the MRCPsych written papers. Paper A covers the scientific and theoretical basis of psychiatry, whereas Paper B contains a critical review section and questions pertaining to clinical topics (Box 2.1). Each paper consists of 150 questions: approximately two-thirds of these are multiple choice questions (MCQs) and approximately one-third are extended matching items (EMIs). One mark is awarded for each correct answer and incorrect responses are not penalized.

MCQs are suited to assessing factual knowledge (Schuwirth and van der Vleuten 2004) and are useful for evaluating large groups of candidates because marking them can be standardized and automated. The style of MCQ used in the MRCPsych examination is the '1 from 5, single best answer type'. This consists of a short question stem and five possible responses from which candidates are asked to select the most appropriate. EMIs are a variant of the MCQ in which candidates are required to select the most appropriate response to a question stem from a list of 10–20 options. By minimizing recognition effect and reducing the chance of selecting correct answers by chance (George 2003), EMIs are considered more useful than MCQs in assessing application of knowledge (Schuwirth and van der Vleuten 2004). They have been cited as the 'fairest' form of written examination and are increasingly the preferred method of assessing undergraduate and postgraduate courses (McCoubrie 2004).

In response to the COVID-19 pandemic the College obtained approval from the GMC to run online versions of the written MRCPsych examination. Since June 2020, candidates

---

Box 2.1 Content of the MRCPsych written examinations

MRCPsych Paper A
- Behavioural science and sociocultural psychiatry
- Human development
- Basic neurosciences
- Clinical psychopharmacology
- Classification and assessment in psychiatry

MRCPsych Paper B
- Organization and delivery of psychiatric services
- General adult psychiatry
- Old-age psychiatry
- Psychotherapy
- Child and adolescent psychiatry
- Substance misuse/addictions
- Forensic psychiatry
- Psychiatry of learning disability
- Critical review

---

have been able to complete papers A and B remotely on the day of the examination using their own electronic devices. In order to ensure that the online written examinations remain secure and robust, the College delivers these using a proctoring system that combines artificial intelligence to monitor candidates' actions, with live proctors who can intervene if the system flags potential causes for concern. To give candidates an opportunity to take comfort breaks, the questions within each of the online written papers are divided into three sections. Candidates have the option of taking a break after completing each section, but are not permitted to return to submitted sections later in the examination. Any time that candidates use for breaks is taken from the three hours allocated for each paper.

The pass marks for the online written papers are calculated by the College's psychometrician using the same methods as previous examinations; whether or not a candidate passes depends on how their performance compares to an absolute standard and not to other candidates (Bowie 2015). In 2020, the requirement that candidates should have passed Paper A and Paper B in order to sit the CASC was waived.

CASC Examination

The CASC tests candidates' clinical skills and applied knowledge in a range of clinical situations. The format of the CASC is similar to an objective structured clinical examination (OSCE) and consists of 16 stations focusing on history taking, examination and patient management (see Box 2.2). Each CASC station lasts seven minutes (not including reading time) and the examination stations include physical and mental state examination, risk assessment and assessment of mental capacity.

In January 2018, the College stopped using linked stations meaning that the CASC is currently divided into two circuits of eight single stations (which must be completed on the

---

Box 2.2 Content of the MRCPsych CASC examination

Circuit 1
- Six stations focused on management
- One station focused on examination
- One station focused on history taking
- Four minutes reading time per station
- Seven minutes to perform the task

Circuit 2
- Four stations focused on examination
- Four stations focused on history taking
- Ninety seconds reading time per station
- Seven minutes to perform the task

---

same day). These stations are internally criterion referenced and the candidate's performance is marked by an appropriately trained examiner. The pass mark for the CASC is the average of the station pass marks for that day; candidates who score highly in some stations cannot use this to compensate for low performance in others. To meet the minimum standard required to pass the CASC, candidates must meet or exceed the total borderline regression score and achieve the passing score in a minimum of 12 stations. No more than two attempts at the CASC are permitted in each calendar year.

Given the risks associated with conducting the CASC in a live venue during the COVID-19 pandemic, the College started implementing an online CASC in October 2020. The blueprint of this examination remains unchanged with each station of the online CASC designed to be suitable for video consultations; any requirement for physical examination is limited to what can be achieved remotely using the online examination platform.

Preparing Trainees for the Written Papers of the MRCPsych Examination

MRCPsych courses should prepare trainees for the written papers of the examination by offering exam practice and ensuring that the College's curriculum for core training is covered by the course content (Box 2.1). It is therefore helpful if teachers on MRCPsych courses supplement their lectures with example MCQs and EMIs.

The critical review component of MRCPsych Paper B does not readily translate into teaching by lecture format. Ideally, it should be taught via smallgroup teaching or in a workshop format that provides trainees with additional opportunities to put their critical appraisal knowledge and skills into practice. Journal clubs are another important teaching forum for developing these skills (Swift 2016).

Preparing Trainees for the CASC Examination

Many course organizers incorporate mock CASC examination as part of their training programme. Organizing these examinations can be time consuming, labour intensive and expensive. During the COVID-19 pandemic, courses have also had to adapt to support trainees preparing for the online format of the examination, for example by taking steps to avoid 'screen fatigue' and encouraging trainees to familiarize themselves with the online examination platforms used by the College.

Preparing mock CASC examinations (either in person or online) requires a pool of suitable examiners and simulated patients. Ideally, examiners should be consultant psychiatrists with experience of examining and/or an interest in medical education. Simulated patients can be sourced from professional acting companies that specialize in medical student/trainee exams; they introduce standardization to the CASC, allow trainees to be examined without fear of upsetting genuine patients (Barrows 1995) and can be sourced to cover specific areas of the curriculum. With appropriate support, patients and carers should also be involved in the development and delivery of mock CASC stations, including people with intellectual disabilities (Soni et al. 2014). Where possible, mock CASC examinations should be modelled on the two-circuit exam currently adopted by the College (see Box 2.2).

Feedback is an integral and important component of mock CASC examinations. It should focus on performance, use non-judgemental language, emphasize positive aspects of performance and suggest areas for improvement (Shrivastava et al. 2014). The mock CASCexaminations delivered by the MRCPsych courses in Birmingham and Keele offer trainees written feedback about their performance at each station, as well as verbal feedback from each examiner and simulated patient. Too many negative comments can instil defeatism and should be avoided, particularly close to the examination itself. However, if an examiner has serious concerns about a trainee's competency, they have a duty to communicate this to both the trainee and the trainee's educational supervisor. Although mock CASC examinations usually take place near to examination sittings, communication skills sessions and exposure to simulated patients should be integrated throughout MRCPsych courses to allow sufficient time for trainees to refine their skills if required.

MRCPsych Courses

The College's core curriculum states that 'It is essential that trainees in Core Psychiatry Training attend an MRCPsych course that comprises a systematic course of lectures and/or seminars covering basic sciences and clinical topics, communication and interviewing skills' (Royal College of Psychiatrists 2010: p. 82). The standards for an MRCPsych course are explicitly stated and include the need for course content to cover the curriculum, course organizers to be given adequate time and administrative support, patient/carer involvement and regular feedback from trainees and teachers. MRCPsych courses also have a number of functions beyond preparing trainees for the examinations and ideally these should complement each other to produce higherquality psychiatrists (Schuwirth 2004).

The College organizes annual meetings of all the MRCPsych course organizers to share good practice. There are currently approximately 30 courses running across the UK (contact the RCPsych for details), which vary widely in their organization and the number of trainees attending (Berrisford and Vassilas 2010). The Birmingham and Keele MRCPsych courses, for example, are each organized by a remunerated consultant psychiatrist with administrative support. Specialist trainees with an interest in medical education are appointed competitively to 'honorary clinical tutor' posts and allocated a year group for which they are responsible. Patients and carers play an important role in delivering lectures, cofacilitating workshops, providing feedback on trainees' communication skills and meeting with the course organizer and honorary clinical tutors on a regular basis.

Course Content

Owing to the resource implications of teaching a large number of trainees, Birmingham and Keele's MRCPsych courses are funded by trainees' study budgets and the majority of course content is delivered via lectures. Although a programme of lectures enables trainees working in different geographical locations to meet and engage in peer support, didactic teaching can also invoke passivity and discourage deep learning (Newbie and Entwistle 1986). Hence, the three-year course integrates smallgroup teaching throughout year one; the learning objectives for these sessions are stated explicitly and their content is supported by a teaching workbook. Although the content of smallgroup teaching sessions is not always exam focused, the shift from teacher-centred and subject-based teaching to interactive, problem-based, student-centred learning is recognized as an advantage in adult education (Newbie and Entwistle 1986).

Online Learning

Online portfolios and internet-based learning have been prevalent within medical education for some time (Cook et al. 2008). Indeed, the College developed its own e-learning resource, Trainees Online (TrOn, at http://tron.rcpsych.ac.uk) in 2014 after recognizing that trainees were preparing for the MRCPsych examination using websites not subject to quality control. Online modules have been shown to increase knowledge, confidence and application of skills (Ruchter et al. 2012). They are also flexible and their content can be tailored to the needs of individual learners (Cook et al. 2008).

Traditional face-to-face teaching methods have not been widely available during the COVID-19 pandemic, creating an urgent need for MRCPsych courses to deliver their content using online platforms. Some of the advantages of using virtual platforms include the ability to record/store teaching sessions (allowing trainees to consolidate their learning), log trainee attendance, collect anonymous feedback and facilitate group discussion through 'chat' boxes. Many platforms also support 'breakout rooms' which allow teachers to deliver small-group teaching (by dividing trainees into smaller interactive groups). Trainees are more likely to accept online learning if it fits in with their expectations and/or offers a perceived advantage over traditional teaching methods (Wong et al. 2010).

Providing online learning is not without its challenges and relies upon trainees having access to appropriate equipment and a reliable internet connection (since technical difficulties can negatively affect learning and cause trainees to disengage). Regular screen breaks also need to be incorporated into courses to ensure the continued engagement of trainees during teaching sessions.

Enhancing the Sociability of Online Teaching Courses

Whilst MRCPsych courses play a principal role in helping trainees to prepare for membership examinations and specialist training, the sociability of the course is arguably as important. This confers particular significance for (1) international medical graduates (IMGs), who may have to assimilate to a new culture, often separated from their friends and family; (2) trainees returning from extended periods of maternity or sick leave, who are likely to re-join with a new set of peers; and (3) trainees who work in standalone psychiatric units, who may feel isolated from their peers. Meeting peers at a weekly teaching group has the potential to enhance a sense of belonging and may help to moderate some of the everyday stresses that trainees experience (GMC 2019a). Assisting trainees to establish connections and foster peer relationships with other trainees across the training programme is therefore crucial.

In 2019, the Birmingham MRCPsych course helped trainees to feel more connected with their peers by piloting a two-day residential event. The West Midlands School of Psychiatry board supported this and Health Education England provided funding. During the event trainees took part in a number of fun and challenging team-building activities to foster peer relationships and promote collaborative working. Higher trainees also participated in the event by facilitating practical and interactive workshops such as 'How to pass membership exams', 'How to develop a winning portfolio' and 'How to impress at Specialist Trainee interview'. Trainees were encouraged to stay overnight to maximize the time they could spend getting to know each other. Attendees reported that the residential event was a unique opportunity to network with core and higher trainees from across the Deanery. They also appreciated learning in a relaxed, informal environment and found the team-building activities an effective way of getting to know their peers.

Since the COVID-19 pandemic there has been an increase in virtual teaching and reduced opportunities for peer support and belonging. It is therefore of paramount importance that MRCPsych courses explore innovative ways of enhancing the sociability of psychiatric training and trainee wellbeing. Online social events and workshops (including trainee wellbeing workshops) can be delivered virtually. Most of the activities that trainees benefitted from during the residential event, for example, could be replicated virtually. Peer relationships can also be nurtured by placing trainees from different year groups together and asking them to undertake team challenges in breakout rooms. Perhaps now, more than ever, there needs to be a renewed focus on trainee wellbeing and support.

Patient Involvement

Patient and carer involvement is mandated in postgraduate training (Fadden et al. 2005). In order to demonstrate meaningful involvement/avoid tokenism, MRCPsych courses must consider their motivation for involving patients and carers, provide them with adequate supervision and prepare teaching opportunities which meet trainees' expected learning outcomes (Dimambro and Doody 2009). Prior to the COVID-19 pandemic, the MRCPsych courses in Birmingham and Keele achieved this in two distinct ways. Firstly, by running workshops led by patients/carers, drawing upon their lived experiences to generate group discussion about relevant topics, such as being detained under the Mental Health Act. These sessions benefit trainees by challenging negative attitudes and raising awareness of the 'patient journey'; they also benefit patients by empowering them and boosting their self-esteem (Repper and Breeze 2007). Secondly, by recruiting patients and carers to assess trainees during communication skills and CASC practice sessions.

Involving patients and carers in the Birmingham and Keele MRCPsych courses has required additional planning during the COVID-19 pandemic. The move away from face-to-face teaching has also excluded those patients and carers who do not have access to electronic devices, a reliable internet connection or confidence to communicate over a screen. One way of overcoming this is to develop a hub where patients/carers can access the necessary equipment/support to continue their involvement in psychiatric training.

Workplace-Based Assessments: Now and in the Future?

Workplace-based assessments (WPBAs) were introduced by the College in 2007 to support the annual review of competence progression (ARCP) by facilitating the multidimensional evaluation of a trainee's longer-term performance (Brown and Doshi 2006). They aim to ensure that trainees are progressing satisfactorily by identifying areas in which doctors require additional or targeted training. However, acting on findings from a Royal College of Physicians pilot study (Pan Cho et al. 2014), a working group on assessment in psychiatry criticized the use of untrained and nonmedical assessors in WPBAs and argued that there was a crisis in postgraduate workplace assessment (O'Leary et al. 2016). Research also shows that the quality and availability of assessor training is variable, with little divergence in assessment scores across domains, poor correlation with free text comments and only half the suggested action points deemed 'specific' and 'achievable' (Gilberthorpe et al. 2016). Trainee perceptions of WPBAs are mixed (Simmons 2013), with Menon et al. (2012) suggesting that negative attitudes have further undermined their effectiveness. There is also evidence that a significant proportion of trainees who do well in WPBAs are persistently failing the CASC examination (Sikdar 2010).

In response to this criticism, the GMC recommended the development of systems to bridge the gap between competence and performance. In 2012, supervised learning events (SLEs) replaced WPBAs in the blueprint of foundation training, removing the application of domain scoring, allowing descriptors of what went well and what could be improved only. Although SLEs were not introduced into psychiatric training, the aforementioned working group suggested that assessment should become more person-centred and develop relevant skills, such as rapport building and written communication. The College's Person-Centred Training and Curriculum Scoping Group (2019) also emphasized the importance of constructive feedback rather than scoring and recommended that trainees should be assessed on their collaborative care planning and reflections of managing value conflicts.

In order to maximize the potential benefits of WPBAs, assessors should follow the seven requirements of effective performance feedback, that is, for the trainee's benefit, not solicited or imposed, timely, specific, descriptive, accurate, not embarrassing and relevant (Brown and Cooke 2009). Although there is no absolute requirement for trainees to gain feedback from patients, there is evidence this can lead to improvement in performance (Murton 2016).

Differential Attainment

Differential attainment is the gap between attainment levels of different groups of doctors and exists across many areas, including MRCPsych examination pass rates. The GMC (2019b) states that 'differentials connected solely to age, gender or ethnicity of a particular group are unfair', with data identifying a persistent gap in attainment between UK-graduated Black, Asian and Minority Ethnic (BAME) trainees and UK-graduated White trainees. Woolf et al. (2016) cite that postgraduate medical training poses risks to trainees from all ethnic groups but that BAME UK graduates and IMGs face additional risks. These risks are interrelated and can be divided into five categories: (1) poor relationships with seniors could lead to fewer learning opportunities and increased mental health problems; (2) perceptions of unconscious bias and anxiety about bias; (3) poorer performance in exams leading to less autonomy in job choice (and increased likelihood of separation from family and peer support networks); (4) perceived racism and fears of being labelled as problematic; and (5) lack of recognition from trainers about environmental stressors (this is especially relevant in medicine where failure is often attributed to a lack of motivation or ability).

The additional risks affecting IMGs include inexperience with UK assessments, cultural differences that impede relationships with colleagues, lengthy times to learn cultural norms and the potential stigma attached to accessing supplementary support. In addition, there is evidence that the UK healthcare system fails to harness the strengths of IMGs (Lagunes-Cordoba et al. 2020) and that anxiety about examination failure, visa difficulties and ineligibility for jobs may add to the challenges facing them. Refugee doctors have been identified as being at a particularly high disadvantage (Cohn et al. 2006).

Since 2010, the GMC has explored the experiences of doctors progressing through postgraduate training and published a series of reports investigating differential attainment and how to tackle it. Roe et al. (2019) identified 10 factors which are important in achieving this aim (see Box 2.3). These factors overlap but can be divided into three main groups: (1) those focusing on the 'working and learning environment'; (2) those focussing on 'who supports learning'; and (3) those focusing on 'what supports learning'. Informal role models and coaching/mentoring by inspirational senior colleagues have been recognized as having particular value (Roe et al. 2019).

This work is of particular relevance to postgraduate training in psychiatry, where 44% of trainees are estimated to be IMGs (GMC 2019b). In an effort to combat differential attainment in psychiatric training the College has appointed an Associate Dean with responsibility for addressing this issue. It has also set up an annual IMG conference and

---

Box 2.3 Successful factors to address differential attainment (Roe et al. 2019)

1. An inclusive workplace that values diversity[a]
2. Treating learners as individuals[a]
3. Working with inspirational senior colleagues[b]
4. The supportive trainer or supervisor[b]
5. Having the support and validation of peers[b]
6. Working arrangements that facilitate learning[c]
7. Maximizing the value of learning[c]
8. Gaining clarity, certainty and support for career choices[c]
9. Support to pass exams or deal with exam failure[c]
10. Personal motivation and drive[c]

   [a] Factors focusing on the working environment
   [b] Factors focusing on who supports learning
   [c] Factors focusing on what supports learning

updated the College website to include a dedicated area for IMGs. The College's Psychiatrists' Support Service provides information on coaching and mentoring, as well as support on dealing with exams. In the minutes of a meeting in January 2020, the College's Psychiatric Trainees Committee (PTC) expressed its commitment to reducing differential attainment and several locality divisions have a list of mentors willing to provide support to IMGs. The role of the College tutors includes taking an overview of trainees' progress and is likely to be important in understanding the impact of differential attainment and developing awareness/resources to tackle it locally.

Conclusion

Changes to the MRCPsych examinations pose challenges for those involved in designing and coordinating psychiatric training, particularly in terms of tailoring the content of MRCPsych courses to those at different stages of the assessment process. It is therefore imperative that these courses are evaluated thoroughly so that they continue to support examination preparation in an effective and efficient manner. Preparing materials for MRCPsych courses, mock examinations and revision courses is time consuming and labour intensive. It is therefore advisable for course organizers to recruit honorary clinical teachers and a pool of senior doctors who can assist with assessment. The involvement of patients/carers in MRCPsych courses is mandatory, but care needs to be taken to ensure that their contribution is worthwhile and not tokenistic. MRCPsych courses should also be willing to adapt to trainees' needs and develop online learning to run alongside the College's TrOn initiative. The digitization of education/training should not be underestimated, and has taken on additional significance as a result of the COVID-19 pandemic. Teaching courses should, however, consider how to mitigate against the reduced sociability of virtual teaching. Attending online or face-to-face social events, such as a residential courses, can help trainees to feel better connected and supported. It is recognized that some trainees do well in WPBAs yet repeatedly fail the CASC component of the MRCPsych examination; it is therefore crucial for educators to be trained in delivering effective performance feedback to psychiatrists at all stages of training. Particular attention needs to be paid to differential attainment and developing skills to tackle this.

References

Barrows HS (1995) *How to Design a Problem-Based Curriculum for the Pre-Clinical Years.* Springer.

Berrisford GS, Vassilas CA (2010) MRCPsych courses: the national picture. *Psychiatrist*, **34**: 301–3.

Bowie P (2015) Papers A & B marking scheme. Royal College of Psychiatrists. Available at: www.rcpsych.ac.uk/training/exams/preparing-for-exams/papers-a-and-b-marking-scheme.

Brown N, Doshi M (2006) Assessing professional and clinical competence: the way forward. *Advances in Psychiatric Treatment*, **12**: 81–9.

Brown N, Cooke L (2009) Giving effective feedback to psychiatric trainees. *Advances in Psychiatric Treatment*, **15**: 123–8.

Cohn S, Alenya J, Murray K, et al. (2006) Experiences and expectations of refugee doctors: qualitative study. *British Journal of Psychiatry*, **189**: 74–8.

Cook DA, Levinson AJ, Garside S, et al. (2008) Internet-based learning in the health professions: a meta-analysis. *JAMA*, **300**: 1181–96.

Dimambro BJ, Doody GA (2009) Service user organisations: an untapped teaching resource. *Psychiatric Bulletin*, **33**: 72–4.

Fadden G, Shooter M, Holsgrove G (2005) Involving carers and service users in the training of psychiatrists. *Psychiatric Bulletin*, **29**: 270–4.

GMC (2019a) Caring for doctors, caring for patients. Available at: www.gmc-uk .org/-/media/documents/caring-for-doctors-caring-for-patients_pdf-80706341.pdf).

GMC (2019b) *The State of Medical Education and Practice in the UK: The Workforce Report*. GMC.

George S (2003) Extended matching items (EMIs): solving the conundrum. *Psychiatric Bulletin*, **27**: 230–2.

Gilberthorpe T, Sarfo M D, Lawrence-Smith G (2016) Ticking the boxes: a survey of workplace-based assessments. *Psychiatric Bulletin*, **40**: 89–92.

Lagunes-Cordoba E, Maitra R, Dave S, et al. (2020) International medical graduates; how can UK psychiatry do better? *BJPsych Bulletin*, **2**: 1–6.

McCoubrie P (2004) Improving the fairness of multiple-questions: a literature review. *Medical Teacher*, **26**: 709–12.

Menon S, Winston M, Sullivan G (2012) Workplace-based assessments: attitudes and perceptions among consultant trainers and comparison with those of trainees. *Psychiatrist*, **36**: 16–24.

Murton CA (2016) The impact of multisource feedback (MSF) including patient feedback on psychiatric trainees. *MedEdPublish*, **5**: 23.

Newbie DI, Entwistle NJ (1986) Learning styles and approaches: implications for medical education. *Medical Education*, **20**: 162–75.

O'Leary D, Al-Taiar H, Brown N, et al. (2016) Workplace assessment in crisis? The way forward. *Psychiatric Bulletin*, **40**(2): 61–3.

Pan Cho S, Parry D, Wade W (2014) Lessons learnt from a pilot of assessment for learning. *Clinical Medicine*, **14**: 577–84.

Repper J, Breeze J (2007) A review of the literature on user and carer involvement in the training and education of health professionals. *International Journal of Nursing Studies*, **44**: 511–19.

RCPsych Person-Centred Training and Curriculum Scoping Group (2019) Training in psychiatry; making person-centred care a reality. *BJPsych Bulletin*, **43**: 136–40.

Roe V, Patterson F, Kerrin M, et al. (2019) *What Supported Your Success in Training?* Work Psychology Group.

Royal College of Psychiatrists (2010) *A Competency Based Curriculum for Specialist Core Training in Psychiatry*. Royal College of Psychiatrists.

Ruchter V, Lindsey C, Graham M, et al. (2012) Use of online modules to enhance knowledge and skills application during an introductory pharmacy practice experience. *American Journal of Pharmaceutical Education*, **76**: 69.

Schuwirth LW (2004) Assessing medical competence: finding the right answers. *Clinical Teacher*, **1**: 14–18.

Schuwirth LW, van der Vleuten CP (2004) Different written assessment methods: what can be said about their strengths and weaknesses? *Medical Education*, **38**: 974–9.

Shrivastava SR, Shrivastava PS, Ramasamy J (2014) Effective feedback: an indispensable tool for improvement in quality of medical education. *Journal of Pedagogic Development*, **4**: 12–20.

Sikdar S (2010) WPBA or CASC/OSCE: where is it going wrong? *Psychiatrist*, **34**: 72–3.

Simmons M (2013) How are workplace-based assessments viewed by UK psychiatry trainees? *Psychiatria Danubina*, **25**: 182–4.

Soni S, Hall I, Doulton P, et al. (2014) Involving people with intellectual disabilities in the assessment of healthcare professionals. *Advances in Mental Health and Intellectual Disabilities*, **8**: 362–9.

Swift G (2016) Are journal clubs useful in teaching psychiatry? *BJPsych Advances*, **22**: 203–10.

Wong G, Greenhalgh T, Pawson R (2010) Internet-based medical education: a realist review of what works, for whom and in what circumstances. *BMC Medical Education*, **10**: 1–10.

Woolf K, Rich A, Viney R, et al. (2016) Perceived causes of differential attainment in UK postgraduate medical training: a national qualitative study. *BMJ Open*. Available at: http://dx.doi.org/10.1136/bmjopen-2016-013429.

Going Beyond 'Good Enough' Teaching in Psychiatric Training

S. Neil Sarkar and Victor Cohn

Introduction

Psychiatrists must seek to make the most of the opportunity offered by the increase in Foundation Programme training posts in psychiatry (see Chapter 15), while continuing to enhance the teaching of medical undergraduate students. We need to create good doctors who are highly professional, good communicators and sympathetic to psychosocial needs of all patients. We also need to improve recruitment to our own specialty.

Medical students prefer to learn general skills rather than specialised ones – this is a 'strategic' outlook that cuts their workload. For a busy foundation year doctor, this problem is further magnified by the added pressure and responsibility of working and the steep learning curve that comes with it. Students' and trainees' views must be balanced with the necessity to teach fundamental principles of psychiatry, otherwise the care of the mentally ill will be compromised through lack of knowledge (Davies 2000; Oakley 2008). Therefore, psychiatrists have a role in teaching all undergraduates generic skills, such as psychosocial aspects of patient care and the doctor–patient relationship, with emphasis on professionalism and good communication. However, as well as this, psychiatrists should appeal to and nurture the interests of psychiatrists of the future by including core psychiatric skills/knowledge in our teaching (Ghodse 2004)

Attitudes to psychiatry significantly improve during teaching programmes (Baxter et al. 2001; Glynn 2006), but interest typically wanes thereafter; one study reported a fall in interest from 10–11% to 3–4% within 1 year (Tharyan et al. 2008). Students' exposure to non-psychiatric specialties in the final year and their focus on what they think they will need immediately after qualifying are likely reasons (Baxter et al. 2001).

Quality of teaching is an important 'modifiable' influence on recruitment, especially for those with neutral views beforehand (Niedermier et al. 2006). Positive attitudes are promoted by direct patient contact, encouragement from consultants and seeing patients respond well to treatment (McParland et al. 2003; Oakley and Oyebode 2008).

A recent survey examining factors influencing career choices among a group of psychiatric trainees and medical students pointed to the powerful role (both positive and negative) of the consultant and role modelling (Paddock et al. 2013). Shah et al. (2011) also investigated factors influencing career choice among foundation trainees (Box 3.1). They found that the psychiatric rotation in the Foundation Programme could improve recruitment by giving trainees work experience in a field they might not otherwise have considered as a career.

Box 3.1 What influences foundation trainees considering psychiatry as a career? (Based on Shah et al. 2011)

Positive factors*

1. Experiences as medical students – finding psychiatric patients interesting, developing an aptitude for the specialty, undergraduate teaching
2. Influence of seniors – role modelling, encouragement, morale
3. Aspects of the work environment – patient contact, general pace of the specialty, team work

Negative factors*

1. Perceived poor prognosis of psychiatric patients
2. Perceived unscientific basis of psychiatry
3. Negative comments made by other specialties

*1, most influential; 2, moderately influential; 3, least influential

Stereotyping and Stigma

Challenging negative stereotypes about psychiatry is a huge motivator for us to create 'ambassadors of psychiatry' through our teaching. Stereotyping is an efficient way of structuring knowledge – it is an effective strategy that cuts the cognitive workload, thus reducing uncertainty related to any novel stimulus (Townsend 1979). It therefore appeals to 'strategic' students (to whom we return later in this chapter).

Stigma in psychiatry is encountered in negative views about psychiatrists as well as their patients. Some have suggested that 'the rejecting voices of others may bring greater disadvantage than the primary condition itself' (Thornicroft et al. 2007). Unfortunately, stigma is common and has an immense impact on patients and a negative influence on recruitment. Stigma is not explicitly addressed in undergraduate teaching, yet we have a duty to tackle it. The problem is magnified by the difficulty of assessing stigma. Mind's 1996 survey on stigma (Read and Baker 1996) revealed that 50% of people with mental illnesses felt discriminated against by medical services, and this theme has been commented on again recently by several teams (Thornicroft et al. 2007; Baker et al. 2016). If parity of esteem between physical and mental health is lacking within medicine, then how can we expect it to exist outside?

Stigmatising attitudes develop in early childhood, so they are difficult to change. Increased knowledge and contact with mentally ill people challenge negative stereotypes, but one negative image can override the cumulative effects of many positive experiences (Byrne 2000). However, as Byrne stated, the starting point in tackling stigma is education, and there are a number of ways in which we can reduce stigma in our teaching of students and trainees. We should therefore acknowledge and address stigma as a separate and important issue in its own right. The more direct contact that students have with both patients and carers, the better. Patients' narratives 'normalise' mental illness and allow patients to be seen as individuals. Students eventually learn that anyone can develop mental illness if there is enough stress, and this lowers the 'them and us' attitude (Gray 2002). Therefore, patients and carers should be involved in training healthcare professionals

(Walters et al. 2007). Home visits allow students to try to understand how a patient lives and behaves in their own environment, culture and context (Walters et al. 2007; Dogra et al. 2008). Additionally, to direct patient interaction, role-play in which students take on the part of patients can be a powerful experience that builds empathy and also reduces stigma (McNaughton et al. 2008).

Ideal Teaching Practice

Role modelling, particularly of senior clinicians, is an important factor that determines career choice and attitudes, so we need to use this to our advantage (Shah et al. 2011; Paddock et al. 2013). We need to demonstrate not only technical skills, but also the right attitude. Ideal teaching practice should therefore counteract negative experiences, whilst building on positives. We need to be enthusiastic about teaching and try to create a relaxed, positive atmosphere with open questions and discussion based on interesting examples. Students might be matched with specific patients, to promote experiential learning. A 'thinking aloud' approach can aid decision making and professionalism (Skånér 2005; Cross et al. 2006). Giving individualised feedback and also asking for feedback to adapt one's own teaching would continually enhance quality (Sluijsmans et al. 2003). A personal narrative explaining what it is like to live the life of a psychiatrist might be an effective way of improving recruitment, as the student or trainee could picture working in the profession themselves (Hashmi et al. 2014; Berkhout et al. 2015).

The essence of teaching ought to be to try to make students/trainees feel important. Foster an environment conducive to learning by not causing students to feel that they are a burden, that their learning is interfering with patient care by intruding on privacy or encroaching on a clinician's time. Students/trainees need instead to be given achievable responsibilities to enable them to feel that they are contributing to patient care, and thus feel accountable and part of a team. Making juniors feel important motivates them to learn more than just how to pass assessments, by promoting deeper learning and professionalism.

Assessments: Limitations and Solutions

Assessment motivates students to learn, but what should the real aim of teaching be – helping students to pass exams or enabling them to be better doctors/psychiatrists (to be competent and professional) (Cantillon et al. 2006)? If we are merely aiming for higher pass rates, we are limited by the validity of assessment (i.e., whether a test predicts that someone will become a good doctor). There is often a balance between validity and reliability (Sweet et al. 2003) and also between what is ideal and what is feasible (van der Vleuten et al. 2012; Hodges 2014). Direct observation of students seeing real patients is valid, but not always practical, hence the use of simulated patients – actors trained to portray signs and symptoms (Schuwirth and van der Vleuten 2003; Dave 2012). However, standardisation of simulation (Sweet et al. 2003; Cantillon et al. 2006) can still cause problems.

Miller's pyramid (Miller 1990) is a well-known framework for assessing clinical competence (Fig. 3.1). Norman (2005) has challenged the simplicity of this framework, and various authors have debated its usefulness: any single assessment (point measurement) implies a compromise on quality criteria, since one method can assess only a part of the pyramid (Norman 2005; Hodges 2006; van der Vleuten et al. 2012). A single method of assessment

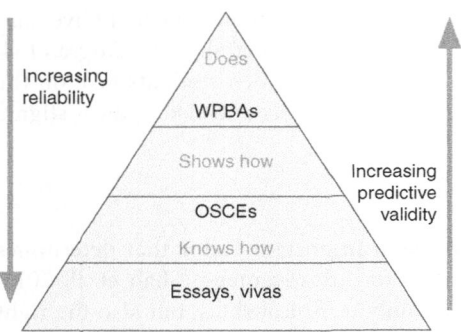

Fig. 3.1 Miller's pyramid amended to show that single assessments often result in a trade-off between reliability and validity. MCQs, multiple choice questions; OSCEs, objective structured clinical examinations; WPBAs, workplace-based assessments.

cannot cover all aspects of competencies of the layers of Miller's pyramid, so we need a blend of methods, including professional judgement (van der Vleuten and Schuwirth 2005).

A competency is the ability to handle a complex professional task by integrating the relevant cognitive, psychomotor and affective skills (van der Vleuten and Schuwirth 2005). It involves knowledge, skills, problem solving and attitudes (Frank and Danoff 2007). In medicine, it has been defined as 'the habitual and judicious use of communication, knowledge, technical skills, clinical reasoning, emotions, values, and reflection in daily practice for the benefit of the individuals and communities being served' (Epstein and Hundert 2002). Too much emphasis on competence-as-knowledge risks creating 'hidden incompetence' – knowledge-smart doctors who have poor interpersonal and technical skills (Miller 1990; Hodges 2006).

WPBAs and Teaching Professionalism

Historically, more emphasis was put on the lower two levels of Miller's pyramid ('knows' and 'knows how'). OSCEs now target the third level ('shows how'), but the development of less standardised, though still reliable, methods of practice-based assessment has led to calls to move assessment back into the real world of the workplace (van der Vleuten and Schuwirth 2005). Workplace-based assessments (WPBAs) for doctors target the highest level ('does') by collecting information in everyday practice, thus improving validity. This method has filtered down to undergraduates (Rethans et al. 2002; Norcini et al. 2003; Wilkinson and Frampton 2004; Cantillon et al. 2006) and the mini clinical evaluation exercise (mini-CEX) is an example for foundation trainees (Ram et al. 1999; Norcini 2003).

Professionalism can be defined as one's professional identity as a doctor (Roberts et al. 2005). It involves 'subordination of one's own interests to those of the patient', that is, humanistic values (Roberts et al. 2005). Professionalism (ethics and communication skills) helps doctors make decisions, especially in psychiatry (Royal College of Psychiatrists 2009; General Medical Council 2013). Psychiatry does not have simple tests of physical parameters for diagnosis. Psychiatrists need skills to engage a patient enough to obtain an accurate history – otherwise even vast knowledge will not allow us to make the right decisions. Certain issues of professionalism are particularly important to psychiatry – detaining/treating patients involuntarily, therapeutic alliances, boundaries, confidentiality, capacity, consent, working with the multidisciplinary team, interagency liaison (Royal College of

Psychiatrists 2009; American Psychiatric Association 2013). Some of these can be easily taught/assessed, but some elements are more difficult.

Teaching professionalism varies owing to the complexity of its components and the limitations of assessment methods. It is learnt largely through an informal process of modelling (Joubert 2006), social constructivism and collaborative learning (Plaice et al. 2002; Joubert 2006), but more explicit teaching is needed. Simulated patients can help to standardise assessment, yet add variety to the students' learning experience by enhancing communication skills in difficult situations, for example involving risk, intrusion and confidentiality (McNaughton et al. 2008; Dave 2012). Observation is by facilitators/peers, but can be videotaped for self-reflection (Ram et al. 1999). Self-reflection and feedback from simulated patients and observers are important for effectiveness. Another possibility is problem-based learning. This method uses a clinical problem to stimulate self-directed learning, which is then discussed in a group, thus enhancing collaborative learning – important in professionalism (Sweet et al. 2003; Cantillon et al. 2006).

The end point in assessments is often seen without an explanation of the route to get there. 'Thinking aloud' to the student in everyday clinical scenarios (Skånér 2005; Cross et al. 2006) might enable them to understand thought processes via a 'decision-making tree'. Equally, feedback should be holistic and not just factual, that is, it should comment on all aspects of professionalism, such as liaising with staff, appearance, dress, punctuality, attitude, legible handwriting and appearing interested, enthusiastic and caring. Role-modelling acts as a blueprint or gold standard for comparison (Plaice et al. 2002; Joubert 2006). Students and juniors should be encouraged to actively observe and discuss a clinician's professional behaviour and interactions with both patients and staff, and then to apply what they have learnt. Direct observation of students (e.g., as they explain diagnosis/prognosis/management) enables individualised feedback on professionalism (Davies and McGuire 2000; Ghodse 2004) and ought to form the bulk of the initial part of any placement. This, in conjunction with modelling, instils confidence and enhances performance for the rest of the placement, and the gains are ultimately far greater than the initial investment of time and effort.

Subjective Judgement in Assessment

Experienced clinicians rely on a gestalt impression, that is, pattern recognition and subjective judgement, for clinical diagnosis (Hodges 2013; Epstein 2007). So, is there a role for holistic supervisor (expert) judgements in student assessment, in the form of subjective global impressions over a specific time frame (Epstein 2007)? Diagnostic, contextual or interpersonal variables might be part of the authentic variability of real practice settings (Epstein 2007). Competence is not fixed/stable, but contextual, constructed and changeable and also at least partly subjective and collective (Hodges 2013). There have been calls for movement away from the purely psychometric model, with the re-examination of the value of subjectivity and judgement (Hodges 2006, 2013; Epstein 2007). Reliance on subjective information and judgement is seen by many as a 'soft option', biased or unfair (van der Vleuten et al. 2012; Hodges 2013) and therefore less reliable. Various authors have discussed ways of increasing the reliability of subjective judgements, for example by increasing the testing time (Hodges 2013), appropriate sampling of raters and simulated patients (van der Vleuten and Schuwirth 2005); increasing the number of judgements and ensuring the independence and diversity (heterogeneity) of raters and sources of information (Eva and

Hodges 2012; Hodges 2013). However, trying to achieve complete objectivity may trivialise the assessment process (van der Vleuten et al. 2012).

Assessment of General Professional Competencies

General professional competencies include an ability to work in a team, metacognitive skills, professional behaviour and the ability to reflect/self-appraise (van der Vleuten and Schuwirth 2005; Hodges et al. 2011). Multi-source ('360-degree') assessments (Epstein 2007) can provide insight into trainees' work habits, capacity for teamwork and interpersonal sensitivity, and it is most effective when it includes narrative comments (as well as statistical data) from credible sources, coupled with constructive feedback and mentoring (Epstein 2007). An example of how this might apply in practice is to undertake a 'friends and family test' to give a global/gestalt impression – such as 'Would you send your friend or family member to this (future) doctor?' If multiple impressions are collected from a wide range of raters (e.g., from the multidisciplinary team, patients and peers), integrated ('jury model') and a narrative feedback is added, this provides robust and valid information (Epstein 2007). Coupled with feedback and mentoring, this will stimulate learning and development (Epstein 2007; van der Vleuten et al. 2012).

Assessment of competencies needs to be increasingly based on qualitative, descriptive and narrative information, but the best way forward is to combine this with quantitative, numerical data (van der Vleuten and Schuwirth 2005). Competencies may be integrated for methods that are not as standardised (e.g., oral exams, mini-CEX). Multiple sources of information from various methods may be used to construct an overall judgement by triangulating information across these sources (van der Vleuten and Schuwirth 2005). Moreover, learning is facilitated when tasks are integrated, and contextualisation (vignette- and problem-based learning) enhances validity (Hodges 2006). Portfolios and log books are now extensively used in both undergraduate and postgraduate medical education, and they include evidence/documentation of, and self-reflection about, specific areas of a trainee's competence and demonstrate professional development.

Strategic Learners

Assessment plays a dominant role in student learning, and has both intended and unintended consequences. For example, end-of-year exams, which rely on recall of factual information, can lead to cramming and surface-level learning (Newble 1983; Epstein 2007). Strategic learners are common in medicine; given the sheer volume of factual information to process in order to become a doctor, students feel overloaded, creating a pressure towards strategic learning. To take more interest or study a topic in depth might mean failing something else, so tight is the balance. Many prefer exams (i.e., surface learning for short-term recall) rather than continuous assessments and study only for the parts of the course that are assessed (Kneale 1997). Cutting corners results in a lack of meaningful understanding or a change in attitude due to cognitive restructuring. Prejudices regarding psychiatric professionals and patients therefore remain, especially as this approach often continues into the post-graduate years

Are We Strategic Teachers?

We can't help thinking that many of us might in fact be 'strategic teachers', such is the juggling act we find ourselves in. We face barriers to teaching, such as lack of time, resources, funding and recognition. Are we in essence merely 'good enough' teachers, as opposed to good teachers? If so, what example is this setting our students and what impact is it having?

Improving the Motivation to Learn

Motivation can be extrinsic or intrinsic. Strategic learners are motivated extrinsically (e.g., by assessment). Intrinsic motivation is mediated by student factors (e.g., previous experience, desire to achieve and curiosity to learn) and enhanced by maximising the learning environment, relevance (e.g., immediate needs/future career) and good teachers (Markert 2001). Maslow's hierarchy of needs indicates that students'/trainees' non-clinical needs must be met first in order to increase their motivation to learn (Maslow 1943). In essence, we can achieve this by making them feel important (i.e., promoting feelings of trust, belonging and self-esteem), as well as attending to their basic physiological needs (e.g., physical safety and comfort). However, this can be difficult owing to lack of facilities in the community (e.g., designated space and IT resources) and wards that can be chaotic and dangerous. Therefore, ground rules must be clear and involve mutual respect and trust. Regular dialogue to ensure that a positive learning environment is being maintained is essential. Pastoral issues must not be neglected (Cantillon et al. 2006).

Self-Regulated Learning

Improving motivation is linked to the promotion of self-regulated learning (SRL). SRL is a complex and highly individual process (Sitzmann and Ely 2011; Zumbrunn et al. 2011), which is essential for life-long learning as a healthcare professional. Factors known to stimulate SRL are social support, the opportunity for guided and independent practice, with the support of feedback and stimulation of reflective practice, and the opportunity to make errors and learn from them (Sitzmann and Ely 2011; Berkhout et al. 2015). It is also influenced by the student's specific goals (Berkhout et al. 2015). It should be maximised by offering students more tailored learning opportunities and support based on recognising each learner's needs, personal goals and narrative (Berkhout et al. 2015). Perhaps this could be aligned to future career aims (Hashmi et al. 2014). If students cannot relate to external goals set by the curriculum, it will deter SRL (Berkhout et al. 2015). Therefore, as Wass et al. (2001) note, 'assessment is the most appropriate engine on which to harness the curriculum'. Formative assessments provide benchmarks to orient the learner and reinforce their intrinsic motivation to learn. However, infrequent summative exams (often at the end of a training block) do not give opportunities to link the results with feedback or inform students' learning needs (Schuwirth and van der Vleuten 2006).

Making the Most of the Learning Environment

The uniqueness of the psychiatric setting should be used to its best advantage (Cantillon et al. 2006). Working within a multidisciplinary team and involving patients and carers/relatives enables students to understand different points of view. This is essential to becoming a psychiatrist (Davies and McGuire 2000). Arranging a mix between general versus specialised and in-patient versus community settings will give students the

> **Box 3.2** Characteristics of good teachers in two dimensions (Beishuizen et al. 2001; Sutkin et al. 2008)
>
> **Ability/cognitive dimension**
>
> * Skills
> * Knowledge
> * Experience:
>
>   clear explanations
>
>   improvisation, anecdotes
>
> **Personality/non-cognitive dimension**
>
> * Humanistic/interpersonal skills
> * Enthusiastic/emotionally activating, charismatic
> * Self-aware

broadest view of psychiatry with which to make an informed career choice or develop sympathetic attitudes to the field (Ghodse 2004). Home visits are an effective way of reducing stigma towards patients (Walters et al. 2007). Ward rounds can be made more useful by highlighting teaching points and giving students tasks to keep them active. Smaller groups enhance collaborative learning and teamwork (Sweet et al. 2003; Cantillon et al. 2006), and one-to-one teaching and feedback are tailored, adaptable and instil enthusiasm as well as enabling modelling (Sweet et al. 2003; Cantillon et al. 2006; Cross et al. 2006). 'Hot-seating', allowing students to see patients alone in clinic before seeing them together, enables experiential learning (Kolb 1984; Kneale 1997). However, this is not always feasible, due to time constraints and a shortage of rooms.

Teachers' characteristics influence students' learning and motivation. We were inspired by those who were enthusiastic and caring. Good teachers create an atmosphere in which students are motivated by intrinsic drives – identifying with and then modelling enthusiasm. The literature points out that the characteristics of good clinical teachers broadly fall into two dimensions: Beishuizen et al. (2001) identify them as the ability and personality dimensions, whereas Sutkin et al. (2008) describe them in terms of cognitive and non-cognitive dimensions (Box 3.2). Although skills and characteristics in the personality/non-cognitive dimension are difficult to teach, they need more emphasis, as they dominate the literature on good medical teaching.

Conclusion

With the recent increase in the number of foundation posts in psychiatry in the UK, we have an excellent opportunity to address problems in psychiatry such as stigma, recruitment and holistic care. However, we need to attend to the basics and turn to the literature on teaching, medical education and psychiatry in order to do this.

We have to motivate medical students and trainee doctors with good teaching and a variety of methods to promote active learning, thus overcoming the culture of strategic learning. As teachers, we need to be knowledgeable, but humanistic qualities need more emphasis. We must also give and receive regular feedback, adapt to students' needs, maximise the learning environment and make students feel important. This will improve deeper learning, enhance professionalism and reduce prejudice against psychiatry. It might even improve recruitment to the field.

More specifically, we should promote positive attitudes towards psychiatry in all students and juniors, even if they do not want to become psychiatrists. This will help to address stigma against psychiatrists and also against our patients. We must remember that students with neutral views are the most likely to have their attitudes modified by good teaching. We should try to identify students who show enthusiasm for psychiatry and should try to maintain their interest until they make their career choices. This could be achieved by mentoring them over time, involving them in research projects and audits, setting up psychiatry interest groups and campaigning for more exposure to psychiatry in the final undergraduate year.

Most importantly, we should look at ourselves and the examples we set. We, as influential individuals, have a huge bearing on the future of psychiatry. We must look beyond our own short-term interest and goals and consider the bigger picture.

Acknowledgements

For information, the original paper on which this chapter is based was: Sarkar SN & Young AH (2017). Going beyond 'good enough' teaching in psychiatric training. *BJPsych Advances*, 23(2), 131–42. doi:10.1192/apt.bp.115.01510. The authors wish to acknowledge with thanks the contribution of Professor Allan Young to the original paper.

References

American Psychiatric Association (2013) *The Principles of Medical Ethics with Annotations Especially Applicable to Psychiatry*. APA.

Baker M, Wessely S, Openshaw D (2016) Not such friendly banter? GPs and psychiatrists against the systematic denigration of their specialties. *British Journal of General Practice*, **66**: 508–9.

Baxter H, Singh SP, Standen P, et al. (2001) The attitudes of 'tomorrow's doctors' towards mental illness and psychiatry: changes during the final undergraduate year. *Medical Education*, **35**: 381–3.

Beishuizen JJ, Hof E, van Putten CM, et al. (2001) Students' and teachers' cognitions about good teachers. *British Journal of Educational Psychology*, **71**: 185–201.

Berkhout JJ, Helmich E, Teunissen PW, et al. (2015) Exploring the factors influencing clinical students' self-regulated learning. *Medical Education*: **49**: 589–600.

Byrne P (2000) *Stigma of Mental Illness and Ways of Diminishing It*. Cambridge University Press.

Cantillon P, Hutchinson L, Wood D (2006) *ABC of Learning and Teaching in Medicine*. BMJ Publications.

Cross V, Moore A, Morris J, et al. (2006) *The Practice-Based Educator: A Reflective Tool for CPD and Accreditation*. John Wiley & Sons, Inc.

Dave S (2012) Simulation in psychiatric teaching. *Advances in Psychiatric Treatment*, **18**: 292–8.

Davies T, McGuire P (2000) Teaching medical students in the new millennium. *Psychiatric Bulletin*, **24**: 4–5.

Dogra N, Anderson J, Edwards R, et al. (2008) Service user perspectives about their role in undergraduate medical training about mental health. *Medical Teacher*, **30**: 152–6.

Epstein RM (2007) Assessment in medical education. *New England Journal of Medicine*, **356**: 387–96.

Epstein RM, Hundert EM (2002) Defining and assessing professional competence. *JAMA*, **287**: 226–35.

Eva K, Hodges BD (2012) Dialogue: Scylla or Charbydis? Can we navigate between objectification and judgment in assessment? *Medical Education*, **46**: 914–19.

Frank JR, Danoff D (2007) The CanMEDS initiative: implementing an outcomes-based framework of physician competencies. *Medical Teacher*, **29**: 642–7.

General Medical Council (2013) *Good Medical Practice*. General Medical Council.

Ghodse H (2004) Psychiatry for tomorrow's doctors: undergraduate medical education. *International Psychiatry*, **3**: 1–2.

Glynn S, Reilly M, Avalos G, et al. (2006) Attitudinal change toward psychiatry during undergraduate medical training in Ireland. *Irish Journal of Psychological Medicine*, **23**: 131–3.

Gray J (2002) Stigma in psychiatry. *Journal of the Royal Society of Medicine*, **95**: 72–6.

Hashmi A, Talley M, Parsaik AK (2014) Individualising psychiatry clerkships to medical student career choice. *Medical Education*, **48**: 1104–5.

Hodges B (2006) Medical education and the maintenance of incompetence. *Medical Teacher*, **28**: 690–6.

Hodges B (2013) Assessment in the post-psychometric era: learning to love the subjective and collective. *Medical Teacher*, **35**: 564–8.

Hodges BD, Ginsburg S, Cruess R, et al. (2011) Assessment of professionalism: recommendations from the Ottawa 2010 Conference. *Medical Teacher*, **33**: 354–63.

Hodges BD, Hollenberg E, McNaughton N, et al. (2014) The psychiatry OSCE: a 20-year retrospective. *Academic Psychiatry*, **38**: 26–34.

Joubert PM (2006) Medical students on the value of role models for developing 'soft skills': 'That's the way you do it'. *South African Psychiatry Review*, **9**: 28–32.

Kolb DA (1984) *Experiential Learning: Experience as a Source of Learning and Development*. Prentice Hall.

Markert RJ (2001) What makes a good teacher? Lessons from teaching medical students. *Academic Medicine*, **76**: 809–10.

Maslow AH (1943) A theory of motivation. *Psychological Review*, **50**: 370–96.

McNaughton N, Ravitz P, Wadell A, et al. (2008) Psychiatric education and simulation: a review of the literature. *Canadian Journal of Psychiatry*, **53**: 85–93.

McParland M, Noble LM, Livingstone G (2003) The effect of a psychiatric attachment on students' attitudes to and intention to pursue psychiatry as a career. *Medical Education*, **37**: 447–54.

Miller GE (1990) The assessment of clinical skills/competence/performance. *Academic Medicine*, **65**: 63–7.

Kneale P (1997) The rise of the 'strategic' student: how can we adapt to cope? In Armstrong S, Thompson G, Brown S (eds.), *Facing up to Radical Changes in Universities and Colleges*, pp. 119–30. Routledge.

Newble DI, Jaeger K (1983) The effect of assessments and examinations on the learning of medical students. *Medical Education*; **17**: 165–71.

Niedermier JA, Bornstein R, Brandemihl A (2006) The junior medical student psychiatry clerkship: curriculum, attitudes, and test performance. *Academic Psychiatry*, **30**: 136–43.

Norcini JJ, Blank LL, Duffy FD, et al. (2003) The mini-CEX: a method for assessing clinical skills. *Annals of Internal Medicine*, **138**: 476–81.

Norman G (2005) Checklists vs. ratings, the illusion of objectivity, the demise of skills and the debasement of evidence. *Advances in Health*

Sciences Education: Theory and Practice, **10**: 1–3.

Oakley C, Oyebode F (2008) Medical students' views about an undergraduate curriculum in psychiatry before and after clinical placements. *BMC Medical Education*, **8**: 26.

Paddock M, Farooq K, Sarkar SN, et al. (2013) Why choose psychiatry? Report on a qualitative workshop. *The Psychiatrist*, **37**: 146.

Plaice E, Heard S, Moss F (2002) How important are role models in making good doctors? *BMJ*, **325**: 707–10.

Ram P, Grol R, Rethans JJ, et al. (1999) Assessment of general practitioners by video observation of communicative and medical performance in daily practice: issues of validity, reliability and feasibility. *Medical Education*, **33**: 447–54.

Read J, Baker S (1996) *Not Just Sticks and Stones: A Survey of People with Mental Health Problems*. Mind.

Rethans JJ, Norcini JJ, Barón-Maldonado M, et al. (2002) The difference in relationship between competence and performance: implications for assessing practice performance. *Medical Education*, **36**: 901–9.

Roberts LW, Warner TD, Hammond KA, et al. (2005) Becoming a good doctor: perceived need for ethics training focused on practical and professional development topics. *Academic Psychiatry* **29**: 301–3.

Royal College of Psychiatrists (2009) *Good Psychiatric Practice*, 3rd ed. (College Report CR154). Royal College of Psychiatrists.

Schuwirth LWT, van der Vleuten CPM (2003) The use of clinical simulations in assessment. *Medical Education*, **37**: 65–71.

Schuwirth LWT, van der Vleuten CPM (2006) A plea for new psychometric models in educational assessment. *Medical Education*, **40**: 296–300.

Shah P, Brown T, Eagles J (2011) Choosing psychiatry: factors influencing career choice among foundation doctors in Scotland. In Brown T, Eagles J (eds.), *Teaching Psychiatry to Undergraduates*, pp. 255–63. Royal College of Psychiatrists.

Sitzmann T, Ely K (2011) A meta-analysis of self-regulated learning in work-related training and educational attainment: what we know and where we need to go. *Psychological Bulletin*, **137**: 421–42.

Skånér Y (2005) General practitioners' reasoning when considering the diagnosis heart failure: a think-aloud study. *BMC Family Practitioner*, **6**: 4.

Sluijsmans DMA, Brand-Gruwel S, van Merrienboer J, et al. (2003) The training of peer assessment skills to promote the development of reflection skills in teacher education. *Studies in Educational Evaluation*, **29**: 23–42.

Sutkin G, Wagner E, Harris I, et al. (2008) What makes a good clinical teacher in medicine? A review of the literature. *Academic Medicine*, **83**: 452–66.

Sweet J, Hutly S, Taylor I (2003) *Effective Learning and Teaching in Medical, Dental and Veterinary Education*. Kogan Page.

Tharyan P, John T, Tharyan A, et al. (2008) Attitudes of 'tomorrow's doctors' towards psychiatry and mental illness. *National Medical Journal of India*, **14**: 355–9.

Thornicroft G, Rose D, Kassam A, et al. (2007) Stigma: ignorance, prejudice or discrimination? *British Journal of Psychiatry*, **190**: 192–3.

Townsend J (1979) Stereotypes of mental illness: a comparison with ethnic stereotypes. *Culture, Medicine & Psychiatry*, **24**: 205–29.

van der Vleuten CPM, Schuwirth LWT (2005) Assessing professional competence: from methods to programmes. *Medical Education*, **39**: 309–17.

van der Vleuten CPM, Schuwirth LWT, Driessen EW, et al. (2012) A model for programmatic assessment fit for purpose. *Medical Teacher*, **34**: 205–14.

Walters K, Raven P, Rosenthal J, et al. (2007) Teaching undergraduate psychiatry in primary care: the impact on student learning and attitudes. *Medical Education*, **41**: 100–8.

Wass V, van der Vleuten C, Shatzer J, et al. (2001) Assessment of clinical competence. *Lancet*, **357**: 845–9.

Wilkinson TJ, Frampton CM (2004)
Comprehensive undergraduate medical
assessments improve prediction of
clinical performance. *Medical Education*,
38: 1111–16.

Zumbrunn S, Tadlock J, Roberts ED (2011)
*Encouraging Self-Regulated Learning in the
Classroom: A Review of the Literature.*
Metropolitan Educational Research
Consortium.

A Guide to Conducting an Online Literature Search for Medical Educators

Riccardo De Giorgi and Patricia Casey

Introduction

Conducting a literature search can be a daunting experience. Most medical educators are in the difficult position of striving for a high-quality search while working in a busy academic and clinical environment.

The practice of research according to the principles of evidence-based medicine (EBM) has been perfected (i.e., has become richer and more complex) over the years, and the same goes for literature searching – an integral and key aspect of EBM (McKeever et al. 2015). However, the thought of dealing with an astonishing amount of literature (more than 55 million records only between the two major databases, PubMed/MEDLINE and Embase (Lefebvre et al. 2021)), would likely overwhelm even the most enthusiastic individual. The task of conducting a literature search thus often seems like a twofold burden that presents both psychological and practical barriers. In this chapter, we intend to lighten this burden by adopting an accessible language and approach. We will describe essential knowledge and examine hands-on basic and advanced strategies for performing an online literature search in the context of medical education.

It should be emphasized that we will not discuss how to conduct a literature search for the specific purpose of writing a systematic review for a specialized journal (e.g., a Cochrane review), for which we refer the reader to more suitable manuals (Higgins et al. 2021) and articles (Atkinson and Cipriani 2018).

Dealing with Psychological Barriers

As trivial as it may sound, getting into the right mindset is the first and most essential step before initiating a literature search. At this stage, breaking down the problem into parts and establishing specific goals is helpful. This is best done by asking yourself some questions and trying to answer them as plainly and fairly as possible.

Do I Have a Specific Clinical/Research Question?

An adequate literature search can only be achieved if it aims to answer a well-defined, detailed question. The meticulous definition of this is critical, as its influence will determine the result of your search. Whether you are conducting a literature search for an article or in preparation for a lecture, a faulty clinical/research question is setting you up for failure. Making inferences from data that cannot answer the initial question is a far too common mistake.

The task of choosing a suitable, evidence-based question might seem intimidating at first. In fact, it is easily addressed by using a simple framework (Davies 2011), such as the

PICO – population, intervention, comparison, outcome – for interventional trials and their meta-analyses. For example, a researcher interested in evaluating the effect of a particular antidepressant in people with depression would ask: 'Is fluoxetine (intervention) more or less efficacious (outcome) than placebo (comparison) in depressed patients (population)?' But if the same researcher started including studies on patients with anxiety disorders too (i.e., a population different from the one originally defined), the search results and all the subsequent findings would be inaccurate. This does not mean that the initial question is set in stone, as it can be further tailored to individual needs: if the same researcher later realizes that studying the anti-anxiety effects of fluoxetine better matches their interest, it may be appropriate to widen the population under consideration. Slight or more substantial variations of this framework can likewise be employed according to the specific requirements of the search. For example, the PECO – population, exposure, comparison, outcome – for observational studies and their meta-analyses; the ECLIPSE – expectation, client group, location, impact, professionals, service – for health policy; or the SPICE – setting, perspective, intervention, comparison, evaluation – for service evaluation. Further frameworks for building a variety of clinical/research question can easily be retrieved online (Davies 2011). There is also the option of tweaking any of the existing frameworks to ensure that it matches your needs (e.g., if your question is unlikely to involve a comparison group, you would just skip it).

Sometime, a clinician may want to conduct a literature review of broader scope, answering a less defined clinical/research question such as 'what is the aetiology of attention deficit hyperactivity disorder (ADHD)?'. In this case, finding an appropriate structuring framework may prove difficult or indeed be too restrictive. This is likely due to the fact that the available frameworks have generally been devised with the intention of obtaining systematic evidence from clinical studies (e.g., interventional trials), which can then be pooled – something that would simply not make sense for the data retrieved from general questions about, for example, 'the causes of ADHD'. It is still possible, however, to obtain high-quality, or even comprehensive and systematic evidence. Firstly, some of the 'further resources' reported below oftentimes provide excellent summaries of studies on topics such as the aetiology of certain disorders (e.g., the *Lancet* 'seminars'). Secondly, some strategies using index terms in specific search engines such as PubMed can be employed to obtain a large number of relevant records – see the Search Tools section below.

This does not mean, however, that no clinical/research questions about diseases' aetiology can be structured in a systematic fashion. For example, a more specific question on the involvement of genes in the aetiology of ADHD could be: 'in the general population (i.e., human, not animal studies – population), which genes (exposure) are responsible for the onset of ADHD (outcome)?'

The importance of framing your question accurately cannot be emphasized enough. Ask yourself: Is it formulated in an unambiguous and understandable fashion? Does it follow a clear structure? Your clinical intuition and common sense will help you reply to these questions objectively and impartially. If the answer to all of them is yes, then proceed. If not, take a step back, and start again.

Does My Search Need to Be Systematic and All-Inclusive?

Since the rise of EBM practices, the types, classifications and descriptions of reviews that can be conducted in the medical field have become a matter of considerable and ongoing debate, often pervaded by overlapping definitions, misused concepts, incorrect terminologies and overall confusion (Grant and Booth 2009). A widespread misconception is that a literature search according to EBM principles must always be as structured and as comprehensive as a search done for a systematic review (e.g., a Cochrane review). However, if the purpose is not to write a systematic review, but for example to gather evidence for a lecture, does the corresponding literature search have to comply with all those rules and boundaries for being considered 'respectable' (i.e., evidence-based)? In this case, a literature search that is thorough, but does not have the ambition of including all the published and unpublished evidence on the topic, seems more appropriate. In other words, the need for all-inclusiveness can be less stringent. But what about the need to be systematic? Some could argue that a literature search for a traditional narrative review does not demand a predefined strategy and therefore might avoid using a framework such as the PICO to formulate the initial clinical/research question. But narrative reviews are still written with the intention of answering a defined, if broader, question, which must be properly established in advance.

In summary, an effort should be made to approach any literature search in a systematic fashion, which means following a clear methodology and a pre-specified plan detailing why certain evidence is privileged over other information. Only then can the search still be called evidence-based.

Do I Need Help?

It may sound like a paradox, but the greater your experience in literature searching, the more you will be comfortable with relying on other parties for help.

The simplest form of support can come from your team in your routine clinical or academic practice. It can range from general advice to more practical tasks delegated to other team members.

A surprisingly often overlooked source of assistance with literature searching are library services, commonly offered by most departments and trusts. Again, the scope of such help varies largely, but most librarians can give enthusiastic and competent guidance, especially when involved at the early stages of a literature search. The library service at the Royal College of Psychiatrists is also a valuable resource for its members wishing to conduct searches. In addition, librarians can provide you with additional, highly skilled training. If access to these services is not an option, a quick search for online resources, such as courses and video tutorials, is a valid alternative; today, their quality is frequently very high, as they often include a myriad of perks such as step-by-step walkthroughs, interactive platforms and even tailored troubleshooting.

Dealing with Practical Barriers

Once the strategies above have been implemented, the reader will be reassured that most of the practical barriers will have started crumbling too. Before jumping into the execution of the literature search, two more issues may still require some attention.

Firstly, it is vital to have ready access to the full texts of the articles that will be retrieved. There is little more frustrating than spending hours trying to navigate some convoluted journal systems for accessing a full text, only to discover that the paper is irrelevant to the initial question. Despite a significant push from major research funders and councils towards shifting the whole publishing model on an 'open access' basis (Schiltz 2018), too many articles remain behind a paywall. University departments tend to use their own platforms to access an extensive assortment of publishers, so this is a good option if you are routinely working in an academic setting. Alternatively, in the UK, belonging to a National Health Service (NHS) trust offers the oftentimes forgotten opportunity to register for an OpenAthens account (https://openathens.nice.org.uk), thus allowing you to reach most of the desired papers. The institutions' own repository may also contain some papers written by its academics. PubMed Central may also be a useful resource for full articles as may Google Scholar. If retrieving 'that' article remains a problem, it is again recommended to ask for help from library services, which in most cases will definitively solve it.

Secondly, and perhaps prosaically, it is important to make time in an otherwise busy schedule to dedicate to the tasks of designing and performing an adequate literature search. This is something that takes varying amounts of time, so set that aside to decide on the question and formulate your search methods using the correct words.

Basic Literature Searching

Having dealt with various kinds of barriers, we can move on to the 'nuts and bolts' of an online literature search.

A first point of access to high-quality information generally involves using resources (e.g., guidelines, local policies, etc.) available electronically or in paper form to most clinicians – see the Further Resources section below for more information. However, these sources may not be able to help with all areas of mental health research: for instance, developments in understanding the aetiology, course and prognosis of psychiatric disorders; mental health services evaluation; and ethics in psychiatric practice, to name but a few, are somewhat more difficult to retrieve.

Luckily, there are several other basic tools that can be used by any clinician, even if entirely new to the practice of literature searching.

Single Citation Matcher

Sometimes, you might know of an article you want to use as a basis for your search but may experience some difficulties retrieving it. Suppose you attend a journal club and one of your colleagues mentions a paper by a particular author on a certain topic, so you decide you would like to know more about it. How do you find it? The single citation matcher tool can help with that. This is a free facility available on the opening page of PubMed under 'Tools'. You simply add in as much information about the citation as is available to you. The name of the author(s) and year of publication along with the journal name are the most useful. The more information you have about the citation, the narrower the search. You need to check that the names of the author and journal are spelt correctly but alternatives are provided as you enter your information. You will then be able to obtain the exact citation and read the abstract.

While the abstracts of the relevant citation and related articles are always available, the papers themselves may not be, unless they are open access, which will be indicated in the search. Otherwise, they will need to be obtained through the university subscription/institutional library (see the section above, Dealing with Practical Barriers).

Google Scholar

Google Scholar is a free and easy-to-use starting point for many literature searches in psychiatry. It can lead to hundreds of relevant papers very quickly, and some full papers are accessible directly through it.

To begin, digit 'Google Scholar' into your web browser and left-click: the Google Scholar browser will appear. One can do either a basic or an advanced search. To run a basic search, you simply type in the search bar the relevant words you want to search. Boolean (linking) operators (Table 4.1), named after George Boole (a nineteenth-century English mathematician), can be used to narrow, broaden or define your search.

An advanced search in Google Scholar automatically includes the Boolean operators and gives the opportunity to provide additional filters, such as the publication dates. Moreover, it not only identifies papers that are relevant to the topic you are researching, but also retrieves information about other papers that have cited these and a list of similar papers. Finally, it provides links to several bibliographic databases and identifies those that are available freely. To perform an advanced search, you need to go on the Google Scholar homepage and look at the top left-hand corner for a symbol with three short horizontal lines: click on this and then on the 'Advanced search' icon so that the relevant page will open.

Clinical Queries Tool

The clinical queries tool is another free implement on PubMed that allows for a basic search to be structured around a specific clinical/research question. Under 'Clinical Study

Table 4.1 Boolean (linking) operators

" "	These are used around words that you want returned in that exact combination you have placed them in; for example, "depressive disorder". If these words did not have quotation marks, you would retrieve all papers with the word depressive and all the papers with the word disorder in them.
AND	This narrows the search; for example, "depressive disorder" AND "anxiety", only papers with both depressive disorder and anxiety will be returned
OR	This expands the search so that papers with either one or the other term will be identified, often used for synonyms; for example, as well as anxiety you may want to include the term generalized anxiety disorder, so you would type anxiety OR "generalized anxiety disorder"
NOT	This identifies a word that you want to exclude; for example, "depressive disorder" NOT "health anxiety" will exclude papers pertaining to health anxiety.
()	These are used to separate different concepts that have been linked with other operators; for example, "depressive disorder" AND (anxiety OR "generalized anxiety disorder") ensures that all the returned papers will contain depressive disorder and either anxiety or generalized anxiety, whereas omitting the parenthesis would result in papers with both depressive disorder and anxiety but also papers with only generalized anxiety disorder.
* or #	These are used to search for alternative forms of the word; for example, suicid* retrieves suicide, suicidal, suicidality.

Categories', five headings can be searched: therapy, clinical prediction guides, diagnosis, aetiology and prognosis; the 'Scope' can be either broad or narrow. The results generated cover three areas pertaining to the question: clinical studies, systematic reviews/clinical practice guidelines and genetics. The results obtained can also be further narrowed using filters such as language, recency of publication, sex, age, etc. Drexel University Libraries has an excellent video tutorial on using this tool.

Advanced Literature Searching

The Search Strategy

When devising and then running a search strategy, two key elements must be considered: the databases that will be searched and the tools that can be used for each database.

Health-Related Bibliographic Databases

Numerous databases are available electronically, each with a slightly different focus, accessibility requirements and sets of rules. Regrettably, there is often some confusion between the concepts of a 'database' (i.e., a repository of references to journal articles, such as MEDLINE) and a 'search engine' (i.e., a retrieval system, such as PubMed, that can access one or multiple databases). This confusion is complicated further because certain databases sometimes have their own search engine (e.g., Embase). In general, we could argue for a lack of clear consensus regarding this distinction – an argument that goes beyond the scope of this chapter and which perhaps only the most veteran search strategists could disentangle. In fact, a perfectly reasonable literature search can be performed with some elementary knowledge of just a handful of health-related bibliographic databases/search engines. As such, the list below is far from exhaustive but should cater for most needs.

PubMed is possibly the most well-known electronic search engine in the world. Its popularity is likely related to the fact that it is free and relatively simple to use. It is not a bibliographic database but provides unrestricted access to the MEDLINE database, which includes over 27 million references from some 5,200 journals. It also covers other citations not yet indexed for MEDLINE (i.e., articles that have not gone through the process of manual indexing by professionals), the full-text articles archived in PubMed Central, and several e-books via Bookshelf, for a total of more than 32 million records (US National Library of Medicine 2020). Although a search via PubMed alone would not normally suffice for the production of a high-quality systematic review, a confident user of this tool would be more than capable of conducting a decent literature search for any other purpose. Hence, we will analyse it in further detail below.

The other most important database is Embase, which can be accessed through its built-in search engine provided by Elsevier, though a subscription is necessary. It contains over 37 million references from some 8,100 journals, comprising several thousand that are not available on MEDLINE (Elsevier 2020), while also having recently included all MEDLINE records (Lefebvre et al. 2021). The latter explains why a growing number of researchers prefer this platform, though the paywall remains a barrier for both independent investigators and institutions. We will provide a more in-depth description on how to search this system in the next subsection.

PsycINFO® is another database worth mentioning for any research in the area of mental health. It contains some five million records from a variety of journals, books and dissertations in behavioural and social sciences (American Psychological Association 2020), which can be accessed for a fee via its own search engine.

It is evident at this point that, aside from MEDLINE via PubMed, most bibliographic databases and search engines may require a separate, paid subscription. A means to bypass this problem is via apposite service providers that have access to multiple databases at the same time. For example, the reader may have heard of the Ovid platform (Wolters Kluwer 2020a), which is subsidized by several academic institutions. This grants access to all the databases mentioned above (MEDLINE, Embase, PsycINFO®) and several more. Although the learning curve for these search interfaces may be steeper, the advantage of using a single tool for all your searches could make it worth it.

As mentioned, many other databases and search engines are available. A literature search focusing on clinical trials should also consider using the Cochrane Central Register of Controlled Trials (CENTRAL) (Cochrane Library 2020). The Cumulative Index to Nursing and Allied Health Literature (CINAHL) is instead more relevant to nursing and allied healthcare professions (EBSCO 2020).

A non-beginner in the field of literature searching may also be aware of platforms such as Web of Science and Scopus. These are citation indexes that can be used for more advanced techniques of forward/backward citation searching (i.e., skimming through articles that cite each other), for which we suggest referring to dedicated manuals (Lefebvre et al. 2021).

When choosing which databases to include in a literature search, the balance between sensitivity (i.e., striving for comprehensiveness) and specificity (i.e., avoiding hundreds of non-relevant records) needs to tip according to the specific needs and aims of that search (see the section above, Does My Search Need to Be Systematic and All-Inclusive?). As a rule of thumb and for most purposes, a high-quality search run on an individual database is far better than several incongruous ones. Therefore, we will now examine those tools that can help to achieve this goal.

Search Tools

Once you have chosen one (or more) database/search engine,[1] there is a number of ways you can go about your search. One could enter some words relevant to their clinical/research question into the search bar and run a basic search. This is called a text-word search. Unfortunately, this simple strategy tends to be quite ineffective, usually returning thousands of irrelevant results. The above-mentioned forward/backward citation searching can be employed for an initial scoping of the literature available on a certain topic, or more frequently as a complementary technique, in addition to a systematic search, to ensure inclusiveness.

The planning tool we recommend using, however, is the so-called concept map (Table 4.2). A concept map allows you to structure your search in a way that is both simple and evidence-based. It is easy to edit and keep track of any changes you make, thus transforming your literature search into a real itinerant process. Finally, it can be applied to any database, or at least eases the translation of a search from one database to another.

A prerequisite for the concept map is, yet again, formulating a clinical/research question according to one of the frameworks presented above. We can practise with our previous

---

[1] Note: for the purpose of this heading, the term 'database' will be used to include both 'search engine' and 'database'.

Table 4.2 Example of a concept map (simplified)
Clinical/research query: Is fluoxetine more or less efficacious than placebo in depressed patients?

#1	P	*Concept*: depressed patients
		Index term(s): - PubMed/MEDLINE: "Depressive Disorder"[Mesh] - Embase: depression/exp
		Keyword(s): "depress*"[tiab] OR "unipolar"[tiab]
#2	I	*Concept*: fluoxetine
		Index term(s): - PubMed/MEDLINE: "Fluoxetine"[Mesh] - Embase: fluoxetine/exp
		Keyword(s): "fluoxetin*"[tiab] OR "Prozac"[tiab])
#3	C	*Concept*: placebo
		Index term(s): - PubMed/MEDLINE: "Placebos"[Mesh] - Embase:
		Keyword(s): "placebo*"[tiab] OR "treatment as usual"[tiab] OR "case management"[tiab]
#4	O	*Concept*: efficacy [Generally not included in the final search, see main text]
		Index term(s): - PubMed/MEDLINE: – - Embase: –
		Keyword(s): –

example, based on the PICO: 'Is fluoxetine (intervention) more or less efficacious (outcome) than placebo (comparison) in depressed patients (population)?'. Here we have four concepts, which might scale down to three if we remember that the 'outcome' is not often included in a search strategy as it tends to be less well defined in articles' titles and abstracts.

Each concept is then probed via two different means: index terms and keywords.

Index Terms

Index terms are essentially tags selected from a controlled, database-specific vocabulary, and then assigned to the articles in a database by professional indexers. As such, this is not an automated process, and therefore requires some time between the article's publication and its indexing. Index terms are also known as MeSH (Medical Subject Headings) on PubMed, or Emtree on Embase. These terms are sometimes identical across several databases, but they are more frequently spelled with subtle differences: for example, for the population concept 'depressed patients', the MeSH is 'depressive disorder', whereas the Emtree is 'depression'. Moreover, index terms are built according to a hierarchical model, with broader and narrower categories that do not always reflect each other in different databases – something to bear in mind when transposing a search strategy from one database to another.

The formal way to find index terms that describe your concepts varies slightly according to the database. On PubMed, you would type your concept into the search bar, then select 'MeSH' in the scroll-down menu before running the search. On Embase, you would click on 'Emtree' before entering your concept in the search bar, then run your search. In both cases, a page will appear (Fig. 4.1) with a number of index terms that likely fit your concept (e.g., for 'depression', they can be 'depressive disorder', 'depressive disorder, treatment-resistant', etc.): choose the one that best matches your clinical/research question. Clicking on the index term will provide a description of the term, which can help with your choice. Moreover, it will show a number of subcategories that may or may not be relevant for your search (e.g., for 'depressive disorder', it could be 'depression, post-partum', 'seasonal affective disorder', etc.).

Running a search of an overarching index term automatically includes all of its subcategories, a method also known as explosion – unless you click on the relevant button that prevents the search from comprising those subcategories (e.g., 'Do not include MeSH terms found below this term in the MeSH hierarchy' on PubMed, 'Explode' on Embase). Whether you decide to explode your index terms or not should be based on your sensitivity versus specificity assessment discussed earlier. Index-term explosion can be indicated differently, via field codes, on the various databases: for instance, "Depressive Disorder"[Mesh:NoExp] shows on PubMed if the term is not exploded, whereas "depression/exp" is seen on Embase for the exploded term.

The index-term page (Fig. 4.1) is also useful for conducting searches that need to answer more general clinical/research questions, such as the previously mentioned 'What is the aetiology of ADHD?' Due to its breadth, it is worth in this case searching only one database – the one you are most comfortable using. On PubMed, you would start by retrieving the index term for ADHD, then click and select the subheading 'etiology' so to limit results to this specific subject: "Attention Deficit Disorder with Hyperactivity/etiology"[Mesh]. The chances are that you will get too many records to screen, so you can use the filters (see below for further information) on the left-hand side of the web page to narrow down your search: for example, you may be interested only in the most recent, highly validated evidence, in which case we would recommend filtering the results to include reviews (whether systematic or not) and books published over the last five years, perhaps only in human studies. Should you continue retrieving too many records for your own perusal, you might add (AND) the index term "Causality"[Mesh], or decide to focus (again, via AND) on a stricter subcategory in the aetiology of ADHD, such as "Genes"[Mesh].

A search that only includes index terms is already quite valid. However, as mentioned before, articles' indexing is a manual process that takes time, so it is conceivable that more recent articles relevant to your search may have not been indexed yet. Furthermore, there is always a small yet reasonable chance of error or tags going amiss. Therefore, once you have taken note of all the index terms matching your three or four concepts, it is time to dig into the keywords.

Keywords

Keywords are nothing but free-text terms that are likely to have been used in certain articles to express a concept: for example, the terms 'Prozac' and 'fluoxetine' for the intervention concept 'fluoxetine'. A number of keywords can be considered for each concept (e.g., 'placebo' could be substituted with 'waiting list', 'watchful waiting', 'treatment as usual', etc.). A mix of common-sense, clinical knowledge and a good thesaurus should be used

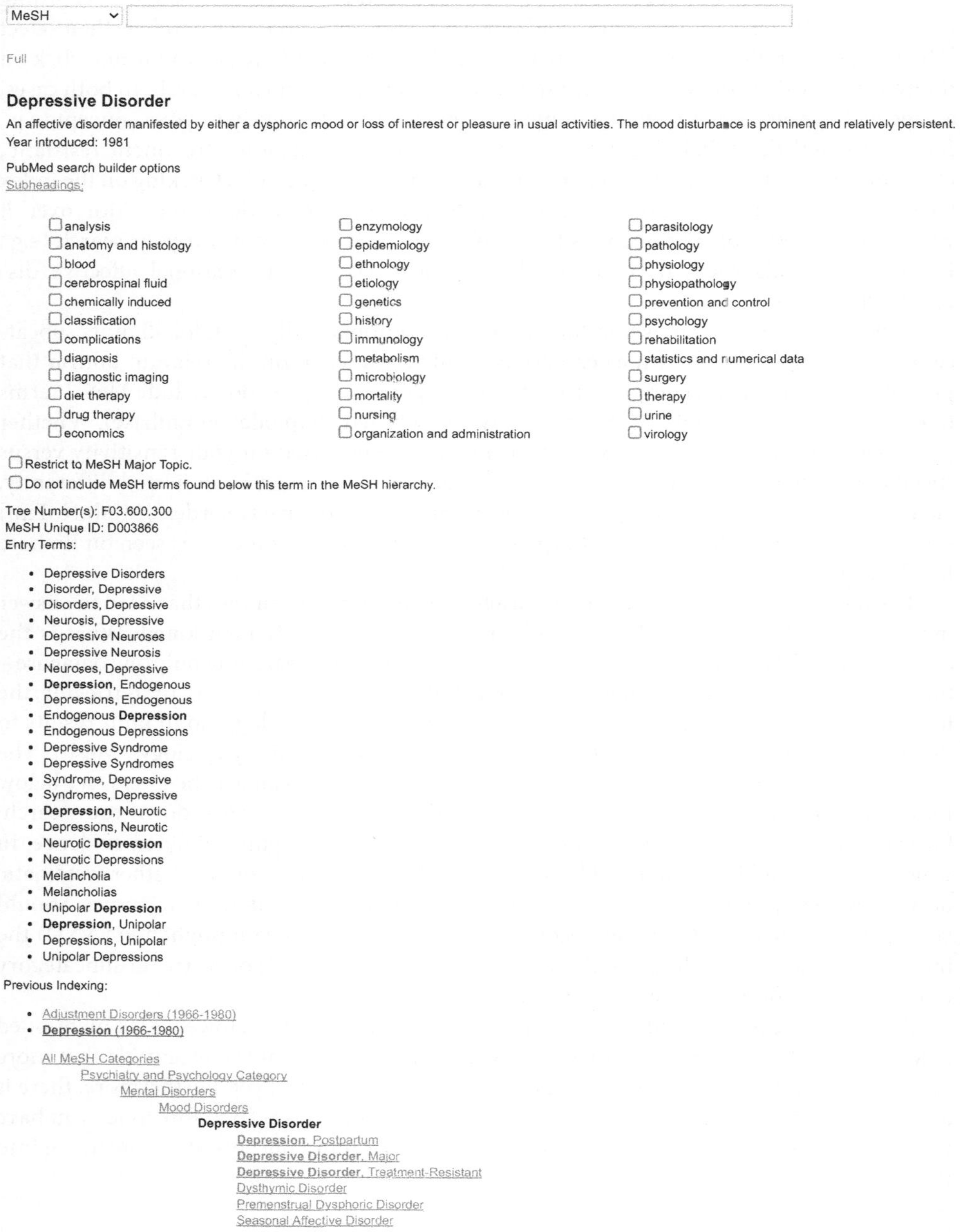

MeSH ⌄

Full

Depressive Disorder

An affective disorder manifested by either a dysphoric mood or loss of interest or pleasure in usual activities. The mood disturbance is prominent and relatively persistent. Year introduced: 1981

PubMed search builder options
Subheadings:

☐ analysis	☐ enzymology	☐ parasitology
☐ anatomy and histology	☐ epidemiology	☐ pathology
☐ blood	☐ ethnology	☐ physiology
☐ cerebrospinal fluid	☐ etiology	☐ physiopathology
☐ chemically induced	☐ genetics	☐ prevention and control
☐ classification	☐ history	☐ psychology
☐ complications	☐ immunology	☐ rehabilitation
☐ diagnosis	☐ metabolism	☐ statistics and numerical data
☐ diagnostic imaging	☐ microbiology	☐ surgery
☐ diet therapy	☐ mortality	☐ therapy
☐ drug therapy	☐ nursing	☐ urine
☐ economics	☐ organization and administration	☐ virology

☐ Restrict to MeSH Major Topic.
☐ Do not include MeSH terms found below this term in the MeSH hierarchy.

Tree Number(s): F03.600.300
MeSH Unique ID: D003866
Entry Terms:

- Depressive Disorders
- Disorder, Depressive
- Disorders, Depressive
- Neurosis, Depressive
- Depressive Neuroses
- Depressive Neurosis
- Neuroses, Depressive
- **Depression**, Endogenous
- Depressions, Endogenous
- Endogenous **Depression**
- Endogenous Depressions
- Depressive Syndrome
- Depressive Syndromes
- Syndrome, Depressive
- Syndromes, Depressive
- **Depression**, Neurotic
- Depressions, Neurotic
- Neurotic **Depression**
- Neurotic Depressions
- Melancholia
- Melancholias
- Unipolar **Depression**
- **Depression**, Unipolar
- Depressions, Unipolar
- Unipolar Depressions

Previous Indexing:

- Adjustment Disorders (1966-1980)
- **Depression (1966-1980)**

All MeSH Categories
    Psychiatry and Psychology Category
        Mental Disorders
            Mood Disorders
                Depressive Disorder
                    Depression, Postpartum
                    Depressive Disorder, Major
                    Depressive Disorder, Treatment-Resistant
                    Dysthymic Disorder
                    Premenstrual Dysphoric Disorder
                    Seasonal Affective Disorder

Fig. 4.1 An example of an index term (MeSH) page on PubMed.

when scoping for potential keywords. Since they are free text, you do not need to change keywords between databases. Also, you can account for word endings (truncation), e.g., suicid* will capture papers that use the word suicide, suicidal, suicidality etc. The symbol that substitutes for letters (wildcards) is database-specific (* or #), so seek further guidance for the database of your choice before applying these strategies to your search. The main advantage of using truncations and wildcards is that it allows you to employ the same keyword for several similar terms that may have been used in a certain article (e.g., 'wom#n' for both 'woman' and 'women'), including potential spelling mistakes (e.g., 'fluoxetin*' for 'fluoxetine' and the incorrect 'fluoxetin').

To avoid generating an unduly elevated number of irrelevant results, we would suggest limiting your keywords search to the title and abstract of the articles that will be screened. This can be achieved by adding to your keyword a field code such as [tiab], which stands for title and abstract (e.g., "depression"[tiab]), or at least [tx] for including most fields but the 'author' and 'affiliation' ones. Again, please note that this list of letters alternatives, field codes, etc. is not exhaustive, so you can refer to more advanced online material once you are a confident user of these basic strategies.

The Concept Map

Any reader might feel a bit lost at this point, and with good reason. Devising a well-structured concept map that includes several index terms and keywords is one of the last steps of any literature search, yet arguably the most demanding. Even a seasoned researcher may doubt themselves: 'Have I selected the most suitable index terms? Is my list of keywords comprehensive enough? What if I end up retrieving thousands of irrelevant results? Or, even worse, no results at all? Maybe my clinical/research question was too broad or too narrow in the first place . . .'. To these fearsome questions we would like to provide two reassuring answers. First, and intuitively, there is no such thing as a 'perfect concept map', let alone a 'perfect search strategy'. As long as your concept map is structured around a good clinical/research question and appropriately documented, you can keep 'perfecting it' until you reach a satisfactory result – that is, a result that matches the goals and expectations you set before starting your search (see the section above, Does My Search Need to Be Systematic and All-Inclusive?). Secondly, we refer you back to another subject discussed earlier, namely 'Do I need help?' You could show your concept map to your team colleagues or librarians and tweak it on the back of their feedback. Moreover, you can compare the search terms you chose for your concept map with those used in well-established search strategies for articles that are known for their robust methodologies, such as Cochrane reviews – look for them in the appendix/supplementary material.

Now that you have honed and polished your search terms (both index terms and keywords) according to the concepts of your clinical/research question, it is finally time to combine them into a viable search string that you can run on your database(s) of choice. The process of unifying the several index terms and keywords which reflect the same concept (e.g., the search terms "Fluoxetine"[Mesh], "fluoxetin*"[tiab], "Prozac"[tiab] for the intervention concept 'fluoxetine') is called nesting, and employs the Boolean (linking) operator (see Table 4.1) 'OR' as well as appropriately placed parentheses '()' to ensure that these terms are kept together: (("Fluoxetine"[Mesh]) OR ("fluoxetin*"[tiab] OR "Prozac"[tiab])). Nested concepts are normally clustered under a unique number (e.g., #1, #5, etc.). These concept-related numbers are combined via 'AND' into a search string that ultimately expresses your clinical/research question. Note that the operator 'NOT' can be used instead for a concept that you do not want included in your search (e.g., NOT "Animals"[Mesh] if you are not interested in animal studies).

An abridged example for ease of purpose: if the population concept is nested in #1 (("Depressive Disorder"[Mesh]) OR ("depress*"[tiab] OR "unipolar"[tiab])), and the intervention concept in #3 (("Fluoxetine"[Mesh]) OR ("fluoxetin*"[tiab] OR "Prozac"[tiab])), the resulting combined search string would be "#1 AND #3" – run this string to finally enjoy your search results.

If, in the end, your search retrieves too many records, you might consider using one of the several filters available on most databases, usually presented on a side menu. For example, the PubMed filter 'Species → Humans' should allow for all non-human (i.e., animal and *in vitro* studies) to be excluded, though unfortunately their reliability is somewhat inconsistent. Filters for specific study designs, such as randomized controlled trials, tend to be more dependable (Lefebvre et al. 2021). Overall, if your literature search does not aim for all-inclusiveness and would benefit from a positive specificity-to-sensitivity ratio, by all means add some filters to your search.

Further Resources

Finally, we would like to recommend some additional resources that would be at best complementary to a literature search conducted for a systematic review, but could easily become essential and save you plenty of time if your search is aimed at anything else.

Once again, start by formulating a clinical/research question, though it may be more loosely defined on this occasion. Unless it is a very specific one, or it refers to concepts or technologies that have only been developed recently, the chances are that some guidelines or manuals have been published on the topic. A list of high-quality, readily available resources is provided in Box 4.1.

Some major medical journals (e.g., the *Lancet*) regularly publish sections called 'seminars' that can provide a valuable overview of a certain topic. Also, Wolters Kluwer publishes a well-established journal, *Current Opinion in Psychiatry*, which comprises easy-to-read review articles focusing only on the most recent evidence on a variety of mental health topics (i.e., only studies published within 12–18 months from the review are generally included). *Evidence-Based Mental Health* is a journal covering clinically relevant research in mental health which is available in paper and online and free to members of the Royal College of Psychiatrists, with a focus on supporting clinicians to learn and apply an evidence-based approach to their own practice.

Systematic reviews are oftentimes an excellent source of comprehensive information. Apart from the above-mentioned Cochrane reviews, several other databases can be consulted. Prospero is an international database for registered systematic reviews. The full protocol of existing systematic reviews is available for reading without charge. This is a rich source of information for those writing on a particular topic.

Box 4.1 Readily available sources of high-quality evidence

- NICE Guidelines – available online, free
- Cochrane library of systematic reviews – available online, free
- Maudsley Guidelines – available as a book and online (if your library has a subscription)
- Evidence Based Mental Health – available in paper and online, free to RCPsych members

Additionally, the front of online interactive platforms for literature searches is an ever-developing one. UpToDate (Wolters Kluwer 2020b) is a subscription-only interface that allows you to quickly retrieve summaries of high-grade, recent evidence in response to specific clinical issues. Similarly, Trip (Trip Database Limited 2021) is a meta-database with a built-in PICO framework used to run a search – both a free and paid version are offered. Scite_ (Scite Inc. 2019), which requires a subscription after a free trial, is a fast-developing tool that uses an innovative Smart Citation algorithm to automatically search for published studies supporting or contrasting the articles referenced in a certain paper.

Conclusion

In this chapter, we have discussed several strategies that medical educators can employ to conduct an adequate literature search. This guide is not to be considered exhaustive: the field of literature searching very much benefits from technological advancements (e.g., utilization of machine-learning approaches), and is thus in constant development. Authors wanting to use their literature search for the purpose of publishing a paper on a specialized journal might need to hone their knowledge and skills via further manuals (Higgins et al. 2021). However, a literature search performed following the methods described in this chapter can provide the backbone to high-quality teaching sessions, assist in writing scientific papers and even inform clinical judgement and decision making.

References

American Psychological Association (2020) APA PsycINFO®. Available at: www.apa.org/pubs/databases/psycinfo?tab=1.

Atkinson L, Cipriani A (2018) How to carry out a literature search for a systematic review: a practical guide. *BJPsych Advances*, 24: 74–82; doi: 10.1192/bja.2017.3.

Cochrane Library (2020) Cochrane Central Register of Controlled Trials (CENTRAL). Available at: www.cochranelibrary.com/central/about-central.

Davies KS (2011) Formulating the evidence based practice question: a review of the frameworks. *Evidence Based Library and Information Practice*, 6: 75–80; doi: 10.18438/B8WS5N.

EBSCO (2020) CINAHL Database. Available at: www.ebsco.com/products/research-databases/cinahl-database.

Elsevier (2020) Embase content. Available at: www.elsevier.com/solutions/embase-biomedical-research/embase-coverage-and-content.

Grant MJ, Booth A (2009) A typology of reviews: an analysis of 14 review types and associated methodologies. *Health Information & Libraries Journal*, 26: 91–108; doi: 10.1111/j.1471-1842.2009.00848.x. PMID: 19490148.

Higgins JPT, Thomas J, Chandler J, et al. (eds.) (2021) *Cochrane Handbook for Systematic Reviews of Interventions, Version 6.2* (updated February 2021). Cochrane. Available at: www.training.cochrane.org/handbook.

Lefebvre C, Glanville J, Briscoe S, et al. (2021) Searching for and selecting studies. In Higgins JPT, Thomas J, Chandler J, et al. (eds.), *Cochrane Handbook for Systematic Reviews of Interventions, Version 6.2* (updated February 2021). Cochrane. Available at: www.training.cochrane.org/handbook.

McKeever L, Nguyen V, Peterson SJ, Gomez-Perez S, Braunschweig C (2015) Demystifying the search button: a comprehensive PubMed search strategy for performing an exhaustive literature review. *Journal of Parenteral and Enteral Nutrition*. 39: 622–35; doi: 10.1177/0148607115593791. Epub 2015 Jun 30. PMID: 26129895; PMCID: PMC4513072.

Schiltz M (2018) Science without publication paywalls: cOAlition S for the realisation of full and immediate open access. *PLoS Medicine*, 15: e1002663; doi: 10.1371/journal.pmed.1002663. PMID: 30178782; PMCID: PMC6122176.

Scite Inc. (2019) Scite_: Smart Citations for better research. Available at: https://scite.ai/home.

Trip Database Limited (2021) What Is Trip? Available at: www.tripdatabase.com/about.

US National Library of Medicine (2020) MEDLINE, PubMed, and PMC (PubMed Central): how are they different? Available at: www.nlm.nih.gov/bsd/difference.html.

Wolters Kluwer (2020a) About Ovid. Available at: www.wolterskluwer.com/en/solutions/ovid/about.

Wolters Kluwer (2020b) UpToDate: evidence-based clinical decision support. Available at: www.wolterskluwer.com/en/solutions/uptodate.

Chapter 5

Writing for Learning and Publication

Peter Tyrer and Andrew Northern

A useful aim for all psychiatrists is to write at least one competent, not necessarily first-rate, article or chapter on a subject on which they have become an expert. 'I am never going to be an expert', we hear some of you say, but this is simply not true. Everyone can become an expert in one area, even it is very tiny indeed. So, for example, if you come across someone in your practice who has the feeling of ants crawling over their skin, commonly called formication (please get the spelling right), and this is severe and troubling, you might want to write a review of 'formication in psychiatry'. You will find about 50 published references on the subject but not very many from psychiatry. You now have a manageable series of papers to examine and can finish up with a scholarly paper pointing out the differences between formication as a symptom of physical disease and psychiatric disorder.

So we are assuming that all people reading this chapter will be thinking, at some point, that they will be writing for publication.

This chapter attempts to give broad advice that all can follow, irrespective of their literary skills. It is separated into four parts:

(1) choosing what you wish to write;
(2) understanding your readership;
(3) creating a story; and
(4) removing what is unnecessary.

Choosing What You Wish to Write

There is no point in writing rubbish. Joan Collins, the actress, socialite and archetypal celebrity, some years ago was invited to write a novel that she probably had no wish to write, but publishers love celebrities and go out of their way to court them. So Joan, always in need of extra revenue, agreed to write a novel called *Hell Hath No Fury*, a line from a William Congreve play of 1697, to which everyone now knows the ending. It was probably the most literate part of the novel, because the publishers blanched when they saw the script, describing it as 'very primitive', 'jumbled and disjointed', 'alarming', 'dated', 'dull' and 'clichéd'. They then refused to give Joan the $1,200,000 advance that had been agreed. But Joan had good lawyers and there was nothing in the contract that said the novel had ever to be published. So she took the publishers to court, and won in 1996, and has done even better in writing about the court case since.

The message here is simple. If you are asked to write something that you have no wish to write, do not accept. You are not likely to be enticed by £1,000,000 or even £100, but money should not come into it. One similar aspect of this problem is the well-known phrase, 'publish or perish', that is often dangled in front of aspiring academics, or even trainees, in their latter years. 'A published paper will help you get the job you want', becomes the message. But if you have nothing to write about, do not be tempted. Like all aphorisms it can be wrong. However, it is worth remembering when an author has had an article refused repeatedly and is getting down-hearted; if they genuinely feel there is something new in the paper then it is probably the writing that has let the author down.

Understanding Your Readership

It is equally unhelpful to think of writing for publication as being only about 'writing up' your work. If you rather think of publishing as being an act of communication through which you are conveying a clear and important message to an audience within, and often beyond, your own disciplinary community, the most important consideration when choosing what to write for any potential publication must surely be: 'What am I contributing here?' The more you engage with and reflect on the literature alongside your day-to-day experiences in your practice and the data you have at your disposal, the more you will start to notice potential contributions you can make.

Rather than aiming frantically to shoehorn everything you are doing into print and hoping that readers will see the relevance, slow down and take the time to carefully curate your knowledge and data from your practice with a view to locating and showcasing the aspects that will have some kind of impact in the context of the existing literature. Perhaps you can address a gap in the literature where little empirical evidence exists. This is the most common motivation behind publishing. Or perhaps you have evidence that supports or contradicts previously published findings. Any of the above are valid reasons to publish. But alongside the research world, remember not to lose sight of the potential impact of your publication on real-world practice. Although it is easy to lose sight of this in the day-to-day demands of your work, motivating yourself to write is much easier when it comes from a conviction that what you write will improve on the status quo and contribute in some way, no matter how small, towards making a meaningful difference to people's quality of life.

If you keep the impact of the paper you are writing on both the research world and the real world at the front of your mind, you will find that you are more focused and efficient at every stage of the writing process. In the early stages, focusing on the contribution and potential impact helps you to prioritize and select which information is essential for a particular paper and which information is disposable. As you edit your text, this bigger-picture view provides a prism through which you can critically read what you have written and notice where your focus has drifted and where content needs to be reorganized or deleted accordingly. Preparing a tightly organized and focused paper with a contribution and potential impact that are made explicit to the reader at every opportunity will only accelerate the peer-review process.

Creating a Story

Writing a scientific article is quite different from writing a novel. You have to follow strict rules and be precise and accurate in your descriptions. But there is one element that is the same. A good article makes a good story. It has an internal logic and structure that makes the reader want to continue to the end. It hangs together and is readily understood, and when you have finished it you should be able to summarize its essentials easily.

So when you have written a first draft, hand it over to some people you know who are not in the scientific field. Ask them if they understand what the paper is about and what it tells them that is new. If they reply after reading, 'this is too complicated for me', you have failed to communicate successfully. We accept there are some subjects, such as advanced mathematics, where a good article is very difficult to follow, but this is not true of psychiatry; every reader should be able to understand.

But there is one caveat to add. Do not let the need to make a good story take away from the data presented in your paper. Data are annoying. They mess up nice hypotheses and get in the way of neat stories, but they should always be king. Do not ignore data when they contradict your views; weave them into the narrative even if you have to add an extra clunky paragraph explaining why they do not fit in. There is great concern among journal editors currently about the influence of ghost writers. These inventive people can make a beautiful silk purse out of a tattered sow's ear of a paper, but they are just concerned with telling a story, so when facts get in the way they are conveniently ignored.

Some trainees are uncertain how many references to insert into a paper. The simple rule is 'add a reference when you are making a statement of probable fact, do not bother if the fact is unequivocal.' So you need to add a reference to the statement 'formication is found in 70% of patients with Parkinson's disease' but not one stating ' formication is the sensation of ants crawling over your skin.' If there is a particularly striking finding reported you may need to add more than one reference.

Misunderstanding on the part of the reader often arises from the writer operating under a prevalent false assumption that the data speak for themselves. Of course, it is important to present the data clearly, but your responsibility in communicating your research goes far beyond merely presenting your data to be interpreted. You, the writer, are responsible for ensuring that the most important implications from your data cannot possibly be missed or misinterpreted by your reader. As most research is now openly accessible online, you need to provide a commentary that complements the data so any potential reader who wishes to access your work can see what is important and what is unimportant, which implications are certain, and which implications are tentative (the verb 'suggest' is very useful for the latter purpose). The commentary should relate the data back to the context of your research aims, your method and the previous findings in the literature. The wider the readership you are aiming for, the more background information you need to provide when discussing implications.

Throughout the publication you are composing, at every stage of the journey that you are taking your reader on, always make it clear to the reader how the information you are providing relates to what has come before and what will come after. An important first step in achieving this is to create appropriate subheadings that show the logical development of the narrative. Learned journals sometimes cavil at this, but all will allow minor subheadings. Remember that, as a research writer, your aim is the opposite to that of the crime novelist, you are not aiming to keep your reader in suspense, but to set up their expectations from the start and meet them with the evidence you provide. A section can therefore start by reorienting the reader with key information from previous sections and even by including explicit statements that help the reader anticipate the content that follows; for example: 'Our objective in this section is to … ', which can be particularly helpful where the section headings deviate from the traditional Introduction–Method–Results–Discussion (IMRaD) or Introduction–Results–Discussion–Methods (IRDaM) formats.

The most useful way to guide the reader and ensure they do not get lost in the text is to focus on the narrative structure of your paragraphs and sentences. The transition between paragraphs and sentences should always be logical and seamless so the reader does not feel like they are leaping from one point to the next. At the paragraph level, readers quickly become confused and distracted if each paragraph does not have a single clear focus. A paragraph may have a more in-depth focus, such as 'discussing the advantages of using a particular treatment', or a broader focus, such as 'comparing the evidence for several different treatments'. In either case, the writer should begin the paragraph by preparing the reader with a clear narrative entry statement that makes the focus of the paragraph explicit. Examples of clear paragraph openings that correspond with the focuses above would be: 'Numerous case reports have indicated the beneficial effects of . . . '; or: 'More recently, two treatments . . . have been trialled with mixed efficacy . . . '.

Likewise, at the sentence level, the reader will be looking expectantly to the beginning of the sentence for guidance on how the information in the sentence fits into the narrative. A skilled writer will organize information in such a way that their sentences pick up on information in the previous sentence and move the reader's understanding forward, particularly when presenting background information, as in the following example: 'Formication is a prevalent symptom in a wide variety of physical and psychiatric disorders. Since diagnosis and treatment of these conditions requires different expertise, dermatologists and psychiatrists need to collaborate closely.' The reference back to the information in the previous sentence, 'these conditions', provides a firm hook that anchors the reader and keeps them tied to the narrative. Remember that once sufficient background information has been provided to establish what is known on the topic, the reader will eventually expect a concession, typically preceded by 'However', to signal a research gap that can be addressed by your work or by future work in the field.

Another key element of the sentence that the reader relies on to interpret the meaning is the main verb. One of the questions we are often asked about writing for publication is whether the writer should use the passive voice (e.g., X was examined) or the active voice (we examined X). Our answer is to first check the editor's guidelines for authors to see if there are any stylistic preferences expressed by the editor, but most importantly to note that effective writing uses both the active and the passive voice. The priority is always being as explicit as possible so that the reader can follow the narrative. Since the passive voice removes the agent from the sentence, it can be useful in certain contexts in a publication, but ambiguous in others. A sentence such as 'Data from patients reporting sensations of formication in psychiatric settings between 2016 and 2020 were retrospectively reviewed' would be effective in a paragraph where the writer is describing their research methods. The reader can follow the narrative easily in this method description as there is no doubt that the agent doing the reviewing here is the researcher authoring the paper. The use of the past tense also helps to indicate this. Do bear in mind, though, when using the passive in this way that packing a lot of information into the subject noun phrase generally makes reading and processing the information a cumbersome task. However, in a different context, such as when writing an abstract, this same example sentence might be ambiguous as the writer is likely to be shifting focus quickly from the background and previous research to describing their own research. In this case it would serve the reader best if the writer chose to switch to the active voice and the present tense to indicate a shift in the narrative: 'Here, we retrospectively review'.

In the example above, there is no doubt in the reader's mind that 'we' refers to the researchers writing the paper, but even when the use of 'we' is permitted by journal editors, you still need to be judicious in how you use it; resolving potential ambiguity is once again the guiding principle. In a sentence presenting background factual information at the beginning of an introduction, such as: 'We recognize the importance of the relationship between the clinician and the patient in increasing the likelihood of a successful clinical outcome', the reader is left to speculate whether 'we' refers exclusively to the researchers, more broadly to all those involved in psychiatric research and practice or, indeed, to the general public as a whole. It would therefore be advisable to avoid 'we' in such instances and shift the focus instead on to the information: 'The relationship between the clinician and the patient is an important factor in increasing the likelihood of a successful clinical outcome', would do the job if it is common knowledge, or you may add language to specify the scope of the statement such as ' . . . is widely recognized as . . . ' or ' . . . has recently been established as . . . ', accompanied by a citation if needed.

On the other hand, it is advisable to use 'we' to give prominence to your contribution to the literature rather than risk burying it with the agentless passive. With this in mind, 'We have developed a new set of guidelines for managing the treatment of patients reporting sensations of formication in psychiatric settings' is a more powerful and less awkward sentence for the reader to process than the passive equivalent: 'A new set of guidelines for managing the treatment of patients reporting sensations of formication in psychiatric settings has been developed', where the key action verb only appears once the reader has navigated a long, complex noun phrase, leaving the researcher's ownership of the guidelines potentially shrouded in ambiguity.

Removing What Is Unnecessary

Mark Twain, a master of prose, once wrote: 'Writing is easy. All you have to do is cross out the wrong words'. He was referring to all writing and, although he was not especially familiar with the vast literature of learned journals, we are sure he would have applied this dictum to these publications also. It is probably even more relevant to modern academic publishing than it was then. A very good exercise for an aspiring author is to complete the abstract of the paper you have written in a learned journal. Anybody who has ever written a scientific article will have struggled with the demand of a 250-word, or even a 150-word, abstract that encapsulates the central components of a paper. What agony goes into that elimination of the phrases that seems to encapsulate 100 hours of research effort, the acid comment that will bowl over your competitors and the complicated statistic that is all-revealing but can only be explained adequately with extra words.

All writing is selective; it chooses what it wants to convey to the reader and omits any parts that are not part of this choice. It is sometimes useful to look at the first sentences of scientific papers that illustrate this.

'We wish to suggest a structure for the salt of deoxyribose nucleic acid (D.N.A.)'. So wrote Watson and Crick in their first sentence on 25 April 1953. This is a classic example of an initial manifesto sentence, precise and informative. It is short, pithy and foreshadows the rest of the short paper that follows, only a few hundred words, but which makes it abundantly clear that they are making a major breakthrough in science. An equivalent in fiction is Tolstoy's first sentence in Anna Karenina – 'all happy families are alike, each unhappy family is unhappy in its own way'. This single sentence tells you all about what is going to follow.

The nearest equivalent that we can find in mental health is the first sentence of David Rosenhan's pioneering paper in 1973, which exploited the cracks in psychiatric diagnosis, particularly the loose interpretation of schizophrenia at that time: 'if sanity and insanity exist, how shall we know them?' Note the use of 'shall', not 'will', illustrating the subtle difference between these words.

So, the first exercise in the summary of a paper (unless it is forced into formal sections such as aims, methods, results and conclusions), is to pick on an arresting sentence to start. If the researcher, with colleagues, has found some interesting data on formication that only apply to psychiatric patients, they could use a sentence such as 'we report here the distinguishing features of formication that enable its medical and psychiatric classification'.

It certainly takes time to tease out the perfect phrasing to use to express a concept. However, once you have the words that make your key concepts clear, the job is complete, and you can weave these words through your paper to create a thread for the reader to follow. You will be surprised how much repetition you find in published scientific papers, until you realize that the repetition is there for a good reason. Those who seek out and read scientific research value the consistency and predictability of the writing above all else so that they can use the writing as a scaffold through which they can easily see the distinctions in the data that are important. Repetition is counterintuitive to less-experienced writers of scientific texts, as they are used to writing to impress and, in some cases, have been formally taught to do so by varying their language. However, unless synonyms are extremely carefully chosen to express a nuanced difference that is important to your narrative, which is rarely the case, they do a disservice to readers of a scientific text. This should reassure you that you do not need to be a poet to become a published scientific research writer. Effective scientific research writers use a necessarily restricted form of language, almost a code, to help their global audience to access quickly the hundreds of hours of labour that went into their research, all in a matter of minutes, without being slowed down or unnecessarily distracted by the writing itself. As George Orwell famously observed, 'good prose should be transparent, like a window pane'.

One of the key differences between experienced and novice writers is that experienced writers are ruthless editors. They do not become too attached to the sentences they produce on their first draft. Effective writing is a process of careful curation and subtraction down to the essentials. Although the information you are communicating is likely to be complex, the writing does not necessarily have to be. Observe how an idea expressed in a 38-word sentence: 'It is not uncommon to encounter sentences which, though they contain a great number of words and are constructed in a highly complex way, nonetheless turn out on inspection to convey very little meaningful substance of any kind', can often be expressed more effectively after being distilled down to eight words: 'Complex sentences do not necessarily contain complex ideas.' Before editing your sentences down, consider whether you need that sentence at all. Might it be more relevant elsewhere or in a separate publication? It can always be stored away in notes, as good work never goes to waste, but it should never be retained in the paper out of sentimentality or because somebody else insisted that it should be there.

Although the end-product is what readers see and remember, writing is essentially first and foremost a process, or even a habit. The best way to manage the process of producing and refining your text is to set a clear and realistic goal for what you can achieve in each session. Remember that writing is an iterative process, so scheduling daily writing sessions with modest goals is likely to produce a better text than ambitiously setting aside a single day to do all your writing. Experienced writers know that the time they are not writing is as important in the process as the time that they are writing. Regularly and purposefully stepping away from your keyboard in between focused writing sessions will help you to see your draft with fresh eyes and to develop and edit your text more efficiently and effectively.

One last point; do not be seduced by the Internet into reproducing large slabs of unnecessary prose into your writing. If you are struggling to find the right words, it is easy to be enticed by the writings of others on Wikipedia or other sites that seem to do the job for you. They don't. They add unnecessary words to your writing, they put you in danger of plagiarism if authors recognize their text in your work and, almost always, they are slightly off the point that you want to make. So, resist the urge to look for shortcuts online, but instead make time in your schedule for writing and discussing your own writing and other writing in your field with your peers.

Developing writing competence is an ongoing lifelong process, but can be accelerated by actively engaging with texts and readers. Seek different perspectives on your writing from readers and note down your own impressions as a reader as you read research texts written by others in your field. Through reading and engaging with texts as an active writer, you will develop a general feel for what works for readers, and this instinct and reader-awareness can be channelled into your own writing. We also recommend the books on science research writing by Hofmann (2014), Mogull (2017) and Glasman-Deal (2020) below, which provide further invaluable practical guidance on writing successfully for publication.

References

Glasman-Deal H (2020) *Science Research Writing: For Native and Non-native Speakers of English.* World Scientific.

Hofmann AH (2014) *Scientific Writing and Communication: Papers, Proposals,* *and Presentations.* Oxford University Press.

Mogull SA (2017) *Scientific and Medical Communication: A Guide for Effective Practice.* Routledge.

Small- and Large-Group Teaching

Anne Worrall-Davies

Introduction

This chapter covers the basics of large- and small-group teaching, including methods of delivery, evaluation, practical tips and assessment methods. It includes evidence from teaching in psychiatry and from medical, and higher, education. The chapter comprises the following sections:

(1) Large-group teaching:

    (a) Why do we teach psychiatry in large groups?

    (b) What is a large group?

    (c) Methods of large group teaching.

(2) Small-group teaching:

    (a) Why do we teach psychiatry in small groups?

    (b) What is a small group?

    (c) Methods of small group teaching.

(3) Evaluation of your teaching.

(4) Assessment of students.

(5) Top tips: preparation techniques for teaching large and small groups.

Large-Group Teaching

Why Do We Teach Psychiatry in Large Groups?

Worrall-Davies wrote about successful small group teaching in 1999, when teachers were moving away from lectures as the cornerstone of teaching psychiatry and towards a much more interactive way of teaching in small groups (Worrall-Davies 1999). Since then, small groups have become the mainstay of delivering professional skills training, though lectures have not seen their demise as was predicted (Mazur 2009; Brown and Eagles 2011). The wide use of virtual learning environments, the explosion of readily available information on the Internet and the global coronavirus pandemic in 2020 and 2021 have exponentially opened up the possibilities for large-group teaching.

Clinical teachers often do not have the choice as to the method of teaching or the size of group. It is an unfortunate fact that large-group teaching fits easily with university and professional bodies' set assessment and examination timetables (Race 2020). This may change in future; changes in examination formats during the coronavirus pandemic led to the introduction of Performance Grade music examinations being held monthly, with students assessed remotely through submitted recordings of their examination pieces (Associated Boards of the Royal Schools of Music 2020).

What Is a Large Group?

A large group constitutes at least 25 students, but in both real-life and virtual settings you may find yourself teaching 300 people (University College London Arena Centre 2019). An additional point to remember is that, if you are delivering a virtual teaching session, the group may be much larger than you had anticipated. It is always worth remembering to ask the organizer beforehand how many people have signed up to join the virtual teaching, so that you can be prepared to adjust the interactive parts of the session to accommodate the larger group size. For instance, if you had anticipated 60 students attending, and had planned a 'virtual hands up' response to questions you pose, you might need to deliver this as a digital poll instead.

Methods of Large-Group Teaching

Nowadays, when there is so much information available readily on the Internet, students do not need to attend lectures in order to access information. This chapter does not consider how to deliver a good lecture; this is covered in Chapter 11. Large-group teaching sessions now have a different purpose, facilitating students to find out about the 'big picture' and to make sense of the current cutting-edge ideas on a topic. Students are very sophisticated about what they hope to gain from a teaching experience. Race (2020) argues that students come to large-group sessions with three questions that they wish to have answered:

(1) What can I now do that I couldn't do before as a result of attending the session?
(2) What is a good example and a poor example in this particular field?
(3) Where does this topic 'fit into' my course module or degree?

Box 6.1 shows examples of each of these for a core psychiatric trainee attending a large-group teaching session on eating disorders in young people.

Box 6.1 What a core trainee in psychiatry might want to gain from a large-group teaching on urgent assessment of the physical health of a young person with an eating disorder

- What can I now do that I couldn't do before?
- Will I know how to assess a very underweight young person who presents in the emergency department when I'm on call?
- What's different about assessing a young person to assessing an adult with an eating disorder?
- What is a good example and a poor example of how to do this assessment?
- What does NICE (the UK's National Institute for Health and Care Excellence) say about managing eating disorders in young people?
- Does the Royal College of Psychiatrists have a position?
- Where does this topic 'fit into' my training?
- Will it help me pass MRCPsych exams?
- Is it relevant to me if I don't become a child and adolescent psychiatrist?

A crucial point to consider from the start is how long a large group of students (face to face, or in a virtual session) can remain engaged on a topic. This will influence how you plan and deliver the teaching. Recent research suggests that the previously held belief that students lose focus after 15–20 minutes is not the case. Students alternate between being focused and disengaged in 'shorter and shorter cycles' as the class progresses, but this pattern can be broken by using interactive techniques to re-engage them (Bunce et al. 2010). You should aim to change task several times during a one-hour session – and if you are teaching for an entire half-day, make sure that there are plenty of short breaks for stretching legs, walking around or getting a drink.

Use the storytelling framework: a beginning, middle and an end. Frame your topic for the session in a couple of introductory sentences on your opening slide and tell students what you are going to cover in the session. Divide the content into three to four sections – 'the middle of the story' – and then have a clear 'ending'. It is often useful to have a short summary at the end of each of the sections of content. Boxes 6.2 and 6.3 present two suggestions for keeping students engaged through repeated changes of task. Box 6.4 has suggestions for other techniques you might use to optimize learning and engagement, and Box 6.5 addresses tackling your nerves beforehand.

It is important to plan your method of delivery in the context of the teaching space. Find out in advance what the seating layout is and if you have an option to alter it from rows of chairs to small circles of chairs, for instance. If tables are not available, it will be impossible to do a task that requires papers to be spread on a table. Likewise, in a remote learning session, you can send small groups of students to pre-selected breakout rooms. There are many good resources online (e.g., Schreyer Institute for Teaching Excellence 2021).

Box 6.2 Suggestion for 50-minute large-group teaching session on emergency assessment of eating disorders

- Get people settled, final tech test, social chat to engage students, get started with an introductory section outlining up to three key issues you want the students to know, understand and be able to put into practice in an assessment. (5 minutes)
- YouTube video clip of young person and their parent talking about their emergency eating disorder assessment appointment (2 minutes). Mini lecture: key symptoms and signs to elicit in history and examination. (8 minutes)
- Show a slide of the physical health data for a hypothetical patient who has several 'red' physical health markers in managing emergencies in eating disorders (MEED) guidance. (Royal College of Psychiatrists 2022). Ask students to work in pairs or fours (dependent on size of group and seating arrangement) or individually if they are accessing remotely to decide: 'Based on these physical health investigations, how concerned are you about this young person's physical health?' (10 minutes)
- Mini lecture: assessing and managing the physical sequelae of eating disorders. (10 minutes)
- Questions. (10 minutes)
- Next steps: the homework, more reading, the student assessment, what will happen in the next session and students completing an evaluation of session. (5 minutes)

Box 6.3 Suggestion for 50-minute large-group teaching session on prescribing in first-episode psychosis

A week ahead of the session, students will have been given the task of researching the type of psychotropic medication used to treat psychosis and to be prepared to discuss in the session.

- Get people settled, final tech test, social chat to engage students; introductory slide outlining up to three key issues you want the students to know, understand and be able to put into practice. (5 minutes)
- Based on the 'flipped classroom' model, get students to work in groups of two to four, discussing what they have learned from their researching, and/or using their experience in psychiatry or other placements, lived experience etc. (7 minutes)
- Students feed back from their groups: psychotropics used for first-episode psychosis – facilitated and guided by teacher. (10 minutes)
- Slido (or similar polling tool) poll based on the session content. (3 minutes)
- Mini lecture: side effects of psychotropics used for first-episode psychosis and screening and intervening for cardiometabolic syndrome. (10 minutes)
- Slido poll based on the mini-lecture content. (3 minutes)
- Questions. (10 minutes)
- Synthesizing poll results and recap of material. (2 minutes)

Box 6.4 Techniques to use in a large-group teaching session

- **Think–pair–share.** Ask a question or pose a problem to the group. After students have had time (e.g., five minutes) to compose a response, ask them to 'pair' with another student to discuss their responses, before sharing with the larger group.
- **Minute paper.** Ask students to spend up to three minutes writing the key 'take-away' message of the teaching session up to that point, plus one or two questions that haven't been addressed. This helps with students' skill in summarizing, as well as highlighting what they may wish to ask you about, or find out through further study.
- **Clicker questions.** Questions are presented in multiple-choice format on the whiteboard, or using polls in MS Teams, or Slido or similar. All students should select a response to the question, and the results can be displayed in real time and then discussed.
- **Mind or concept map.** Ask students to draw a mind map (or use alternative visual/creative method to summarize what the lecture has covered, then ask students to compare with a partner.

Small-Group Teaching

Why Do We Teach Psychiatry in Small Groups?

Small groups are ideal for promoting meaningful learning and teaching professional skills and competencies. Educational research describes three distinct student learning styles: surface, deep and strategic (Entwhistle 1998; Entwistle and Ramsden 2015). Students who employ surface learning assimilate material by rote learning and are often not fully engaged in their educational journey. Nonetheless, there are some situations in medicine

> **Box 6.5** Taking control of your nerves
>
> 'I dreaded being asked to teach large groups because my voice would go squeaky and my throat so dry, and sometimes no sound came out of my mouth when I tried to speak! My consultant suggested I think about voice coaching. I love theatre and so I joined a local theatre group – not only have I learnt some great techniques for speaking in public, but I've got a new outside interest and friendship group too! Win-win!'
>
> 'I get to the teaching room ahead of schedule and just spend a few minutes practising some breathing exercises – it really makes such a difference.'
>
> 'I took up running recently and it has reduced my general anxiety massively. I'm much more in control of my body, my breathing and my performance when I'm chairing meetings or teaching.'

and psychiatry when much factual material must be memorized. Surface learning results in good immediate recall of material; however, deep learning sets a better longterm pattern of recalling and applying new material. Students who use the deep learning approach look for meaning in what they learn and are curious and critical about the material and its connections to other parts of their curriculum. Strategic learners combine both techniques depending on what is required of them. Many other factors affect the way students learn (Biggs and Tang 2011), including their physical and mental health, motivation, educational background, current environmental situation and the teaching environment (Gijbels et al. 2014).

What Is a Small Group?

Small-group teaching is a rather broad term without a clear definition. It covers tutorials, seminars and small problem-based learning classes – the size of the 'small' group may vary from a handful of students to 20–30 participants.

Methods of Small-Group Teaching

The small-group setting provides an ideal opportunity for teachers to facilitate active learner participation and to encourage students to try out new ways of learning, out of their comfort zone. For many of the psychiatric concepts and ideas that we teach, deep and strategic learning styles are the most desirable to inculcate in psychiatrists. Although the teaching methods discussed later in this chapter can promote deep learning, it should be remembered that, for some students, surface learning is the more natural method, and many may attempt to convert interactive sessions into fact-gathering sessions because this feels more comfortable. You yourself may be a natural surface learner, making teaching styles aimed at promoting deep learning inherently more difficult for you to deliver. This is a topic that you could usefully bring to your peer group or one to one supervision. There are a variety of styles and techniques you can use (Box 6.6); reflect carefully on which might best suit you, your material and your students.

Poor attendance and engagement issues are more obvious and more problematic in a small group than in a large group. If 3 students in a group of 10 are absent or not engaged, it can be difficult both to deliver the planned session and to ensure that the others do remain

---

Box 6.6 Examples of some small-group teaching techniques

- **Case-based discussion**. Presentation of case followed by group discussion. There should be a clear aim of the presentation, for instance, to consider a diagnostic or therapeutic dilemma. The discussion should focus on answering the posed question or dilemma.
- **Buzz group**. Brief, two-minute discussion of a clear question or topic, done in pairs. Ideas generated are fed back and discussed by whole group.
- **Syndicate task**. Mini-project work done by individuals or two to four students together, reported back to the whole group. This might include 'homework' between the small group sessions.
- **Thought shower/brainstorm**. Rapid idea generation from whole group. Idea received with no criticism by tutor and collated. Discussion and evaluation of collated ideas by whole group.
- **Role play**. Small groups of students act out vignettes- some students may play observers of the role-play, leading to discussion by whole group.
- **Fish-bowl exercise**. Small group, two to four students discuss or present a topic in front of the remainder of the group who watch and then discuss. The small group then acts as 'observer' to the remainder of group who re-present the topic.
- **Round**. Each participant talks in turn.
- **Pyramid**. Start in pairs, then work in groups of four, then eight, 16 etc. until the whole small group is involved in the task.

---

engaged. Race (2020) considers some of the reasons why small groups go wrong and how to tackle the issues. The University of Wisconsin-Madison (2021) provides a useful resource on 'helping groups to get results' with descriptions of unhelpful group behaviours. Many of these will be familiar to you from working therapeutically with groups: late arrival, non-attendance, not working, disrupting the group, dominating the group, a silent group. Box 6.7 summarizes some of these issues and how to address them.

A good small-group teacher facilitates communication between students, and between students and their teacher. Tutor interventions can be divided (Brown and Eagles 2011) into authoritative (prescriptive, informative and confronting) and facilitative (cathartic, analytic and supportive). Authoritative interventions tend to shut down dialogue in teaching sessions, whereas facilitative ones encourage dialogue. Most psychiatrists will be accustomed to using facilitative interventions clinically. Listening and responding to students is very similar to listening and responding to a patient or family. It is important to be able to show the students that you are actively listening to what is being said – nonverbal signs are useful, as are prompts, and encouraging 'mmm-mmm' sounds. It is worth taking some time to consider how you ask questions. Is your questioning clear, encouraging and open enough to facilitate discussion?

Questions may be asked to gather information, to join in, with little expectation of correct and incorrect responses:

(1) recall–observation–thought: divided as to whether the question elicits a recalled fact, encourages an observation on a topic or invites a discursive comment;
(2) open or closed: inviting an extended response or a yes–no answer, respectively;

> **Box 6.7** Some unhelpful small-group behaviours and how to address them
>
> - **Persistent late arrival.** Agree ground rules at the start of the module. Don't be late yourself. Don't make sarcastic/unkind remarks to latecomers. Take time to find out if there is a problem leading to late arrival.
> - **Non-attendance by some/all students.** Make sure that you don't cancel sessions. Ensure the sessions are relevant; check out with students if the teaching is what they want and, if not, how you could modify it to make it so. If your organization allows, take an attendance register.
> - **Some students not working.** Get students engaged from the start with a quiz; check out with repeated non-workers if they have a problem (personal, professional).
> - **Student(s) disrupting the group.** Consider why this is happening; check out with the student(s) in a break; collaboratively re-set the group ground rules.
> - **A student dominating the group.** Support the group to reflect as a whole on whether it is functioning; use the 'form–storm–norm–perform' cycle to help them with this; discuss privately with the dominant student.
> - **The silent group/student.** Consider whether you are talking too much or being too authoritative; check with the student privately if there is a problem.

(3) encouraging–threatening: respectively providing or preventing a safe enough environment for an answer to be attempted; and

(4) clear–confused: confused questions have more than one question embedded in them, or are ambiguous.

Threatening and confused questions are clearly to be avoided, just as they are in clinical practice. As clinicians, we generally tend towards open questions rather than closed, to elicit more authentic information. But remember that sometimes the occasional closed questions have their purpose too; there are situations when a yes or no answer is required.

Evaluation of Your Teaching

Whilst it is good practice to have a range of teaching methods that you are comfortable with, it is also important to know when to use each one. It is easy when you discover a 'new' method to want to use it at all opportunities, leaving your students unsure whether you are teaching a psychiatry topic or delivering a masterclass in innovative teaching practices! The best way to avoid such mistakes is through self-reflection, student evaluation and peer observation of teaching sessions. All clinicians are used to reflecting on the content and process of clinical sessions, and it is only a matter of habit to reflect on the content and process of a teaching session. Being a 'reflective teacher' uses the same skills as being a good clinician. Why did it seem to go badly after a good start? What could I have done to encourage the students to talk more? What can I do next time to avoid running over time? A useful framework might be

- What went well and why?
- What went badly and why?
- What could I do to improve next time?

More detail, outside the scope of this chapter, can be found in Brown and Eagles 2011.

Peer observation is another important way of assessing your performance as a teacher. Setting up a group of colleagues to sit in on each other's' teachings is a non-threatening way of organizing peer observation. Remember that most of us actually perform better than we think we do. A useful framework to use is 'plan–observe–reflect–review' (Butcher et al. 2019). The 'plan' stage ensures that you know what you want from the observation. Do remember to check with students whether they are comfortable with you recording or having another person present before you start. Your observer might count the number of each type of question or might record the student responses to different type of questions. It is helpful to the observer if they have a checklist to use or you ask them to answer a specific question such as 'Do I talk too much?' or 'Did I get the key points across?' It is helpful to ask your observer to answer specific questions about the teaching, or to do focused tasks, such as timing the proportions of a session in which you and the students are talking. Self-reflection with the observer is crucial, so make sure you have time for this, immediately afterwards ideally.

Assessment of Students

Student assessment is just as important as the design or method of your teaching. You have a responsibility to your students to assess them in a fair and appropriate way, and also to uphold the integrity of the organization or institution to which the students belong (Butcher et al. 2019). Race (2020) goes as far as to state that his chapter on assessment is the most important in his book. Certainly, you need to spend a significant proportion of your teaching preparation time considering whether the content and method of delivery will lend themselves to the mode of assessment. In some circumstances, assessment will not be determined by you, for instance, if you are teaching on a Member of the Royal College of Psychiatrists (MRCPsych) course. However, in other circumstances you will be responsible for both the teaching and the assessment.

Assessment can be diagnostic, summative or formative. A diagnostic assessment is completed at the start of the students' learning process and helps both the teacher and student understand how much they already know or understand about the topic. A formative assessment takes place in the middle of a course or module and gives students and teachers feedback on student progress; it should not be used to contribute to the overall end assessment. The summative assessment takes place at the end of a course or module and provides a measure of whether the student has achieved their learning goals or not. Formative assessment is used extensively in current postgraduate psychiatric training with 360-degree feedback and workplace-based assessments being core components (Brown and Eagles 2011).

Helping students to understand what is required of them in an assessment and giving them stress-free 'practice runs' are an important part of a teacher's role (Lowe 2007; Race 2020) and enable students to develop 'assessment literacy' (Higher Education Academy 2012). Not all psychiatric trainees are the same; medical undergraduate training is delivered very differently around the world, so don't assume that every student is wholly familiar with the UK approach to psychiatric training and assessment of competencies.

Top Tips: Preparation Techniques for Teaching Large and Small Groups

Even the best teachers need to refine their delivery technique and need practice. Actors rehearse intensively before going out on stage; stand-up comedians in a live improvized act will have rehearsed much of their material and the way that they deliver it beforehand. They also modify their material based on the reaction it gets.

This is one of the reasons that observation of your teaching can be really helpful; your observer can highlight what you do really well, as well as give pointers for what you could improve on. Ask a colleague whose advice and judgement you value, and offer to observe them in return–peer review is an excellent way to learn. Before being formally observed, you can 'self-assess' your own delivery through the video function on a smartphone. See if you can pick out what works well and what doesn't. Do you look enthusiastic? Are you talking to the students or reading crib notes? Do you give clear instructions about the task you are asking them to undertake? You can then check this out by sharing with a friend or partner, before moving on to more formal observation of your teaching. Race (2020) provides a detailed checklist for new teachers in higher education; and there is a superb online resource (University of Cambridge Local Examinations Syndicate 2021), explaining the educational theory behind the importance of reflection on your teaching.

My main top tip is that it is (nearly) impossible to over-prepare. Teaching preparation takes time – a rule of thumb is that it may take up to eight hours from start to finish to prepare a one-hour group session, if this is a new topic that you have not taught before. Some basic but top tips for preparation are:

(1) **Prepare, practise and relax**. Have at least one practice run-through, ideally to others, but you will gain much from rehearsing either in front of your smartphone, or to a mirror (Cantillon 2003). Make sure that you give yourself some space the night before: don't stay up anxiously drafting and re-drafting the material. Give yourself plenty of time on the day to get to the teaching venue or to access the digital platform. Don't sit up worrying about what might go wrong. 'Rain check' yourself just before the teaching, and don't overdo the caffeine intake. And finally, be prepared to enjoy yourself! This matters so much – if you convey enthusiasm for your subject you will not only help your students want to learn, they will be more likely to ask questions and extend their understanding.

(2) **Prepare your background**. Make sure that you know as much as you can find out about the group you will be teaching. Are they all psychiatric trainees? What do they know about this subject already? What do they as a group bring in terms of life experience to the teaching? All student are individuals, and bring different learning needs and preferences, different experiences of training and education, different life experiences (Butcher et al. 2019). Being culturally aware and sensitive as a teacher is crucial to ensure that all students, regardless of colour, gender, age or disability, can access your teaching and learn. The diverse classroom is a more efficient, effective and creative vehicle for learning. Levine and Stark (2015) showed that making learning spaces accessible to all students, specifically non-majority groups, benefits all students though enhanced problem solving, creativity and decision making. The third McKinsey report (McKinsey & Company 2020) showed that boardroom effectiveness was directly correlated with diversity: 'the greater the representation, the higher the likelihood of outperformance',

and this is equally true of the teaching room. Get to know your students through informal conversations before and after the teaching slot and encourage them to share their professional and personal experiences in the group, not only to foster individual confidence and engagement, but also to enrich the learning experience of the whole class. There is much added value to be gained for students – and for you as the teacher – by drawing on students' diverse backgrounds, such as lived experience or experience of practising psychiatry in another country, if they are willing to share these in the group.

(3) **Prepare your teaching space**. Get to the room ahead of time. If the room is empty, you can quickly familiarize yourself with it and set it up as you want. If it's occupied, don't feel hesitant about knocking on the door five minutes before your session starts; the previous teacher should know to finish on time.

(4) **Prepare your method**. Your chosen way of delivering the group teaching should ensure that the material can be understood and applied by your students. Contrary to what has been written previously, current educational research suggests that tailoring the method of teaching delivery to fit with each individual student's preferred learning style does not improve learning outcomes and may in fact be unhelpful (Rohrer and Pashler 2012; Aslaksen and Lorås 2018; Newton and Salvi 2020).

(5) **Prepare your material**. Butcher et al. (2019) have an excellent chapter 7 on learning resources and handouts. Ensure your material is culturally inclusive; and that your examples, if local or UK-bound, are understandable and relevant to psychiatrists who have trained overseas.

(6) **Prepare the tech**. Have a back-up and a back-up to the back-up. Even if your previous experience is that the Wi-Fi signal in your teaching room is good, don't rely on it – make sure you have a Plan B, such as piggybacking off your phone, etc.

(7) **Prepare for questions**. There is nothing worse than being asked a question that you feel completely unprepared for, so think ahead about what you might be asked and make yourself a list with brief points you might want to include in your answer. Remember, though, that it is impossible to anticipate all the questions that students might ask about the topic; you don't have to know the answer to every single one. The situation is exactly the same as duty of candour in the clinical situation when you don't know the answer to give to a patient. It is better to say 'I can't answer that right now' than to give a wrong answer, particularly since there is bound to be somebody in the room who knows that you are winging it! The sign of maturity is to say: 'I don't know the answer right now – I will need to go look at that', 'It's complicated – I will post it up on the VLE [virtual learning environment]' or 'A great question – let's talk about that in more detail next time'.

(8) **Prepare for the nerves**. As psychiatrists, we are entirely comfortable with working with small groups of people. Our clinical careers are centred on going to professionals' meetings, multiagency meetings, family meetings, etc. So small-group teaching comes more naturally to many of us, in a way that large-group teaching doesn't. Of course, there will always be some people who love, and thrive, on engaging a large group. But for those who don't, there are many ways to build confidence. We know intellectually that these are all normal physiological reactions to anxiety; add the pressure of knowing that you are talking to several hundred people – who in your imagination, will see you 'make a mess of it' and you can expect to feel very anxious indeed! The answer is simple: preparation and practice. Use breathing exercises, mindfulness or

meditation – whatever works for you. Consider voice or drama classes if you want to improve your vocal delivery and 'stage presence' (see Box 6.5).

(9) **Prepare your story.** You should view a teaching session as telling a story. Stories, at their very best, not only convey information in a recallable way, they change beliefs and attitudes. Telling a story makes a connection between the narrator and the audience. At the basic level, stories make us human. We learn many lessons from stories. If you think about this, then your teaching takes on a whole new meaning. The two important things are to have a good story to tell; and to tell it well. Have a clear story structure: beginning, middle and end. Use mapping and flagging techniques to guide the students through the 'story'. Begin with a clear introduction to introduce the topic; for example, 'Today, I'm going to talk about' or 'In the next 50 minutes we are going to learn the basics in . . . '. Then 'map' out the 'route' that the session is going to follow. 'First . . . then . . . finally . . .'. You may wish to help students remember where your teaching topic fits in a module or course, such as, 'You'll remember that last week Sara talked to you about . . . ' When you are changing direction or moving on to a new point, remember to 'flag' it to the group so that they know; for example, 'Having reviewed the research . . . let's move on to think about . . .'.

(10) **Prepare to learn something new!** The best teachers are honest and humble enough to know that they are only there to guide students on the journey; they are not the fount of all knowledge.

References

Aslaksen K, Lorås H (2018) The modality-specific learning style hypothesis: a mini-review. *Frontiers in Psychology*; doi: https://doi.org/10.3389/fpsyg.2018.01538.

Associated Boards of the Royal Schools of Music (2020) Performance Grades. Available at: https://gb.abrsm.org/en/performancegrades/ (accessed 11 April 2021).

Biggs JB, Tang C (2011) *Teaching for Quality Learning at University*. Open University Press.

Brown T, Eagles T (2011) *Teaching Psychiatry to Undergraduates*. Royal College of Psychiatrists.

Bunce DM, Flens EA. Neiles KY (2010) How long can students pay attention in class? A study of student attention decline using clickers. *Journal of Chemical Education*, **87**: 1438–43.

Butcher C, Davies C, Highton M (2019) *Designing Learning. From Module Outline to Effective Teaching*. Routledge.

Cantillon P (2003) ABC of learning and teaching in medicine: teaching large groups. *British Medical Journal*, **326**: 437.

Entwhistle N (1998) Approaches to learning and forms of understanding. In Dart B, Boulton-Lewis G (eds.), *Teaching and Learning in Higher Education: From Theory to Practice*, pp. 72–101. Australian Council for Educational Research. Available at: www.researchgate.net/publication/245459885_Approaches_to_learning_and_forms_of_understanding.

Entwistle N, Ramsden P (2015) *Understanding Student Learning*. Routledge.

Gijbels D, Donche V, Richardson JTE, et al. (2014) *Learning Patterns in Higher Education. Dimensions and Research Perspectives*. Routledge.

Higher Education Academy (2012) A Marked Improvement Transforming Assessment in Higher Education. Available at: www.advance-he.ac.uk/knowledge-hub/marked-improvement-transforming-assessment-higher-education-assessment-review-tool.

Levine S, Stark D (2015) Diversity makes you brighter. *The New York Times*. Available at: www.nytimes.com/2015/12/09/opinion/diversity-makes-you-brighter.html.

Lowe J (2007) Assessment that promotes learning. Available at: www.schreyerinstitute.psu.edu/pdf/Assessment_That_Promotes_Learning.pdf.

Mazur E (2009) Farewell, lecture? *Science*, **323**: 50–1.

McKinsey & Company (2020) Diversity wins: how inclusion matters. Available at: www.mckinsey.com/featured-insights/diversity-and-inclusion/diversity-wins-how-inclusion-matters.

Newton PM Salvi A (2020) How common is belief in the learning styles neuromyth, and does it matter? A pragmatic systematic review. *Frontiers in Psychology*; doi: https://doi.org/10.3389/feduc.2020.60245.

Race P (2020). *The Lecturer's Toolkit*, 5th ed. Routledge.

Rohrer D, Pashler H (2012) Learning styles: where's the evidence? *Medical Education*, **46**: 634–5.

Royal College of Psychiatrists (2022) Managing emergencies in eating disorders, College Report CR233. Available at: https://rcpsych.ac.uk.

Schreyer Institute for Teaching Excellence (2021). Flexible teaching strategies. Available at: www.schreyerinstitute.psu.edu (accessed 11 April 2021).

University College London Arena Centre for Research-based Education (2019) Large group teaching: how to teach and manage large groups of students and where to find further resources. Available at: www.ucl.ac.uk/teaching-learning/publications/2019/aug/large-group-teaching.

University of Cambridge Local Examinations Syndicate (2021) Getting started with reflective practice. Available at: www.cambridge-community.org.uk/professional-development/gswrp/index.html.

University of Wisconsin-Madison (2021). Facilitator toolkit: a guide for helping groups get results. Available at: www.nj.gov/education/AchieveNJ/teams/strat14/FacilitatorToolKit.pdf.

Worrall-Davies A (1999) Successful small group teaching. *Advances in Psychiatric Treatment*, **5**: 376–81.

Whys and Hows of Patient-Based Teaching

Monica Doshi and Nick Brown

Introduction

The traditional medical education system has produced scientifically grounded and clinically skilled physicians who have served medicine and society. Sweeping changes launched around the turn of the millennium have revolutionized undergraduate and postgraduate medical education across the world (Gutierrez et al. 2016; Shelton et al. 2017; Samarasekera et al. 2018). Training has moved from being time-based to become more outcome-based, with a move away from the apprenticeship model to a more structured and systematic approach, emphasizing learning and development of skills.

Competency-Based Learning

The new competency-based learning emphasizes outcome in the form of performance. This is judged on what a doctor does, that is, performance of tasks, how these tasks are approached and the level of professionalism shown (Harden et al. 1999).

For psychiatry, consideration of what constitutes 'good clinical care' and the working life of the consultant are fundamental to understanding the desired outcomes of training. The Royal College of Psychiatrists, in its published curriculum documents, discusses how competency-based training and learning leads to the achievement of a range of interlinked intended learning outcomes in order to produce 'Consultant Psychiatrists for practice in the UK to the level of CCT registration and beyond' (Royal College of Psychiatrists 2010).

The emphasis is on teaching clinical skills, necessitating the development of patient-based approaches to learning. Many will feel that patient-based teaching is what they have always used. This may be true but as we move to systematic approaches there is a need to be more efficient and focused. Patients present according to their clinical need, not to the individual's training need; thus, care is required in the selection of patients for teaching in order to ensure the prescribed range of learning outcomes are achieved. There needs to be an accompanying attitudinal shift from an objective and distant biopsychosocial model towards more awareness of the impact of illness on patients and carers.

Fundamentals of Patient-Based Teaching

Patient-based teaching is the teaching of clinical skills using real patients. There are significant advantages but also challenges in delivery (Box 7.1). It offers lifelike preparation and has direct relevance to the trainee's future (Spencer 2003), that is, their day-to-day performance as a doctor. The skills a trainee learns from one patient are transferable to contact with others (Dent 2001). For example, if a trainee learns competently to assess

> **Box 7.1** The advantages and shortfalls of patient-based teaching
>
> **Advantages**
>
> Learning occurs in the context of real clinical practice
>
> Opportunities for role modelling
>
> Teaches transferable skills
>
> Increased learner motivation
>
> Increased professional thinking
>
> Integration of clinical skills including communication skills, problem solving, decision making and professional ethics
>
> **Shortfalls**
>
> Requires careful planning to avoid ad hoc nature
>
> Decline in availability of patients
>
> May not easily be able to cover the entire curriculum
>
> May be difficult to supervise and deliver
>
> Conflicting pressures of teaching and service delivery

suicidal ideation in an individual with depressive disorder they may use this learnt skill for assessing suicidal ideation in people with other disorders.

Patient-based teaching enables direct feedback from the patient (Ferenchick et al. 1997) and offers the opportunity for shadowing (see the section on teaching models below), in which trainees can observe a humanistic approach from an experienced clinician and learn from this (Dent 2001).

Numerous aspects of patient assessment and management can be taught by patient-based teaching (Ramani 2003). For example, communication skills can be practiced in discussing a therapeutic intervention with a patient (Rees 1987; Janicek and Fletcher 2003); clinical reasoning and decision making (Jolly et al. 1998); clinical ethics (Seigler 1978) and appropriate attitudes (LaCombe 1997). Interpersonal skills such as empathy, sensitivity and communication can be learnt by observation and shadowing or by performance under supervision with feedback.

The General Medical Council advocates early contact with patients for medical students, that they experience 'a range of specialties, in different settings, with the diversity of patient groups that they would see when working as a doctor' and that they experience 'an opportunity to support and follow patients through their care pathway' These standards came in to force in January 2016 (General Medical Council 2015). The idea is that students and trainees can learn on real patients under appropriate supervision for their level and ability.

The Changing Patient Base

Opportunities to teach with in-patients have been declining for some time. There are opportunities for patient-based teaching in out-patient and other community settings but this is not always easy to observe and supervise. Teaching can conflict with the pressures and current models of service delivery and the funding arrangements for medical education in

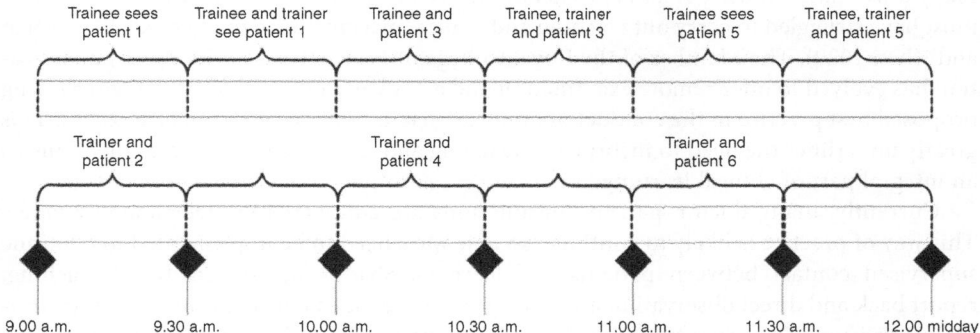

Fig. 7.1 Wave scheduling. Reproduced from Cox, K. Planning Bedside Teaching:1. Overview. *Medical Journal of Australia*, 158, 280–282, 1993. © John Wiley and Sons.

the National Health Service (Dave et al. 2010). One way of fitting teaching time into a clinic schedule with minimal impact on the number of patients seen is to apply 'wave scheduling' (Fig. 7.1), a technique suggested by Ferenchick et al. (1997).

Simulated (or Standardized) Patients

Any reduction in numbers of real patients may necessitate a need to supplement by the judicious deployment of simulated patients in teaching without losing a patient-centred ethos and approach (Hearn et al. 2019). The rapid advances using simulated patients and simulation technology that have occurred in many fields of medicine have been slower to take root in psychiatry. It was the best part of two decades before simulated patients began to appear in psychiatric medical education (Eagles et al. 2007). The current state of knowledge in psychiatry suggests that there is a considerable range of current and further potential value, including delivery of full longitudinal histories (Eagles et al. 2001a, b, 2007; Dave 2012). The use of simulated patients may offer a relatively straightforward, albeit not cheap, way of compensating for some of the lack of opportunity that is now present in daily clinical practice. A variety of curriculum outcomes may be covered, including communication, diagnostic, psychotherapeutic and clinical reasoning skills (Eagles et al. 2007; Brenner 2009).

Virtual Patients

A step on from simulated patients may be virtual patients. These are defined by the Association of American Medical Colleges (AAMC) as "a specific type of computer-based program that simulated real-life clinical scenarios: learners emulate the roles of healthcare providers to obtain a history, conduct a physical exam, and make diagnostic and therapeutic decisions' (AAMC 2007). The use of virtual patients has shown some early promise in undergraduate teaching of psychiatry (Combs and Combs 2019) and may have a part to play in the new world of medical education.

The Impact of the Pandemic

As the coronavirus (COVID-19) pandemic became more and more pervasive, so the effect on medical education began to take effect. The disruption has already been widespread and many universities in the UK and abroad have moved to conduct assessments remotely, and most have struggled to carry out teaching and clinical placements in many specialties (Mian and Khan 2020). The Member of the Royal College of Psychiatrists (MRCPsych) qualification has evolved to offer remote examination and a body of literature is emerging regarding proposed best practice in the conduct of remote consultations (Ramkisson et al. 2020). This greatly underlines the need to incorporate teaching and assessment of remote consulting as an integral part of clinical learning.

Currently, many doctor–patient consultations are conducted via telephone or video. This way of practice is likely to continue, so new ways need to be implemented to continue supervised contact between patients and learners. Shadowing, patient-based teaching, report back and direct observation are all possible using video consultations with appropriate supervision. The advantages are that it is acceptable to students and their supervisors and can sometimes offer better feedback to the learners (Darnton et al. 2020). However, there may be inherent biases in that there are limits on the range of examination possible, and delivery platforms will require patients to have the appropriate technology, thus favouring socially advantaged patients (Darnton et al. 2020).

Therefore, imaginative ways have needed to be found, including the use of telemedicine, such as providing patients (real or simulated) with a tablet in an isolated examination room, enabling communication with a learner and trainer without risking exposure to the pathogen and the waste of protective equipment (Hollander and Carr 2020).

If the effects of the pandemic persist, or new threats emerge, consideration will need to be given to the embedding of such techniques for teaching and learning, assessment and examinations. Telepsychiatry has been shown to have the potential to include simulated patients (Kennedy and Yellowlees 2003) so there is something to build upon.

Teaching Models

There are numerous ways in which psychiatrists can teach trainees using real patients (Box 7.2). Trainers must be familiar and comfortable with each of these as all of them can and should be deployed for the fullest learning to occur. Some methods require one-to-one sessions and others are suitable for small-group teaching.

Shadowing (Role-Modelling)

Shadowing, or role-modelling, enables trainees to learn from the behaviour of a senior clinician in consultations with patients – the clinician's attitude to the patient, their professional approach, their handling of difficult situations and how they negotiate treatment plans. This works well when a good example is set. Should the senior clinician not have a professional approach then the students' learning might be misguided. Another problem with shadowing is that the learning is passive – it relies on the students' motivation to observe and reflect on what is happening.

Patient-Centred Teaching

In contrast to shadowing, patient-centred teaching is an active technique in which trainees are allocated patients at the start of their placements. They assess the patients and follow their progress during treatment. They are encouraged to present their findings, interpret investigation results and be involved in discussions about patient management. They

Box 7.2 Models for patient-based teaching

Shadowing
The trainee shadows a senior, usually consultant, and learns by observation

Patient-centred
The trainee is allocated patients and follows their progress from start to end of an episode of illness

Reporting back
The trainee assesses the patient and reports back to the trainer

Direct observation
The trainer observes the trainee's performance directly

Video recording
The trainee's interview with the patient is video recorded and later discussed with the trainer (and potentially peers for group learning)

Case conference
A case is presented to, and discussed by, a wider audience, which may be multiprofessional

supplement what they have learnt by background reading. They are actively involved in their learning by being encouraged to review their patients regularly and contribute to clinical discussions.

The Report-Back Model

The trainee sees the patient alone for assessment, for example to take a history. They report back to the trainer, presenting their findings, their views on the diagnosis (problem solving) and appropriate management (judgement). They are given constructive feedback by the trainer.

Direct Observation

The trainer sits in on the trainee's interview with a patient to observe the trainee on a set task (e.g., discussing with a patient a change of treatment). After the interview, the trainer gives feedback on the trainee's performance. This is a useful technique for learning isolated skills but less appropriate for teaching clinical judgement or problem solving.

Video-Recorded Interviews

This technique was first employed in the 1970s (Gask 1998). There are several ways in which this can be used (Vassilas and Ho 2000). For example, the trainee(s) and trainer may watch stored tapes of doctor–patient consultations and use them as a basis for discussion.

Alternatively, the trainee may tape an interview with a patient. The patient's full consent is required as per the General Medical Council guidelines (General Medical Council 2012), which were updated in March 2013. The video is viewed with the trainer (and perhaps with other trainees), after which the content is discussed and feedback given. This is a useful way of learning and refining consultation and communication skills.

The sessions are more successful when there is a clearly defined purpose or agenda, such as learning the assessment of mood and associated communication skills.

Case Conferences

A case is presented to a wider (sometimes multi-professional) audience and interesting or challenging aspects are discussed.

Doing Patient-Based Teaching

The key to a successful patient-based teaching session is good preparation on the part of the trainer. With good preparation, the curriculum can be systematically covered. Topics taught are not dependent on chance, as in the traditional apprenticeship model (Ramani 2003). It may seem obvious, but it is essential to define what is to be taught, to whom and how.

Planning must include the anticipation of numbers and required resources, for example, how many students there are, how large the room is, what equipment is available and whether or not other staff will be present.

A. Selection of Patients

The choice of patients to be used in teaching requires careful consideration. Janicek and Fletcher (2003) emphasize the importance of attending to the patient's comfort as the first step in teaching at the bedside. The patient's clinical condition must not be detrimentally affected by the teaching. They must have the capacity to give consent, and full consent must be obtained. Thus, the patient should be told what is likely to happen during the session – how many trainees to expect, what the aims of the session are, what the trainees will do, how long it is likely to take and how they can stop the session if they want to. The patient must be informed that there might be discussion that does not relate to themselves or their condition and that their confidentiality will be maintained. They should be given the opportunity to ask questions at the end of the session. It is important to clarify how they wish to be addressed during the session.

Obviously, the trainer must know the patient and their condition. The selection of patients requires that teaching can fulfil curriculum objectives. Some clinicians have lists of patients who are willing to participate in training. This makes it easier to plan teaching and cover the curriculum.

Trainers worry that patients participating in teaching could find it stressful, upsetting or detrimental to their health. However, research suggests that most patients like being involved in this way (Wright 1974; O'Flynn et al. 1997; Lynöe et al. 1998). Patients report that they learn about their condition, feel special and experience increased self-esteem. They also value the opportunity to use their illness to benefit others; for example, a review from Newcastle found that patients saw themselves as offering facilitation in the development of students' attitudes and professional skills (Stacy and Spencer 1999).

B. Defining Learning Outcomes

Before beginning the teaching, the trainer should define the desired learning outcome (the aim) and set objectives for the teaching session that will achieve this aim. Learning needs and outcomes for a trainee in the first six months of training are different from those of a more experienced learner. Similarly, the needs of a psychiatric trainee differ from those of a trainee for general practice. By knowing the experience and career aims of the trainee, the learning session can be pitched at the right level and the clinical content suitably selected. It is important not to overwhelm the trainees and attempting to cover too much will result in little being retained. Clarify what the trainees should gain from the teaching. What should they know and be able to do at the end of the session? How should their attitudes change? E.g., should they improve their understanding of the impact of illness on the lives of patients and their families?). A trainer could encourage trainees to take responsibility for their own learning by asking them to set their own learning outcomes (within the context of the curriculum). This approach can enhance the trainees' motivation to learn.

Well-written objectives contain four elements:

- a description of the learner;
- the behaviour that they will demonstrate (e.g., be able to inform the patient of the benefits and risks of treating vs. not treating depression in pregnancy);
- the conditions in which they will demonstrate the learning (here in a follow-up of a pregnant woman with depressive episode); and
- the degree in which they can do this (e.g., in a sensitive and supportive manner).

These points enable the trainer to set the content and select appropriate teaching strategies for the teaching session. The resulting objectives give clear guidance to the trainee of what is expected and therefore direct their learning.

This fictional case example is used as a basis to describe how to undertake patient-based teaching.

> Mrs. K is a 26-year-old married woman who was assessed by a trainee as a new patient in an outpatient clinic. She is 22 weeks gestation and has a history of recurrent low mood. She was prescribed sertraline 50 mg daily and had remained well on this for two years prior to being pregnant, stopping the medication when she discovered she was pregnant. She presents with gradual lowering of mood, early morning wakening, decreased appetite, low energy and a lack of motivation. She is experiencing hopelessness, thinks she is not a good mother and that her four-year-old daughter will be better without her. She will not do anything to jeopardize her unborn baby but does not feel that she is bonding to him/her. She has no thoughts or intention to harm her daughter.
>
> The case has been fully discussed with the trainer who has summarized that she is suffering with a relapse of her depressive disorder secondary to stopping the medication. The plan is to restart her on the sertraline and to refer her for cognitive behavioural therapy. She will need basic investigations as a baseline at starting the treatment and to exclude other causes for her low mood.

For the fictional case example above, the aim (a broad statement describing the general goal of the teaching) could be: 'The trainee will learn how to manage a pregnant woman suffering with depressive disorder.' And this gives rise to the objectives of the session as follows, where an objective is a specific intended learning outcome. Examples for this case may include any or all of the following: 'The trainee will sensitively and supportively:

(1) Inform the patient that she is suffering with depression.
(2) Explain the need for treatment.
(3) Explain the benefits of treatment of depressive disorder in pregnancy.
(4) Explain the risks of not treating depression in pregnancy.
(5) Explain the risks of taking antidepressants in pregnancy.
(6) Explain the need to rule out other causes for her low mood, namely, anaemia, low B12 and folate; thyroid dysfunction.
(7) Explain the referral for cognitive behavioural therapy including the process and the timescale.
(8) Do all of the above in a supportive manner allowing the patient time to process the information and to ask questions.'

C. Session Design and Planning

There are essentials in the design of sessions. One is an understanding of the experiential learning cycle (Box 7.3; Kolb 1984). Another essential is a sound knowledge from trainer and trainee of the relevant curriculum content. An understanding of the processes of instructional events (Box 7.4; Gagné et al. 1992) learning from patients which is well described by Cox (Cox 1993a–h; see also Fig. 7.2) will then assist in drafting a plan (see Curzon 1997, p. 277).

D. Starting the Session

Before any training session begins, the trainee should be told the aim and objectives of the session. They should be made aware of the baselines such as the time available with the patient and the need to be courteous and empathic.

Box 7.3 Experiential learning cycle

1. Concrete experience – experience of a new situation
2. Reflective observations – reflection on the experience
3. Abstract conceptualizing – formation of concepts and generalizations
4. Active experimentation – testing the concepts in new situations

---

Box 7.4 The eight events of instruction (after Gagné et al. 1992)

1. Gain the trainee's attention
2. Inform the trainee of the objectives (intended learning outcomes)
3. Stimulate recall of previous knowledge – to confirm that they have the required background knowledge for the level of learning
4. Communicate stimulus material to them – a potted patient history
5. Give learning guidance – tell them how to go about the assigned task
6. Elicit the performance
7. Give feedback on the performance
8. Enhance retention and transfer of what has been learnt – suggest activities to build upon the learning

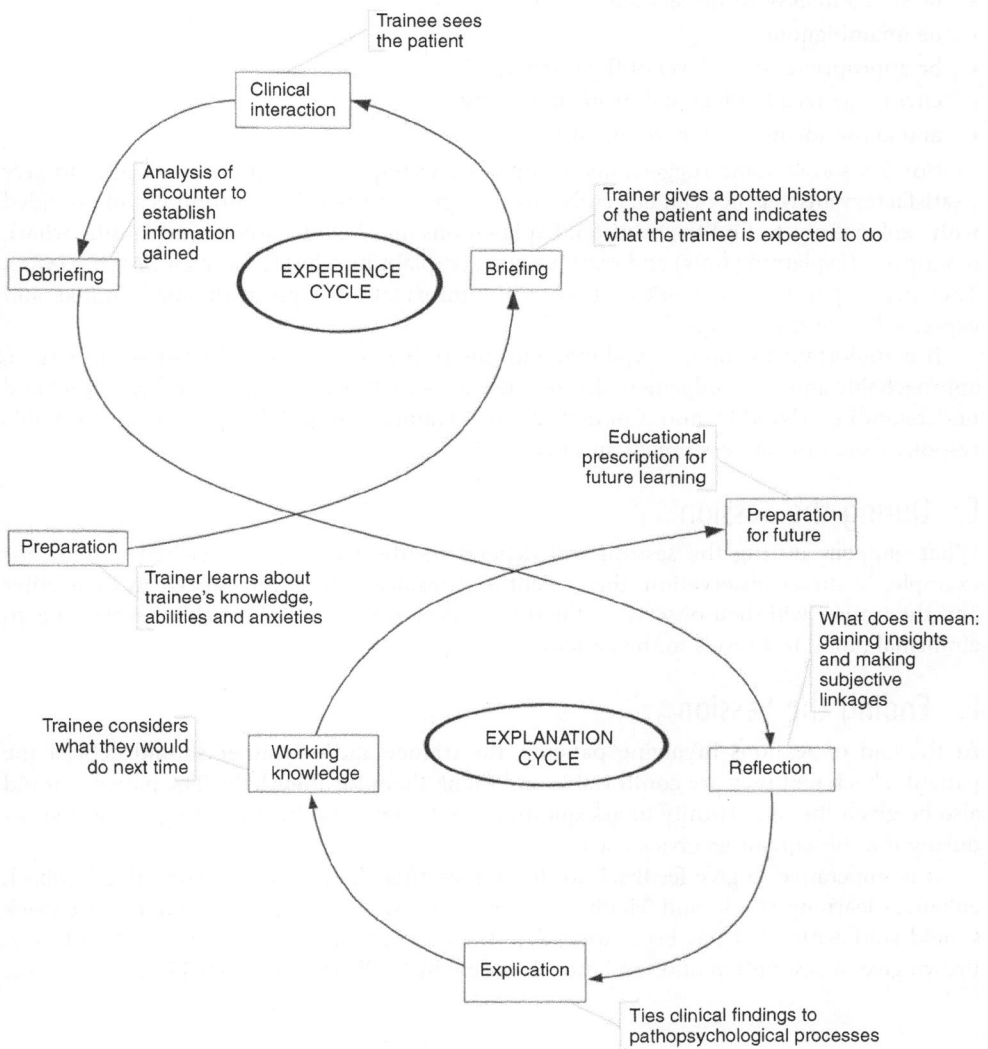

Fig. 7.2 Experiential learning cycle.

Trainees will need certain theoretical knowledge before they can learn clinical skills, and the trainer should question them to ensure that they have this. Without such knowledge the trainee will not have a successful encounter with the patient.

By asking questions the trainer is also encouraging the active involvement of the trainee. People who learn actively rather than by passive observation gain a deeper understanding and better retention of what they have learnt. They have increased motivation, curiosity and interest. Questioning encourages logical and analytical thinking.

Formulating questions requires skill. Generally, questions should:

- be short and easy to remember;

- be stated in easy-to-understand language;
- be unambiguous;
- be appropriate to the level of the learner;
- encourage recall of fact and problem solving;
- and allow adequate time for an answer.

Box 7.5 shows some suggestions for our case example. If the trainee struggles to give a satisfactory answer they can be gently directed, given hints, offered prompts and provided with explanations to find the solution. Explanations may be interpretive (explaining what), descriptive (explaining how) and reason-giving (explaining why) (Brown and Atkins 1988). They are important and work best when the information is given in small chunks and expressed in clear language.

It is important to enhance and maintain the trainee's motivation by being supportive, approachable and non-judgemental. Good teachers are those who are friendly, helpful and understanding (Newble and Cannon 2001). Trainees should be praised for suitable responses because success breeds success.

E. During the Session

What happens during the session will depend on the teaching model being used. For example, in direct observation, the patient and trainee will be introduced to each other and the trainer will then observe as the trainee performs a set task, such as explaining an abnormal blood test result to the patient.

F. Ending the Session

At the end of sessions involving patients, the trainee and/or trainer should debrief the patient, check that they are comfortable and thank them for their help. The patient should also be given the opportunity to ask questions and might also be asked to give their views during the subsequent feedback stage.

It is imperative to give feedback to the trainee after the session. Constructive feedback enhances learning (Rolfe and McPherson 1995) and should be given promptly. Feedback should start with what has been done well, then areas that could be improved and how. Brown gives a description of several models for giving feedback in Chapter 12 of this volume.

Box 7.5 Appropriate preliminary questions relating to the case example

- What factors have contributed to this woman's relapse?
- What do you think her diagnosis is?
- What symptoms of depression is she experiencing?
- What are other symptoms of depression?
- What physical issues could present with depressive features?
- What are her current risks?
- What are the treatment options available to her?

N.B. Not all trainees will be expected to know the risks and benefits of treating depression during pregnancy but these points can be covered in a teaching session before he/she sees the patient. This will depend on their level of training.

Trainees must be encouraged to reflect on what they would and would not do given a similar encounter in the future. They should recap on what they have learnt and be encouraged to seek clarification on aspects they have not understood. Trainees must then be given activities to build on what they have learnt, for example further reading or another patient to see.

The trainer also needs to reflect on the session – what went well and what was less successful. This helps to identify how things might be done differently next time in order to improve their teaching.

Small-Group Teaching

The case example depicts a one-to-one teaching session. In the future, clinical training might have a greater emphasis on small-group teaching. This can have the advantage that individuals learn not only the basic skills but also to work with others as part of a team. Trainers need to be aware of the difficulties of small-group teaching and strategies to deal with them. A particular problem arises during sessions where one trainee is performing the task and the others are observing. It is common for the observers to 'switch off' and become passive onlookers, and this may be exacerbated in teleconferencing sessions. They can be actively involved by being set specific tasks, for example to give feedback at the end. Difficulties can also occur with the dynamics of the group (Jaques 2000; Quinn 2000) and some suggestions for dealing with these are shown in Table 7.1.

Patients as Teachers

In recent decades, the involvement of patients has become common practice in medical education (Wykurz and Kelly 2002) Patients and their narratives have moved beyond being subjects for 'learning material' in clinical training. A considerable body of literature is emerging describing the role of patients as teachers to learners as well as in the design of curricula (Towle et al. 2010; Dijk et al. 2020).

Patients have taken the roles of teachers of a range of clinical skills, including history taking and the physical and mental state examination, as well as feeding back life experiences and acting as assessors giving formative feedback and summative feedback (e.g., during OSCE examinations) (Dijk et al. 2020). In psychiatry, there is a long history of involving patients as teachers (Casement 1985). Ikkos gave an early description of the successful involvement of patients from a local service user group as teachers of interview skills (Ikkos 2003). Furthermore, experience from primary care of patient participation in undergraduate

Table 7.1 Strategies to deal with problems of group dynamics during small-group teaching (Quinn 2000)

Problem	Strategy
Hogging the limelight	Praise the individual for input, and request that others are given a chance to answer. Invite others to comment
Everyone speaking at once	Praise them for wanting to contribute, exert control, try to use humour
Conflict within the group	Accept that people have different views. Remind members to question theories not individuals
Reluctance to participate	Build each individual's confidence, gently encourage participation, ask the group members to take it in turns to contribute

teaching suggests potential therapeutic benefit including raised self-esteem and empowerment for most, although some distress for others, perhaps caused by a poor student interview technique (Walters et al. 2003). Jha struck a cautionary note in a systematic review of the involvement of real patients in medical education, which highlighted issues around ethics and psychological impact for patients (Jha et al. 2009).

In psychiatry, whilst the available literature is varied in approach, the current state of knowledge about the involvement of patients and carers in medical education is generally positive albeit with little information on ethical consequences (Miller et al. 2016).

Conclusion

The shift towards a competency-based model of education and learning in medicine and psychiatry continues at all levels of learning. One of its characteristics is a move from the apprenticeship model of learning towards a training based on well-planned, systematic, curriculum-based teaching sessions. The skills learnt are subject to workplace-based assessments, with successful trainees graduating from one level of training to the next.

There will be increasing levels of supervision, direct observation and assessment of trainees as they work. Learning based on patient contact will remain at the core of medical education, and a patient-based approach in medical training will enable trainees to develop professional and humanistic skills alongside medical knowledge. The changing landscape of clinical service delivery requires both trainers and trainees to actively consider, at all times, the opportunities and resource requirements for patient-based teaching in a variety of community and in-patient settings.

It is axiomatic that in order to ensure the quality of the teaching and assessment they deliver, trainers themselves need formal training in techniques of contemporary medical education, including session planning, setting objectives, assessing performance and giving feedback. However, in a rapidly evolving clinical and educational environment, everyone involved in training will need to tap into the huge potential for learning that involves remote-learning methodology such as teleconsulting as well as simulated and even virtual patients. Solutions will need to be found to address the potential conflict between the pressures of service provision and the delivery of good-quality training. Training organizations will need, as a matter of urgency, to invest effort, resource and formal research into best practice and will have to consider the place of small, patient-based groups alongside traditional one-to-one clinical sessions. Their use in other specialties shows a range of possibilities that suggests that investment should reap rewards

References

AAMC (2007) Effective use of educational technology in medical education. Colloquium on educational technology: recommendations and guidelines for medical educators. Available at: https://store.aamc.org/downloadable/download/sample/sample_id/111/.

Brenner AM (2009) Uses and limitations of simulated patients in psychiatric education. *Academic Psychiatry*, 33: 112–19.

Brown G, Atkins M (1988) *Effective Teaching in Higher Education*. Methuen.

Casement P (1985) *On Learning from the Patient*. Tavistock.

Combs CD, Combs PF (2019) Emerging roles of virtual patients in the age of AI. *AMA Journal of Ethics*, 21: E153–9; doi: 10.1001/amajethics .2019.153.

Council of the European Union (1993) Council Directive 93 / 104 / EC. Concerning certain aspects of the organization of working time. *Official Journal of the European Community*, L307: 18–24.

Cox K (1993a) Planning bedside teaching: 1. Overview. *Medical Journal of Australia*, **158**: 280–282

Cox K (1993b) Planning bedside teaching: 2. Preparation before entering the wards. *Medical Journal of Australia*, **158**, 355–7.

Cox K (1993c) Planning bedside teaching: 3. Briefing before seeing the patient. *Medical Journal of Australia*, **158**: 417–18.

Cox K (1993d) Planning bedside teaching: 4. Teaching around the patient. *Medical Journal of Australia*, **158**: 493–5.

Cox K (1993e) Planning bedside teaching: 5. Debriefing after the clinical interaction. *Medical Journal of Australia*, **158**: 571–2

Cox K (1993f) Planning bedside teaching: 6. Reflection on the clinical experience. *Medical Journal of Australia*, **158**, 607–608

Cox K (1993g) Planning bedside teaching: 7. Explication of the clinical experience. *Medical Journal of Australia*, **158**: 789–790.

Cox K (1993h) Planning bedside teaching: 8. Deriving working rules for next time. *Medical Journal of Australia*, **159**: 64–5.

Curzon LB (1997) *Teaching in Further Education. An Outline of Principles and Practice.* Continuum.

Darnton R, Lopez T, Anil M, Ferdinand J, Jenkins M (2021) Medical students consulting from home: a qualitative evaluation of a tool for maintaining student exposure to patients during lockdown. *Medical Teacher*, **43**: 160–7.

Dave S (2012) Simulation in psychiatric teaching. *Advances in Psychiatry*, **18**: 292–8.

Dave S, Dogra N, Leask SJ (2010) Current role of service increment for teaching funding in psychiatry. *The Psychiatrist*, **34**: 31–5.

Dent JA (2001) Hospital wards. In Dent JA, Harden RM (eds.), *A Practical Guide for Medical Teachers*, Churchill Livingstone, pp. 98–108.

Dijk SW, Duijzer EJ, Wienold M (2020) Role of active patient involvement in undergraduate medical education: a systematic review. *BMJ Open*; doi: http://dx.doi.org/10.1136/bmjopen-2020-037217.

Eagles JM, Calder SA, Nicholl KS, Walker LG (2001a) A comparison of real patients, simulated patients and videotaped interview in teaching medical students about alcohol misuse. *Medical Teacher*, **23**: 490–3.

Eagles JM, Calder SA, Nicholl KS, Sclare PD (2001b) Using simulated patients in education about alcohol misuse. *Academic Medicine*, **76**: 395.

Eagles JM, Calder SA, Wilson S, Murdoch JM, Sclare PD (2007) Simulated patients in undergraduate education in psychiatry. *Psychiatric Bulletin*, **31**: 187–90.

Ferenchick G, Simpson D, Blackman J, et al. (1997) Strategies for efficient and effective teaching in the ambulatory care setting. *Academic Medicine*, **72**: 277–80.

Gagné RM, Briggs LJ, Wager, WW (1992) *Principles of Instructional Design*. Harcourt Brace Jovanovich.

Gask (1998) Small group interactive techniques utilizing video feedback. *International Journal of Psychiatry in Medicine*, **28**: 97–113.

General Medical Council (2012) *Making and Using Visual and Audio Recordings of Patients.* General Medical Council .

General Medical Council (2015) Promoting excellence: standards for medical education and training. Available at www.gmc-uk.org/education/standards-guidance-and-curricula/standards-and-outcomes/promoting-excellence.

Gutierrez CM, Cox SM, Dalrymple JL (2016) The revolution in medical education. *Texas Medicine*, **112**: 58–61.

Harden RM, Crosby JR, Davis MH (1999) *An Introduction to Outcome Based Education* (AMEE Guide no. 14). Association for Medical Education in Europe (AMEE).

Hearn J, Dewji M, Stocker C, Simons G (2019) Patient-centered medical education: a proposed definition. *Medical Teacher*, **41**: 934–8.

Hollander JE, Carr BG (2020) Virtually perfect? Telemedicine for Covid-19 (2020). *New England Journal of Medicine*, **382**: 1679–81.

Ikkos G (2003) Engaging patients as teachers of clinical interview skills. *Psychiatric Bulletin*, **27**: 312–15.

Janicek RW, Fletcher KE (2003) Teaching at the bedside. *Medical Teacher*, **25**: 127–30.

Jaques D (2000) *Learning in Groups*. Kogan Page.

Jolly B, Harris D, Peyton JWR (1998) Teaching with patients. In Peyton JWR (ed.). *Teaching and Learning in Medical Practice*, Manticore Europe, pp. 155–70.

Jha V, Quinton ND, Bekker HL, Roberts TE (2009) Strategies and interventions for the involvement of real patients in medical education: a systematic review. *Medical Education*, 43: 10–20.

Kennedy C, Yellowlees P (2003) The effectiveness of telepsychiatry measured using the Health of the Nation Outcome Scale and the Mental Health Inventory. *Journal of Telemedicine and Telecare*, 9: 12–16.

Kolb DA (1984) *Experiential Learning: Experience as the Source of Learning and Development*. Prentice Hall.

LaCombe MA (1997) On bedside teaching. *Annals of Internal Medicine*, 126: 217–20.

Lynöe N, Sandlund M, Westberg K, et al. (1998) Informed consent in clinical training – patient experience and motives for participating. *Medical Education*, 32: 465–71.

Mian A, Khan S (2020) Medical education during pandemics: a UK perspective. *BMC Medicine*, 18: 100.

Miller C, Pradeep V, Mohamad M, et al. (2020) Patients and carers as teachers in psychiatric education: a literature review and discussion. *Irish Journal of Psychological Medicine*, 37: 126–33.

Newble D, Cannon R (2001) *A Handbook for Medical Teachers*. Kluwer Academic Publishers.

O'Flynn N, Spencer J, Jones R (1997) Consent and confidentiality in teaching in general practice: survey of patients' views on presence of students. *BMJ*, 315: 1142.

Quinn FM (2000) *The Principles and Practice of Nurse Education*. Stanley Thomas.

Ramani S (2003) Twelve tips to improve bedside teaching. *Medical Teacher*, 25: 112–15.

Ramkisson R, Dave S, Abraham S, et al. (2020) Remote psychiatric consultations: top tips for clinical practitioners. *Progress in Neurology and Psychiatry*, 24: 20–5.

Rees J (1987) How to do it: take a teaching ward round. *BMJ*, 295: 424–5.

Rolfe I, McPherson J (1995) Formative assessment: how am I doing? *Lancet*, 345: 837–9.

Royal College of Psychiatrists (2010) A competency based curriculum for specialist training in psychiatry. Available at: www .rcpsych.ac.uk/docs/default-source/ training/curricula-and-guidance/general_psy chiatry_curriculum_march_2019.pdf? sfvrsn=9e53c99a_6.

Samarasekera DD, Goh PS, Lee SS, Gwee MCE (2018) The clarion call for a third wave in medical education to optimize healthcare in the twenty-first century. *Medical Teacher*, 40: 982–5.

Seigler M (1978) A legacy of Osler. Teaching clinical ethics at the bedside. *JAMA*, 239: 951–6.

Shelton PG, Corral I, Kyle B (2017) Advances in undergraduate medical education: meeting the challenges of an evolving world of education, healthcare and technology. *Psychiatric Quarterly*, 88: 225–34.

Spencer J (2003) ABC of learning and teaching in medicine: learning and teaching in the clinical environment. *BMJ*, 326: 591–4.

Stacy R, Spencer J (1999) Patients as teachers: a qualitative study of patients' views on their role in a community-based undergraduate project. *Medical Education*, 33: 688–94.

Towle A, Bainbridge L, Godolphin W, et al. (2010) Active patient involvement in the education of health professionals. *Medical Education*, 44: 64–74.

Vassilas C, Ho L (2000) Video for teaching purposes. *Advances in Psychiatric Treatment*, 6: 304–11.

Walters K, Buszewicz M, Russell J, Humphrey C (2003) Teaching as therapy: cross sectional and qualitative evaluation of patients' experiences of undergraduate psychiatry teaching in the community. *BMJ*, 326: 740.

Wright HJ (1974) Patients attitudes to medical students in general practice. *BMJ*, 1: 372–6.

Wykurz G, Kelly D (2002) Developing the role of patients as teachers: literature review. *BMJ*, 325: 818–21.

Simulation-Based Learning in Psychiatric Training

Anna Ludvigsen, Sridevi Sira Mahalingappa
and Subodh Dave

Introduction

This chapter is an updated version of a previous article on the use of simulation in psychiatry training (Dave 2012). Professor Dave's observation that changes in the delivery of psychiatric care, such as ward closures and the creation of specialist teams, might limit the availability of direct patient contact for trainees was prescient. What was, however, unimaginable at the time of writing the article was the effect that a global pandemic such as COVID-19 would have on the provision of clinical training by limiting access to clinical placements (Lucey and Johnston 2020). These factors have increased the urgency and pressure for those concerned with the delivery of training to create and deliver simulation-based learning (SBL), often online. Many educators may have found themselves wishing for a guide on how to produce psychiatry-orientated SBL experiences. The focus of this chapter will therefore be on how to create and deliver such SBL programmes, based on the authors experience of doing so, often with limited resources, in the setting of a typical, UK-based, medical education centre.

Role plays, which can be considered a form of experiential learning through simulation, are excluded from this review but are covered comprehensively by Eagles and Calder (2011). Ward-based, or *in situ*, simulation is covered in detail by Martin et al. (2020). Working with patients who directly share their own experiences in order to educate trainees is also not covered by this review. This important part of clinical education is covered in a literature review by Miller et al. (2020).

Historical Context

There is a long history of SBL in medicine. In the 1800s, the French midwife Madame Angélique Marguerite Le Boursier du Coudray was commissioned by King Louis XV to teach women safer childbirth practices in an effort to lower rising infant mortality rates. She achieved great success and developing teaching techniques which included the use of life-size, anatomically accurate models of the female pelvis and foetus (Gelbart 1999).

The noted medical educator and neurologist Howard Barrows recognized the value of simulated patients to not only portray physical symptoms but also psychological ones (Barrows 1993). Actors were given characteristics such as 'hostile patient', 'seductive patient', 'patient hates physician' and 'patient from another culture'. This foray into simulating psychological characteristics of patients was the first attempt at using actors to teach issues relevant to psychiatry. It is indeed, therefore, an anomaly that the formal use of standardized or simulated patients in psychiatric education seems to have been delayed by another two decades (Eagles et al. 2007), although this trend is now reversing (Attoe et al. 2016).

Historically, there was little guidance for medical educators on how to provide psychiatrically focused SBL and so standards varied greatly between centres and even among clinical educators within the same department. Published in 2016, the document entitled 'Simulation-based education in healthcare: standards framework and guidance' (Association for Simulated Practice in Healthcare (ASPiH) and Health Education England 2016) aims to address this problem and provides an invaluable resource when creating SBL programmes.

What Is Simulation?

There is no generally agreed definition of SBL. Often, people think it is dependent on the use of expensive specialist equipment and high-fidelity sets but this is not necessarily the case. Professor Gaba of the Center for Immersive and Simulation-based Learning at Stanford University, describes simulation as a 'technique, not a technology, to replace or amplify real experiences with guided experiences, often immersive in nature, that evoke or replicate substantial aspects of the real world in a fully interactive fashion' (Gaba 2007). In other words, simulation is a method to be applied, rather than a technology that can be purchased and used 'out of the box'. Designing and providing a successful programme requires investment in terms of thought, time and resources. Despite having many advantages, SBL is also not a panacea that solves all training requirements, including that of direct clinical experience. However, when used judiciously, SBL can play an important part in medical education, which makes the required outlay in resources worthwhile both from a pedological and resources perspective (Aggarwal et al. 2010).

Common Factors in Simulation

Although SBL programmes vary greatly, they share common factors: generally, a participant will enter a situation that resembles real life in which they can interact with their surroundings and other people in a natural way. They will do so to complete a specific task assigned by a facilitator, who will observe the participant and then help them to make sense of what happened during the simulation as part of the debrief.

The following factors should be considered when planning a simulation programme:

- There must be a plan for the session with clearly defined learning outcomes, which are mapped to the curriculum appropriate to the learner group.
- How will the scenario be created?
- Who will facilitate the session?
- How will the debrief work?
- Who will represent the patient or carer and how will they be briefed at the start, and debriefed at the end of the session? Will they give feedback to the participants and if so how?
- How will the session be evaluated?
- What physical resources are required, such as rooms, audio-visual equipment, props (if used)?

When Is Simulation the Appropriate Tool to Use in Order to Meet Intended Learning Outcomes?

The intended learning outcomes (ILOs) will determine if SBL is the best tool for the job and, if so, will also suggest the way in which the technique of simulation may be applied.

Educational theory such as Blooms taxonomy should be applied to the ILOs (ASPiH and NHS Health Education England 2016). In psychiatric simulation, ILOs are likely to fall into cognitive, affective, human factors and person-centred domains (psychomotor skills are less likely to feature than in 'hands-on' medical and surgical simulations, though certain physical examination skills may be an exception). Simulation can be used to help participants practise, refine and develop skills and attitudes. It can also be used to test a candidate's competence in these domains. Formative assessments in particular are significant drivers of learning. Participants' learning requirements and pre-existing subject knowledge should also be taken into account when determining if SBL is the most appropriate and efficient way of meeting their needs. For example, there is little point in setting up a simulation session in which participants are instructed to carry out a technical task such as conducting a mental state examination (MSE) if the candidates do not know how to do that. Placing them in such a situation might be very demoralizing for the participant and would be a waste of simulation resources. However, once participants have acquired baseline knowledge about how to do an MSE, through lectures, seminars or self-directed learning, then SBL can be used to allow the participant to practice applying that knowledge in a setting that acts as a proxy for real life. One major advantage of simulation is that it can be possible to record interactions, play them back to participants as part of the debrief, encourage reflection on what could have been done differently and then allow the participant to re-enter the simulation and make another attempt, armed with the knowledge gained during the debrief. Once technical knowledge has been acquired simulation can be used to assess a candidate's competence in applying that knowledge (exams such as objective and structured clinical examinations are examples of this).

SBL can extend beyond the practice and examination of technical skills to touch on parts of clinical education that are often difficult to define or indeed teach. For example, when considering person-centred care, the clinician's ability to show empathy and compassion towards their patients is paramount (Mezzich et al. 2016) and of particular relevance to training in psychiatry (Person-Centred Training and Curriculum (PCTC) Scoping Group 2018). ILOs that focus on the clinician's ability to demonstrate person-centred skills are increasingly being included in many undergraduate and postgraduate curricula such as the General Medical Council's 'Outcomes for graduates' (General Medical Council 2018), last updated in 2020, and the Royal College of Psychiatrists' 'Core training in psychiatry' (Royal College of Psychiatrists 2013), last updated 2020. While some have queried whether such skills can be taught (Brenner 2009) other findings suggest that involving patients in medical education increases person-centredness among trainees (Rees et al. 2007) (Moore et al. 2017). Psychiatric SBL is well suited to involving patients in the design and delivery of sessions, as is described below. Such co-produced programmes, when coupled with an appropriate debriefing model, can be used to encourage self-reflection and the development of empathy in junior doctors (Ludvigsen et al. 2015), especially if participants receive feedback from the actor. This feedback can be qualitative or structured, in role or out of role (Eagles et al. 2001).

Developing a Plan for the Session and Creating a Simulation Scenario

In order to 'replicate substantial aspects of the real world' (Gaba 2007, p. 126) there needs to be a predetermined plan outlining the rules of the world which is to be created and entered into by the actor and participant/s. The starting point for this should be the ILOs. Clinical learning outcomes require clinically plausible simulation scenarios. 'Buy-in' to the fidelity of a simulation has less to do with creating a set that cannot be distinguished from reality and everything to do with matching the level of fidelity required for the ILOs (Scerbo and Dawson 2007) and the quality of the debrief (Whilhelm 1991). The 'rules of engagement' for the session should be explained to participants at the start of the session, together with ground rules that promote a safe learning environment. It is advisable to treat participants with the same level of regard as we expect them to demonstrate towards the patients and colleagues, thus modelling the intended learning outcomes

The simulation scenario should address the following components:

- specific context (who the participant is during the simulation, e.g., a core trainee working for the liaison team);
- setting (where the simulation is taking place, e.g., in the emergency department);
- clinical information (relating to the patient); and
- instructions to both the actor and the participant (e.g., what their respective tasks during the encounter are).

In addition, participants should be made aware of how they can interrupt or end the scenario, if they need to, and any limitations to how can they interact with the set (e.g., if can they use the phone that happens to be in the corner of the room to call for senior advice or speak to a relative).

Creating clinical scenarios requires input from someone with the relevant clinical training and experience and may also include input from individuals who have experience of the situation from a different perspective, especially that of the patient or carer. By triangulating these divergent viewpoints during the creation of a scenario, depth and nuance and a more holistic, person-centred approach can be adopted (Attoe et al. 2017, Ludvigsen et al. 2020). For example, if the ILO states that the participant should be able to conduct a MSE under challenging circumstances, then the scenario should reflect this. The designer might ask themselves, and core trainees, what the situation would be in which a junior doctor might carry out an MSE under challenging circumstances.

This might result in a scenario such as: 'You are a core trainee working in liaison psychiatry (context) and are asked to see a patient who has been admitted to a surgical ward (setting). They are waiting for surgery following a fractured leg sustained after a fall from a building. The nursing staff report that they have been behaving strangely and appear to be responding to unseen stimuli and are becoming increasingly agitated (clinical context). Carry out an MSE (instructions).'

Following a Debriefing Model

A debriefing model is a tool that facilitators use to help participants get the most out of the session. The form that model takes is dependent on the ILOs and the purpose of the session. For example, if the aim of the simulation is to assess the participant's competence at carrying out a specific task, such as in an examination, then all that may be required is a mark sheet. If, however, the intention is to coach performance or encourage reflection then something more is required. Why use a debriefing model? It functions as a container for the session, creates consistency between sessions and different facilitators, and is reassuring for the participants because, once explained to them, they will know what to expect. This can do a lot to allay performance anxiety, which can be a serious limitation to learning. Several clinical debriefing models exist such as the Diamond debriefing model (Jaye et al. 2015), the advocacy enquiry model (Rudolph et al. 2006) and the Lederman model (Lederman 1992), among others. Facilitators should receive training in how to use a model, and online, as well as face-to-face, courses are available. For example, the commonly used Diamond debriefing model, originally designed for use in acute medical emergency scenarios, involves three distinct phases: a description of what happened during the simulation, an analysis of the events described and a discussion of how the things learned could be applied in future practice. Table 8.1 illustrates the debriefing model developed by the Nottinghamshire Healthcare Simulation Centre. It has been adapted from the Diamond debriefing model to allow for more didactic teaching of knowledge (e.g., differentials of depression) as well as a greater emphasis on reflection around the thoughts and feelings that may arise during the simulation ('the simulation is an excuse for the debrief and group discussion' is a common phrase used by the facilitators). Facilitator 1 is usually a clinician with basic training in facilitation, facilitator 2 is a member of the simulation faculty.

Facilitators

Who should facilitate simulation? This will depend on the learner group, the ILOs and facilitator availability. Clinical aspects of a course must be addressed by someone qualified to do so. It is important that facilitators are familiar with the scenario and debriefing model, timings and arrangements for how to address any concerns or problems that may arise during the session. Not all facilitators necessarily have to be doctors. Clinical nurse educators, medical educationalists, allied health professionals and, importantly, patients and carers can all be excellent facilitators provided they have sufficient training and support.

Table 8.1 Nottinghamshire reflective debriefing model

Phase	Facilitator task
PREBRIEF Patient-focused Facilitator 1	Establish a joint group understanding of clinical problem and what needs to be covered. Ensure the participant knows what they need to do and how to do it. Make lists of differential diagnosis and 'to do'.
SIMULATION	
CLINICAL DEBRIEF 1 Patient-focused Facilitator 1	Capture new clinical information to ensure the group has a shared understanding (without going into explanation). Highlight anything important that was missed by the scribe/group.
REFLECTIVE DEBRIEF Participant-focused Facilitator 2	To bring to light any difficulties encountered during patient interactions, especially things not often discussed (e.g., feeling irritated with the patient, not knowing what to say, finding it difficult to ask about suicide, etc.). Think 'mini-Balint' group.
CLINICAL DEBRIEF 2 Patient-focused Facilitator 1	Use differentials and 'to do' lists to reformulate what the group thinks is going on and what else should to happen before the consultation is concluded.

Having more than one person facilitating a session, for example a clinician and someone experienced in facilitation who can lead the session, often works well. It is an advantage if facilitators have themselves participated in the type of simulation they are delivering. Ideally, facilitators-to-be will take part in a 'train-the-trainer' session during which they themselves will be participants in a simulation, taking the hot seat and undergoing a debrief before being taught the fundamentals of facilitation, and will have an opportunity for observed practice with feedback.

What Is a Simulated Patient?

Simulation centres that provide programmes which cover acute medical and surgical emergencies have at their disposal increasingly realistic and complex mannequins that mimic a wide array of physiological dysfunction (at a cost). Although artificial intelligence programmes that can imitate people who are experiencing psychopathology are undoubtedly on the horizon, most psychiatric simulation programmes work with actors to simulate patients. The term 'simulated patient' has been used interchangeably at times with 'standardized patient', a term coined by the Canadian psychometrician Geoffrey Norman (Collins and Harden 1998). Various other terms have been used, such as patient instructor, programmed patient, patient educator, professional patient, surrogate patient, teaching associate and volunteer patient. All of these terms are sometimes encompassed in the umbrella term 'standardized patient', which is defined as a simulated/actual patient trained to present their symptoms in a standardized way to provide a student with an opportunity to learn or to be evaluated. 'Simulated patient' is then defined as a person without any real clinical signs or symptoms, trained to portray certain physical signs or symptoms or to play a particular role to facilitate teaching or assessment (Ker and Bradley 2007). This is to be contrasted with role-play patients, where either the learner or the teacher plays the role of a patient to facilitate teaching. With standardized patients, the focus is on consistency of presentation over time settings, which conveys a product 'superior to the inconsistencies of the real patient' (Brenner 2009). In this chapter, the focus is on simulated patients, who are trained to play a role.

Involving Simulated Patients in Psychiatry Teaching

Assessment

Simulated patients are rapidly becoming the norm in both undergraduate and postgraduate summative and formative examinations (Wallace et al. 2002). Here, we focus on psychiatric teaching but readers interested in the use of simulated patients in assessment are directed to an informative articles by Hodges et al. (2002), Johnston et al. (2013) and the Heath and Care Professions Council (2014).

Teaching

Simulated patients have been used in two broad areas of psychiatric teaching: (a) to expose trainees to a wider range of diagnoses and psychopathology; and (b) to teach advanced communication skills relevant to psychiatry (Tysinger et al. 1997; Edinger et al. 1999; Brenner 2009; Neale 2019). Medical students have ranked the use of simulated patients enacting psychopathology as one of the most useful learning experiences in their placements (Hall et al. 2004). Simulated patients portraying schizophrenia have been successfully used to teach the MSE (Birndorf and Kaye 2002) and those enacting delirium to teach liaison psychiatry skills (Chur-Hansen and Koopowitz 2002). They have also been used to teach clinical skills related to the assessment and the management of patients misusing benzodiazepines and opiates (Taverner et al. 2000). Students have praised the use of simulated patients to help them understand psychiatric symptoms (Krahn et al. 2002) and to teach clinical skills in psychopathology in a round-robin interviewing format (Gay et al. 2002).

The addition of a simulated patient psychiatric examination in the teaching programme has been shown to help improve interviewing and interpersonal skills (Bennett et al. 2006). Simulated patients have also been useful in teaching complex skills such as psychotherapy, where using real patients would be ethically complicated (Trudel 1996). Videotaped encounters with simulated patients have proved to be a useful teaching tool to train residents in basic psychotherapeutic skills (Klamen and Yudkowski 2002), and international videoconferencing using simulated patients has been used to teach clinical skills relevant to transcultural psychiatry (Ekblad 2004). Simulated patients have been used to teach psychosocial matters not directly related to, but relevant to, psychiatry, such as breaking bad news with empathy (Quest et al. 2002) and taking a good sexual history and providing HIV counselling (Haist et al. 2004). Haist et al. also used simulated patients in a workshop to teach residents about the assessment and management of domestic violence (Haist et al. 2003). Similarly, Clay et al. (2000) have used a standardized family to teach clinical skills to medical students.

Simulated patients have been used to teach clinical governance issues, which are also relevant to psychiatric practice. An example is the use of simulated patients to teach medical students, the clinical skills needed in discussing medical errors with patients (Halbach and Sullivan 2005). Similarly, simulated hospital admission has been used to increase empathy among medical students (Wilkes et al. 2002). Box 8.1 summarizes the role of simulated patients in teaching skills and attitudes relevant to psychiatry.

Box 8.1 A basic simulated-patient case scenario to teach learning outcomes in depression

Training plan – to be completed by facilitators before the session

Session title:	Depression scenario
Duration of session:	Three hours
Learner group:	Medical students
Number of participants:	Eight; participants will enter the simulation in pairs, one acting as the doctor and one as the observer/scribe
Tutor/s:	One clinical; one simulation faculty
Pre-course preparation/ requirements:	Psychiatry induction; taught classes on MSE and affective disorders
Resources required:	Actor, facilitators, 2 rooms, AV equipment (2 laptops with MS Teams, internet access, projector)

Step 1 – Learning outcomes

Identify learning outcomes (what is to be learned as a result of this lesson):

Learning outcome	Learning activity	Evidenced by
To be able to elicit a history of depression – ILO from university curriculum	Pre-simulation revision of diagnostic criteria for depression Discussion of how to ask a patient about important symptoms Participation or observation of simulation Participation in debrief and group discussion	Participation in simulation and debrief
To be able to carry out a risk assessment and, in conjunction with the patient, compile a safety plan – ILO from university curriculum	Pre-simulation revision of diagnostic criteria for depression Discussion of how to ask a patient about risk and design a safety plan Participation or observation of simulation Participation in debrief and group discussion	Participation in simulation and debrief
Be able to explain things clearly, in a practical way, giving me choices while being clear about the future – ILO from patients	Participation or observation of simulation Participation in debrief and group discussion Feedback from actor	Participation in simulation and debrief

Step 2 – Learning plan

Methodology structure of session:

Topic	Duration	Delivery method
Welcome, introduction, icebreaker and ground rules	15 minutes	Small-group seminar
Revision of depression and components of risk assessment	20 minutes	Small-group seminar/ didactic teaching
Simulation and debrief (divided into four 25-minute segments and 15-minute break)	115 minutes	Simulation and debrief
Summary and feedback from actor	25 minutes	Small-group seminar

(cont.)

Topic	Duration	Delivery method
Participants complete feedback forms	5 minutes	
Total	180 minutes	

Step 3 – Assessment

Consider if there will be an assessment of pre-course knowledge followed by a post-course assessment in order to provide evidence of whether or not learning has taken place/specific ILOs have been achieved.

Step 4 – Evaluation

Create a post-course participant feedback questionnaire.

Step 5 – Actor's brief

(please note, if a scenario has been co-produced with stakeholders, a more nuanced and detailed actor's brief would typically be created than this)

Background

Sam, 35, medical secretary, divorced three years ago. Living with daughter Tanya, four years old.

History and presenting problem (simulated patient's brief)

You are here to see a psychiatrist because your general practitioner (GP) referred you, and your family forced you to come. Your GP has been treating you for depression for the past six months but nothing seems to be getting better. Your boss has spoken to you sharply on a couple of occasions in the past few weeks and since then you have lost any remaining part of your confidence. Your sleep is disturbed and you wake early. You feel as if you can no longer enjoy yourself even if you go out with friends, which you used to love to do.

You do not feel like cooking or eating but force yourself to cook for Tanya, you think you've lost some weight. You don't sleep well, have lost your energy and feel that you are neglecting the housework and Tanya. Indeed, you are beginning to feel that you must be a bad mother because of this and wonder if Tanya would be better off with a more competent mother. You are now beginning to wonder whether you were responsible for the divorce and you are plagued by ruminations on little things in the past. You feel you are barely functioning at work, can't concentrate and are worried about losing your job, which would worsen your already perilous financial situation. You just can't imagine that things will ever get better again and you will ever go back to being your old self. At home, you feel exhausted looking after Tanya. You are impatient with her and then feel guilty. You do have friends but looking after Tanya has meant that it's been difficult to find time with them. You are close to your family but still find it hard to talk about your innermost feelings. Sometimes you feel as if you just want to stop feeling like this and have thought about taking an overdose but you know you will not do it because of Tanya. You have been taking the antidepressants the GP has prescribed and tried a short course of cognitive behavioural therapy (CBT) but nothing seems to help.

Attitude to treatment

You know that the doctor or the counsellor can't change the realities of your troubles (financial, relationships, etc.) so they can't help you.

'I can't imagine how medicines or talking to someone would help, as ultimately these are my problems and I need to sort out the mess I've created' (referring to marriage breakdown).
If asked more ...
You and your husband were basically incompatible – he liked golf and expensive holidays, you enjoyed theatre and a more sedate lifestyle. After Tanya, you also lost interest in sex and you drifted apart pretty rapidly after that. You often wonder whether you should have just put up with his absences abroad and his infidelities.

Approach to interview

You interact logically with the interviewer and are willing to be convinced of the benefits of medication or therapy, although you have little hope that they will make any difference as you cannot understand how your mood can change if your stresses continue.

Step 6 – Instructions to participants

You are a junior doctor working for a community mental health team. You are going to see a patient called Sam Jones who has been referred by her GP with a six-month history of depression, which does not seem to be responding to medication or CBT.

Doctor's tasks, which might be decided by the group during the pre-brief or suggested by the facilitator, depending on the format of the simulation, are, for example, the following:

(1) elicit the history of her depression
(2) carry out a risk assessment
(3) explain referral to the crisis resolution and home treatment team

Observers' tasks

(1) Use the ICD–10 criteria to establish the diagnosis (e.g., mild/moderate/severe depression)
(2) Comment on specific examples of statements or non-verbal behaviour that enabled or hindered therapeutic engagement
(3) Use a structured approach to assessing risk, and present your findings to the group

How to Involve Simulated Patients in Psychiatric Teaching

As already discussed, simulated-patient scenarios need to be tailor-made to deliver the curricular learning outcomes but they also need to be realistic. Simulated patients need not be professional actors but ought to be credible and consistent in their role and available when required. It is also important that they do not have a hostile attitude to psychiatry or to medical education (Cleland et al. 2010). Faculty members, therefore, need to be actively involved in the design, delivery and quality assurance of the scenarios, even when an agency is used for recruitment. Developing good working relationships between actors and facilitators is invaluable. Competent, reliable and experienced actors should be treated as valued members of the simulation team.

Ideally, each participant should have a one-to-one session with a simulated patient in a simulated environment such as an out-patient clinic. Limited budgets, however, can be stretched by using small groups with rotating hot seats and active observation (see examples of student and observer tasks in Box 8.1). The small group (8–10 students) can then benefit from peer, teacher and simulated-patient feedback. When interspersing simulated-patient scenarios with didactic teaching, it is preferable to start with didactic teaching and the simulated-patient interaction can then follow (Eagles and Calder 2011). Box 8.1 provides an example of a simulated patient scenario.

Novel Uses of Simulation

Covert simulated patients in out-patient clinics often go unidentified (Hoppe et al. 1990) and this offers a way to enhance experiential learning for trainees. Technology for tele-psychiatry can easily incorporate simulated patients operating remotely (Kennedy and Yellowlees 2003).

Gaming technology, as is available on videogame consoles, offers the possibility of virtual clinical scenarios whereby user choice will result in varying clinical outcomes. Such simulations have been trialled in internal medicine (Issenberg et al. 2003) and virtual psychiatric scenarios are now commercially available (e.g., VirtualCaseCreator; http://vccweb.health.bcu. ac.uk). Simulated high-fidelity mannequins are now routinely used in medical education but have had limited use in psychiatric education. Incorporating psychiatric content into the scenarios for, for example, an unresponsive patient (mannequin) following tricyclic antidepressant overdose can be used to teach not only resuscitation skills but also the acute management of a suicidal patient. SBL also lends itself to the delivery of multi-professional learning. Akroyd and colleagues designed and evaluated a SBL programme that focused on the multidisciplinary team approach to seclusion reviews (Akroyd et al. 2021). Well-equipped simulation skills centres with video feedback and one-way screens can optimize learning from the re-creation of a difficult ward review or a multidisciplinary team meeting (Srinivasan et al. 2006).

Conclusion

SBL has become an established part of psychiatric medical education and there is a growing evidence base for its utility in teaching and assessment. It appears that psychiatric SBL is finally catching up with medical and surgical specialities. The task for those designing and delivering psychiatric simulation is now to adopt a consistent approach based on recognized standards of quality in SBL such as those described by ASPiH and Health Education England (2016). This should be done in a way that recognizes and incorporates the innovative work that has quietly taken place in many teaching centres by the early adopters of SBL in psychiatric medical education. Psychiatrists, allied healthcare professionals and medical educators can contribute to the development of more person-centred and psychologically orientated simulation practice, especially by partnering with patients, carers and actors. In this way it will be possible to train tomorrow's doctors and psychiatrists in ways that not only encompass the necessary technical skills but also explore the affective, cognitive and other person-centred skills.

References

Aggarwal R, Mytton O, Derbrew M, et al. (2010) Training and simulation for patient safety. *BMJ Quality & Safety*, **19**: i34–43.

Akroyd M, Allison J, Booth S (2021) Multidisciplinary, simulation-based training to improve review of seclusion. *The Journal of Mental Health Training, Education and Practice*, **16**: 224–37.

ASPiH and NHS Health Education England (2016) *Simulation-Based Education in*

Healthcare: Standards Framework and Guidance. Association for Simulated Practice in Healthcare (ASPiH)and NHS Health Education England. Available at: http://aspih.org.uk/wp-content/uploads/2017/07/standards-framework.pdf.

Attoe C, Billon G, Riches S, et al. (2017) Actors with intellectual disabilities in mental health simulation training. *Journal of Mental Health Training, Education and Practice,* **12**: 272–8.

Attoe C, Kowalski C, Fernando A, Cross S (2016) Integrating mental health simulation into routine health-care education. *The Lancet Psychiatry,* **3**: 702–3.

Barrows H (1993) An overview of the uses of standardized patients for teaching and evaluating clinical skills. *Academic Medicine,* **68**: 443–51.

Bennett A, Arnold L, Welge, J (2006) Use of standardized patients during a psychiatry clerkship. *Academic Psychiatry,* **30**: 185–90.

Birndorf C, Kaye M (2002) Teaching the mental status examination to medical students by using a standardised patient in a large group setting. *Academic Psychiatry,* **26**: 180–3.

Brenner AM (2009) Uses and limitations of simulated patients in psychiatric education. *Academic Psychiatry,* **33**: 112–19.

Chur-Hansen A, Koopowitz L (2002) Introducing psychosocial and psychiatric concepts to first year medical students using an integrated biopsychosocial framework. *Education for Health,* **15**: 305–14.

Clay M, Lane H, Willis S, et al. (2000) Using a standardised family to teach clinical skills to medical students. *Teaching and Learning in Medicine,* **12**: 145–9.

Cleland J, Abe K, Rethans J (2010) The use of simulated patients in medical education: AMEE Guide No 42. *Medical Teacher,* **31**: 477–86.

Collins J, Harden R (1998) AMEE Medical Education Guide No. 13: real patients, simulated patients and simulators in clinical examinations. *Medical Teacher,* **20**: 508–21.

Dave S (2012). Simulation in psychiatric teaching. *Advances in Psychiatric Treatment,* **4**: 292–8.

Eagles J, Calder S (2011) Teaching with simulated patients and roleplay. In Brown T.,

Eagles S. (eds.), *Teaching Psychiatry to Undergraduates.* Royal College of Psychiatrists, pp. 230–44.

Eagles J, Calder S, Nicoll KS, et al. (2001) A comparison of real patients, simulated patients and videotaped interview in teaching medical students about alcohol misuse. *Medical Teacher,* **23**: 490–3.

Eagles J, Calder S, Wilson S (2007) Simulated patients in undergraduate education in psychiatry. *Psychiatric Bulletin,* **31**: 187–90.

Edinger W, Robertson J, Skeel J, et al. (1999) Using standardized patients to teach clinical ethics. *Journal of Medical Education,* **4**: 6.

Ekblad S, Manicavasagar V, Silove D, et al. (2004) The use of international videoconferencing as a strategy for teaching medical students about transcultural psychiatry. *Transcultural Psychiatry,* **41**: 120–9.

Gaba DM (2007) The future vision of simulation in healthcare. *Simulation in Healthcare: The Journal of the Society for Simulation in Healthcare,* **2**: 126–35.

Gay T, Himle J, Riba M (2002) Enhanced ambulatory experience for the clerkship: curriculum innovation at the University of Michigan. *Academic Psychiatry,* **26**: 90–5.

Gelbart N (1999) *The King's Midwife: A History and Mystery of Madame du Coudray.* University of California Press.

General Medical Council (2018) Outcomes for graduates. Available at: www.gmc-uk.org/education/standards-guidance-and-curricula/standards-and-outcomes/outcomes-for-graduates.

Haist S, Wilson J, Pursley H (2003) Domestic violence: increasing knowledge and improving skills with a four-hour workshop using standardised patients. *Academic Medicine,* **78**: S24–6.

Haist S, Lineberry M, Griffith C, et al. (2004) Improving students' sexual history inquiry and HIV counseling with an interactive workshop using standardized patients. *Journal of General Internal Medicine,* **19**: 549–53.

Halbach J, Sullivan L (2005) Teaching medical students about medical errors and patient safety: evaluation of a required curriculum. *Academic Medicine,* **80**: 600–6.

Hall M, Adamo G, McCurry L, et al. (2004) Use of standardized patients to enhance a psychiatry clerkship. *Academic Medicine*, **79**: 28–31.

Health and Care Professions Council (2014) *Standards of Education and Training*, HCPC.

Hodges B, Hanson M, McNaughton N et al. (2002) Creating, monitoring, and improving a psychiatry OSCE: a guide for faculty. *Canadian Journal of Psychiatry*, **26**: 134–61.

Hoppe R, Farquhar L, Henry R, et al. (1990) Residents' attitudes towards and skills in counseling: Using undetected standardized patients. *Journal of General Internal Medicine*, **5**: 415–20.

Issenberg SB, McGaghie WC, Petrusa ER, et al. (2005) Features and uses of high-fidelity medical simulations that lead to effective learning: a BEME systematic review. *Medical Teacher*, **27**: 10–28.

Jaye P, Thomas L, Reedy G (2015) 'The diamond': a structure for simulation debrief. *Clinical Teacher*, **12**: 171–5.

Johnston JL, Lundy G, McCullough M, Gormley GJ (2013) The view from over there: reframing the OSCE through the experience of standardised patient raters. *Medical Education*, **47**: 899–909.

Kennedy C, Yellowlees P (2003) The effectiveness of telepsychiatry measured using the Health of the Nation Outcome Scale and the Mental Health Inventory. *Journal of Telemedicine and Telecare*, **9**: 12–16.

Ker J, Bradley P (2007) *Simulation in Medical Education: Understanding Medical Education.* Association for the Study of Medical Education.

Klamen D, Yudkowski R (2002) Using standardized patients for formative feedback in an introduction to psychotherapy course. *Academic Psychiatry*, **26**: 168–72.

Krahn L, Bostwick J, Sutor B, et al. (2002) The challenge of empathy: a pilot study of the use of standardized patients to teach introductory psychopathology to medical students. *Academic Psychiatry*, **26**: 26–30.

Lederman L (1992) Debriefing: toward a systematic assessment of theory and practice. *Simulation in Gaming*, **23**: 145–60.

Lucey C, Johnston S, 2020. The transformational effects of COVID-19 on medical education. *Journal of the American Medical Association*, **324**: 1033–4.

Ludvigsen A, Bachra J, Rastall J, Junaid K 2020. Collaborating with carers to create a simulation scenario for medical students. *BMJ Simulation and Technology Enhanced Learning*, **6** (supplement 1): A40.

Ludvigsen A, Dave S, Thomas R (2015) The effects of post-graduate psychiatry training on junior doctors' attitudes towards and confidence in managing patients with psychiatric presentations. *European Psychiatry*, **30**: 1016.

Martin A, Cross S, Attoe C (2020). The use of *in situ* simulation in healthcare education: current perspectives. *Advances in Medical Education and Practice*, **11**: 893–903.

Mezzich JE, Botbol M, Christodoulou GN, Cloninger RC, Salloum IM (2016) Introduction to person-centered psychiatry. In Mezzich JE, Botbol M, Christodoulou GN, Cloninger RC, Salloum IM (eds.), *Person Centered Psychiatry*. Springer International, pp. 1–15.

Miller C, Pradeep V, Mohamad M, et al. (2020) Patients and carers as teachers in psychiatric education: a literature review and discussion. *Irish Journal of Psychlogical Medicine*, **37**: 126–133.

Moore L, Britten N, Lydall D, et al. (2017) Barriers and facilitators to the implementation of person-centred care in different healthcare contexts. *Scandinavian Journal of Caring Sciences*, **31**: 662–673.

Neale J (2019) What is the evidence for the use of simulation training to teach communication skills in psychiatry? *Evidence-Based Mental Health*, **22**: 23–5.

Person-Centred Training and Curriculum (PCTC) Scoping Group (2018) *Person-Centred Care: Implications for Training in Psychiatry CR215*, Royal College of Psychiatrists.

Quest T, Otsuki J, Banja J, et al. (2002) The use of standardized patients within a procedural competency model to teach death disclosure. *Academic Emergency Medicine*, **9**: 1326–33.

Rees C, Knight L, Wilkinson C (2007) User involvement is a sine qua non, almost, in medical education: learning with rather than just about health and social care service users. *Advances in Health Sciences Education Theory and Practice*, **12**: 359–90.

Royal College of Psychiatrists (2013). *A Competency Based Curriculum*, Royal College of Psychiatrists.

Rudolph J, Simon RE, Dufresne RL, Raemer DB. (2006) There's no such thing as 'nonjudgemental' debriefing: a theory and method for debriefing with good judgement. *Simulation in Healthcare*, **1**: 49–55.

Scerbo MWP, Dawson SM (2007) High fidelity, high performance? *Simulation in Healthcare: The Journal of the Society for Simulation in Healthcare*, **2**: 224–30.

Srinivasan M, Hwang J, West D, et al. (2006) Assessment of clinical skills using simulator technologies. *Academic Psychiatry*, **30**: 505–15.

Taverner D, Dodding C, White J (2000) Comparison of methods for teaching clinical skills in assessing and managing drug-seeking patients. *Medical Education*, **34**: 285–91.

Trudel J (1996) Simulated patients for the teaching of basic psychotherapeutic techniques: a practical guide. *Annals de Psychiatrie*, **11**: 14–18.

Tysinger J, Klonis L, Sadler J, et al. (1997) Teaching ethics using small-group, problem-based learning. *Journal of Medical Ethics*, **23**: 315–18.

Wallace J, Rao R, Haslam R (2002) Simulated patients and objective structured clinical examinations: review of their use in medical education. *Advances in Psychiatric Treatment*, **8**: 342–8.

Whilhelm J (1991) Crew member and instructor revaluations of line orientated flight training. Available at: https://ntrs.nasa.gov/citations/19920062328.

Wilkes M, Milgrom E, Hoffman J (2002) Towards more empathic medical students: a medical student hospitalisation experience. *Medical Education* **36**: 528–33.

Chapter

9

Running Journal Clubs in Psychiatry

Geraldine Swift and Joshua Bellevue de Sylva

Introduction

'Job plans must include dedicated time for academic and educational activities such as attending journal clubs', declare the eligibility criteria for the Member of the Royal College of Psychiatrists (MRCPsych) examinations (Royal College of Psychiatrists 2021, p. 12). Journal clubs also meet the requirements for continuing professional development (CPD) for UK consultant and staff grade and associate specialist (SAS) psychiatrists as defined in College guidelines (Royal College of Psychiatrists 2015). Since the critical review paper was introduced into the MRCPsych examinations in 1999, journal clubs have been seen as one of the main opportunities to teach these skills in psychiatry, and the curriculum for core training in psychiatry requires trainees to present a journal club annually. However, Glasziou's complaint that 'Many journal clubs are boring because the articles are quickly trashed as poor research and nothing changes' (Glasziou 2007) is not uncommon. Can journal clubs promote understanding and practice of evidence-based medicine (EBM) principles? Are they helpful in learning critical review skills required to pass academic exams such as MRCPsych Paper B? What aspects of journal club design influence effectiveness in these areas (Box 9.1)?

What Are the Aims of Psychiatric Journal Clubs?

The first, and perhaps most crucial step in designing a journal club is to agree clear goals and objectives that meet the needs of the target audience.

Keeping Up with the Literature

The literature on psychiatric journal clubs remains sparse and most evidence has to be extrapolated from other branches of medicine or social sciences and from research into educational theory. Traditionally, journal clubs have been viewed as a way of supporting

---

Box 9.1 Key factors for journal club success

- Regular and anticipated meetings
- Clear long- and short-term aims
- A trained facilitator taking responsibility for the club and providing continuity
- Enthusiastic participation by senior staff
- Including a social component to the club
- Integrating best research evidence with clinical expertise and an understanding of patients' wishes and needs

clinicians and trainees in keeping up with current literature and research. In the nineteenth century, Sir James Paget described 'a small room over a baker shop near the Hospital-gate where we could sit and read the journals and where some, in the evening, played cards' (Linzer 1987). Over the next 100 years, journal clubs became a regular part of higher and continuing medical education across all specialties, including psychiatry, where almost all training programmes in the UK and the USA now have regular journal club meetings to discuss recent papers (Taylor and Warner 2000).

With the development of online publishing, accessing research online has in some ways become much easier, but the sheer quantity of published material makes it difficult to pick out the needles of high-quality papers in the haystack of offerings. No one can possibly keep up with all the literature published: we need methods to find research that is valid and applicable.

Acquiring Skills in Evidence-Based Medicine

To provide such an approach, researchers at McMaster University in the USA proposed the concepts of EBM as a way of 'systematically finding, appraising and using contemporaneous research' (Rosenberg and Donald 1995: p. 1122). These can be summarized in four steps (Box 9.2):

EBM is now understood to be the best way of ensuring that a clinician's opinion, potentially limited by knowledge gaps or biases, is supported by evidence from the scientific literature. As EBM evolved, journal clubs aspired to the more specific goal of helping clinicians, and in particular trainees, to acquire the skills necessary to adopt this approach. EBM clubs covering all four steps outlined by Gilbody (1996) and integrated with clinical work may be seen as the gold standard of journal clubs. In an EBM journal club, the presenter describes a clinical scenario, formulates a question emerging from it, demonstrates the search strategy to find relevant, reliable research, appraises a relevant paper and considers how applicable it is to their initial scenario.

Journal clubs traditionally last one hour, but covering all the steps set out by Gilbody is difficult in this brief time. Some EBM clubs are therefore run in cycles over two–four weeks (Table 9.1). The challenge with running a journal club over several weeks is that the audience may vary depending on leave, rest periods and so on, which can make it difficult to maintain momentum.

Running an EBM journal club relies on having facilitators with appropriate skills to formulate questions and teach search strategies. Many busy clinicians do not feel confident in these areas (Warner and King 1997), particularly if they are required to demonstrate these skills in front of an audience of peers and trainees. Accessing additional training (Box 9.3) can help to make this a less daunting task and enable confidence to develop.

Box 9.2 Gillbody's four steps of EBM (Gilbody 1996)

1. Formulate a clear clinical question regarding patient care
2. Search the literature for relevant clinical studies
3. Evaluate ('critically appraise') evidence for effectiveness and usefulness
4. Implement useful findings in clinical practice

Table 9.1 Typical EBM journal club schedule

Week 1	Week 2	Week 3
• Audience describe recent clinical situations that involved uncertainty • Agree scenario of greatest interest • Formulate research question	• Live literature search • Select paper(s) of greatest relevance	• Critical appraisal of selected paper • Consider how it relates to clinical practice

---

Box 9.3 Training to support facilitators of journal clubs

Consider attending a course in EBM or the teaching of EBM: the Centre for Evidence-Based Medicine in Oxford offers recommended training. (www.cebm.ox.ac.uk)

Refresh knowledge of statistics:
• Review the syllabus for the MRCPsych Paper B critical review component. The 2011 syllabus remains current and includes basic biostatistics. (Royal College of Psychiatrists 2011)
• Nikolau offers a useful summary article covering commonly used statistics (Nikolaou 2016).

Seek additional training in relevant platforms:
• Local IT departments may be able to offer this
• Digital Learning Solution's IT Skills pathway (part of Health Education England) offers courses on different office365 software including Microsoft Teams (www.dls.nhs.uk/Home)
• www.support.microsoft.com offers all sorts of information and guides (including videos) for all their applications, including Microsoft Teams

Passing the Critical Review Component of the MRCPsych Exam

Many training programmes include critical review in their syllabus: it is hoped that through studying this area, trainees develop a greater commitment to EBM throughout their career. A key aim for many psychiatric journal clubs has become to support psychiatric trainees in passing the critical review component of their exams.

In the UK, a critical review component accounts for one-third of marks in the MRCPsych Paper B exam. The improvement in recruitment to psychiatry in the UK in recent years means that many training schemes now have a large group of enthusiastic participants who are focused on acquiring the skills and knowledge to pass their exams. The syllabus for the critical review topic theoretically covers all four steps of EBM, but in practice the emphasis in the exam tends to be on critical appraisal, as assessing the ability to formulate questions and conduct literature searches does not lend itself easily to a formal examination process.

In contrast to clubs that cover all four steps of EBM, those that focus on the critical appraisal of a specific study are relatively easy to run: there is an agreed process and trainees are often encouraged to work their way systematically through a series of questions (known as critical appraisal tools) such as those suggested by the Critical Appraisal Skills Programme (CASP: https://casp-uk.net/). Use of critical appraisal tools has been consistently reported as a feature of successful journal clubs (Gottlieb et al. 2018).

Learning theory reminds us that the majority of students will focus their learning on the demands of the exams facing them so it is perhaps not surprising that clubs that teach to the exam are popular. However, even where the key aim of a journal club is to support trainees to pass the MRCPsych exams, the longer-term requirements of professional practice need to be considered. The risk of over reliance on CASP is that it is possible to report diligently on each aspect without feeling confident to give an overall judgement on the quality of the paper and its applicability to clinical practice. To embed lifelong habits of using research, journal-club facilitators and senior participants need to support the audience in stepping beyond critical appraisal tools to understand the article in the context of local clinical practice and current research.

Other Aims: Professional Development and Bonding

A challenge with having exam success as a primary aim for a psychiatric journal club is that it may not engage potential audience members. Senior clinicians are likely to be less interested in attending journal clubs if the format does not relate to the dilemmas they encounter in routine practice, and educational meetings where senior staff are absent tend to be less positively rated by trainees (Heilligman and Wollitzer 1987). Many trainees based in psychiatry are in their foundation years or are working in psychiatry as part of general practice training: education targeting a specific psychiatric exam may appear less relevant to them too. It is important to find ways of meeting the learning needs for these potential participants.

Cave and Clandinn (2007) describe a journal club that focused on books rather than research papers. The books chosen were written by physicians, 'stories of their lives, the lives of their patients and the clinical problems with which they live'. They give the example of a discussion on *The Anatomy of Hope* by Groopman (2005). Jerome Groopman, a professor of medicine at Harvard, writes of his personal and professional struggle to balance the needs of nurturing hope with those of being truthful and realistic in discussing prognosis with patients and friends facing serious illness. This journal club was attended by doctors ranging from trainees to highly experienced consultants and it aimed to foster links between participants and help doctors develop different ways of understanding relationships between colleagues and between doctors and patients. Discussing such works may seem unusual in the context of a journal club, but the authors quote Sackett (1997) as including in his principles of EBM, 'individual clinical expertise that incorporates "thoughtful identification and compassionate use of individual patients' predicaments, rights and preferences in making clinical decisions"'. Such a journal club format can therefore be considered to relate to the fourth step of EBM, namely how to understand and apply the research evidence in the context of the individual patient.

Once a consensus has been reached in terms of the aims of the journal club, the next step is to ensure that it meets regularly and consistently – what characteristics help with this?

Longevity, Attendance and Engagement

Early studies of journal clubs' effectiveness considered the factors associated with high attendance rates and 'the avoidance of periodic abandonment' (Alguire 1998; Deenadayalan et al. 2008). Smaller teaching programmes, having one person taking responsibility for the club and providing continuity as facilitator, discussing original research and providing food were all seen as important. The consistent and enthusiastic participation of senior staff was particularly commented on in psychiatry training programmes, with trainees appreciating the opportunity to meet more experienced colleagues with clinical and research backgrounds (Yager et al. 1991).

Attendance in the Twenty-First Century: Virtual Journal Clubs

Over the past decade, changes in workplace practices make earlier literature on journal club attendance more difficult to apply to current situations. Within medicine, the European Working Time Directive and other developments have limited the total number of hours that can be worked and made rest periods obligatory. In most specialties, including psychiatry, this has meant a move from an on-call system to a shift system. 'Mandatory' attendance is thus harder to implement as trainees are required to rest before and after each shift: the combined effect of the numbers on the rota, compulsory rest days and annual leave means that many trainees are not available to attend teaching sessions. Furthermore, there has been a perceived increase in the intensity of the workloads of psychiatry trainees and consultants (Harrison 2007) that makes it harder for both to carve out time to attend teaching sessions, especially as these can be at a considerable distance from the work base. Finally, the change in attitude towards drug company sponsorship has meant that providing food at any meeting is less common than it was. Linked to these challenges, there has been increased interest in virtual journal clubs, both synchronous and asynchronous, since the early years of this century and this has escalated rapidly since the COVID-19 pandemic.

Twitter and Other Social Media Platforms

With increased internet connectivity and the evolution of social media, Twitter journal clubs started becoming more popular from about 2013 onwards. The general format is where a moderator tweets out a link to an article, encouraging others to read it and publicize it further. At an agreed time, there is a live discussion, with the moderator posting comments and questions to encourage discussion; in turn, others reply, using specific hashtags to distinguish between different conversational threads. Often, Twitter clubs have a subsequent asynchronous element – that is, after the live club, others can continue to read the threads and post comments. Over the subsequent few days, comments posted on Twitter with the relevant hashtag are summarized by the moderator and published (see Fig. 9.1).

In 2015, Roberts carried out a systematic review of Twitter journal clubs, emphasizing their advantages in 'facilitating traditional journal club requirements while also reaching a global audience, and participation of discussion with study authors and colleagues' (Roberts 2015). These benefits still hold true today and some clubs are significantly successful – for example Nephjc is now seven years old and regularly attracts more than 200 active participants contributing over 1,000 tweets (statistics from www.symplur.com). For psychiatrists interested in setting up such a club, Lin and colleagues have written a helpful account of the steps involved (Lin et al. 2015).

However, of the 24 twitter clubs identified by Roberts across a range of specialities (including one in psychiatry – #psychjc), only two were still active in 2021 (Roberts 2015). The lifespan of a Twitter journal club appears to be short and to relate to the enthusiasm of

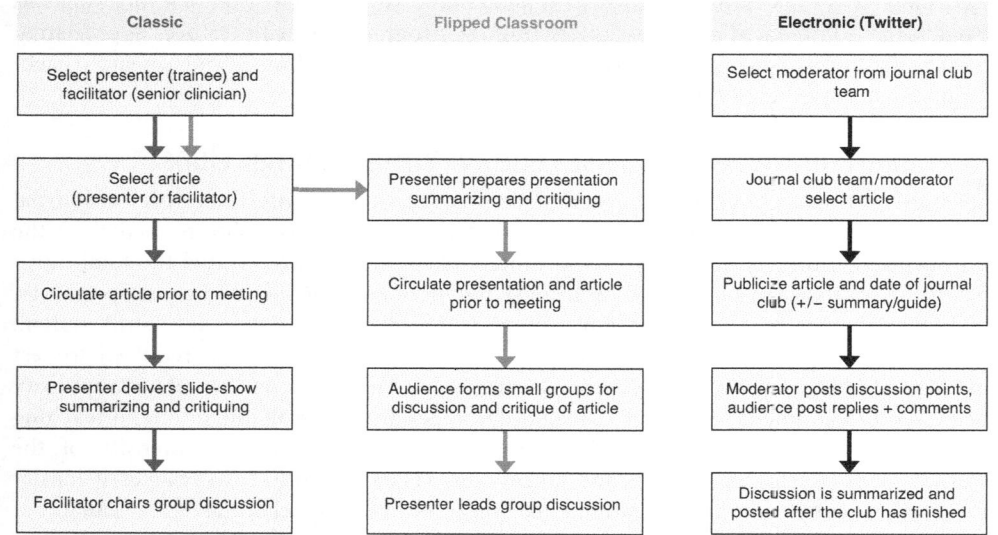

Fig. 9.1 Examples of common journal club formats.

the moderator. The requirements of the Twitter platform in terms of 280 characters, and the challenge in following different threads of discussion, may have limited its popularity.

Other social media platforms such as Facebook, YouTube and wikis have been used for remote journal clubs but also struggle to achieve longevity. It seems that the social aspect of meetings may be an important component of a club's success unless participants are particularly well motivated.

Within psychiatry, we have not identified any current, regularly held, online national or international journal clubs that attract large audiences. Wiki Journal Club summarizes and reviews landmark articles across specialities; the psychiatry area includes important studies such as SADHART but, at the time of writing, there was just one review published in the last three years. The Mental Elf is an independent psychiatry site where individuals post critical appraisals of articles as part of their overall aim of promoting evidence-based psychiatry. The Cochrane Schizophrenia Journal Club produce teaching packs to support journal clubs. See Box 9.4 for details.

Overall, online psychiatry journal clubs seeking to attract audiences beyond a particular teaching programme do not seem to be long lived. However, their archives offer useful resources to facilitators of local clubs with publicly accessible commentaries on a range of papers (Box 9.4).

Journal Clubs During and Beyond COVID-19

Pandemic Restrictions

Following the need for social distancing as part of the COVID-19 pandemic, there was a dramatic pivot to online learning across all areas of medicine: generally, colleagues meeting each other remotely as part of a routine academic programme (Daniel et al.

> **Box 9.4** Resources for journal clubs
>
> **Local Resources**
> - **Seek to engage** academic psychiatrists and other professionals in the journal club: consider clinical psychologists, NHS trust librarians, researchers, local statisticians or look to develop collaboration with an academic journal
>
> **Virtual Resources (free!)**
> - The Mental Elf (www.nationalelfservice.net/mental-health/)
> - The Cochrane Schizophrenia Journal Club (https://schizophrenia.cochrane.org/journal-club)
> - Wiki Journal Club (www.wikijournalclub.org/wiki/Main_Page)
>
> **Useful Books**
> - *The Doctor's Guide to Critical Appraisal* (5th ed., 2020) by Narinder Gosall and Gopal Gosall
>   - The authors run the Superego Café Revision courses, published by PasTest.
> - *Critical Reviews in Psychiatry* (3rd ed., 2005) by Tom M. Brown and Greg Wilkinson
>   - Published by the Royal College of Psychiatrists under the Gaskell imprint (now RCPsych Publications)
> - *50 Studies Every Psychiatrist Should Know* (2018) edited by Ish P. Bhalla, Rajesh R. Tampi and Vinod H. Srihari
>   - Part of Michael E. Hochman's Series, *50 Studies Every Doctor Should Know*, published by Oxford University Press
> - *Get Through: MRCPsych Paper B: Mock Examination Papers* (2016) by Melvyn W. B. Zhang et al.
>   - Useful selection of questions used to build below list of high-yield topics, published by CRC Press (Taylor & Francis Group)

2021). A flurry of publications described these changes to online learning: there were not any papers specifically examining journal clubs but, anecdotally, these underwent the same changes. Nearly all of the papers published described teaching sessions that were exclusively or partially synchronous – that is, where participants gathered in real time, thus offering the possibility of interacting with colleagues. To date, most of the evaluations of these changes in medical education have described the reaction of trainees and educators rather than evaluating the learning or whether it influenced practice.

Although concerns about isolation during the pandemic have been widely acknowledged, online clubs are not always experienced as meeting the need for interaction. Facilitators in St Georges Hospital in London (Mark et al. 2020) noted that, in their journal club, participants often turn off their screen cameras: although numbers attending appear high, it is a challenge to encourage participation.

Beyond COVID-19

As restrictions are eased, a consensus is emerging that much routine teaching will continue to include a significant online element and therefore facilitators will need to pay particular attention to learner engagement (Gordon et al. 2020). Mechanisms encouraging discussion and interaction include the use of breakout rooms, chat features, electronic hand-raising, virtual whiteboards and live online polling using tools such as Mentimeter. Another novel approach has been the use of online games such as Kahoot, which allow educationalists to create quizzes, surveys, jumbles and discussions.

Faced with audiences who feel 'Zoomed out' it is also worth thinking about more general strategies to improve engagement. The single most important aspect is the ability to create a welcoming, safe space where 'learning is social, collaborative, and not hampered by hierarchical boundaries' (McGlacken-Byrne et al. 2020: p. 240).

The 'flipped classroom' format is a concept intended to increase participation, which has been borrowed from general educational theory. In a flipped classroom, the focus changes from the person presenting the paper to the whole audience (see Fig. 9.1). An example would be a reverse critical appraisal journal club, where a clinical question is posed and the audience is asked to design a study that would best answer it (Stallings et al. 2011). The ensuing discussion then informs the subsequent critical appraisal of the chosen article. This approach helps the audience recognize the challenges faced by the researchers; however, it is more demanding of the facilitator's abilities in critical appraisal and this is the kind of format where the participation of local academics and researchers would be helpful for facilitators (Box 9.3). Stallings' club was held face to face but it should work equally well online, ideally using breakout rooms to encourage participation.

Franquet and colleagues describe another model of a flipped classroom where trainees are given an article and asked to create multiple-choice, exam-style questions (Franquet et al. 2016). A quiz generated from the questions acts to consolidate the learning, and participants learn from seeing how their question is understood or misinterpreted by colleagues. Moreover, this approach results in a bank of questions which can be used in the future.

A simpler version is to ask the audience to answer the kinds of statistical questions often posed in critical review exams (Swift et al. 2001). The nominated presenter reads the paper in advance and decides on a list of questions similar to those asked in an exam. At the meeting, those attending are divided into small groups, given the paper to read and allocated several questions. Each group has 20 minutes to decide on answers to the questions, and they then present their conclusions to the large group. Such an approach needs planning over an academic year to ensure key areas of the critical review syllabus are covered (Table 9.2).

Currently, many training schemes are planning to offer a mixed approach where local trainees can come in person and those working further away can log in remotely. Supporting facilitators to develop the necessary expertise is essential: this includes building on skills in EBM and critical appraisal (given that many of the approaches to improve engagement require more in-depth knowledge of EBM than traditional clubs), developing confidence in online teaching and support from medical education administrative staff (see Box 9.3).

In terms of EBM and critical appraisal expertise, Daniel et al. (2021) emphasized the impressive strides in collaboration that the pandemic has fostered, and it may be possible for journal clubs to seek external expertise through links with journals or academic institutes. An example of this was the collaboration between the *British Journal of Psychiatry* and Manchester medical students to launch live virtual clubs (Nabavi and Geers 2020). Several authors have also commented on how academic institutes can provide a cost-effective way of

Table 9.2 Common topics and 'high-yield' areas in MRCPsych Paper B critical appraisal questions (topics in bold are considered highest yield)

Be able to calculate:
- **Absolute/relative risk**
- **Prevalence/incidence**
- **Sensitivity/specificity**
- Odds ratio
- Number needed to treat

Be able to interpret:
- **Confidence interval**
- **P-value and alpha**
- Correlation coefficient
- Standard deviation
- Standard error of the mean
- Validity
  (face, internal, criterion, predictive, concurrent, construct, convergent, divergent, incremental)
- Reliability
- Hazard ratio
- Power

Be able to interpret:
- Forest plot
- Box and Whisker plot
- Kaplein–Meier curve

Know the applicability of:
- **Significance tests**
  (paired/unpaired t-tests, Chi-squared test, Fischer's exact test, ANOVA, Kruskall–Wallis test, Mann–Whitney U-test, McNemar's test, Wilcoxon signed-rank, Z-test, sign test,)
- **Correlation tests**
  (**Spearman**, Pearson, Kendall, Kappa)
- Regression analysis
  (linear, logistic, meta, Cox)

Be able to identify and define:
- **Types of study**
  (cohort, case–control, randomized controlled trials, meta-analysis, observational, qualitative, crossover, cross-sectional, blinded, open label, cost analysis, etc.) including level of research evidence hierarchy
- **Types of bias**
  (observer, recall, selection, Berkson, Neyman, volunteer, misclassification, etc.)
- **Hypothesis testing**
  (type one error, type two error)
- Sample size
- Confounders
- Types of sampling
  (cluster, convenience, quota, snowball, systematic, random, stratified, judgement, etc.)
- Types of randomization
  (simple, block, stratified, covariate, cluster, etc.)
- Types of data
  (continuous, interval, nominal, ordinal, ratio, parametric, etc.)
- Intention to treat

building research capacity by collaborating with local groups and individuals (Western Cape HPSR Journal Club Team 2020; Thakurdesai et al. 2018).

With regards to online teaching, many senior staff continue to feel nervous about presenting or chairing online, especially where this involves newer technology such as online voting or use of breakout rooms. Daniel et al. (2021) remarked that there seems to have been little attention paid so far to the learning needs of faculty in acquiring these new skills and this may be worth considering. In the meantime, support from an administrator familiar with the online platform can be very helpful; where teaching is a weekly event, this has become a significant element in medical education staff's job plans.

Whether synchronous or asynchronous, local or global, the key to longevity and active engagement in journal clubs seems to be their ability to enable a sense of connectedness among participants. McGlacken-Byrne et al. (2020: p. 237) remind us to 'Foster a safe learning environment, in which all participants can articulate areas of uncertainty, ask "low level" questions, and share personal perspectives without fear of ridicule or censure.'

Effectiveness of Journal Clubs

In assessing the effectiveness of journal clubs, the main outcomes that have been considered relate to: skills and knowledge of critical appraisal specifically or EBM more generally; impact on clinicians' behaviour; effect on the care offered to patients; and impact on patient outcomes. Systematic reviews of critical appraisal teaching point to a reasonably consistent picture (Ebbert et al. 2001; Coomarasamy and Khan 2004; Honey and Baker 2011; Horsley et al. 2011). The number of high-quality studies is limited, but it seems likely that teaching critical appraisal is associated with a small but demonstrable improvement in critical appraisal knowledge and skills. It is not clear that there is any change in attitudes (e.g., about the need to conduct literature searches) or in behaviour. There are no convincing studies looking at the impact of teaching critical appraisal on patient outcomes.

Setting Up or Revitalizing a Journal Club

A decade ago, Horsley et al. (2011) called for a high-quality, multi-centre, randomized controlled trial on the teaching of critical appraisal and journal clubs. In the intervening years, no such research has been carried out and this reflects the difficulties in studying the effect of education on patient outcomes. COVID-19 has brought further challenges in understanding how the change to online learning will impact on outcomes. In the meantime, tutors and others responsible for organizing and delivering journal clubs need to take heart from the evidence that these clubs do improve knowledge and skills in critical appraisal.

When setting up or revitalizing a psychiatry journal club (see Table 9.2), consider carefully the aims and intended audience; in particular, decide whether the primary aim is acquiring critical appraisal skills or shaping clinical practice. As Gottlieb et al. (2018) point out, these aspects are not mutually exclusive but one often predominates.

Where the primary focus is on acquiring critical appraisal skills and passing relevant exams, pay particular attention to the syllabus. Consider how the club can support trainees in preparing for their exams and explore the possibility of involving a statistician. If colleagues locally do not feel confident in critical appraisal, try approaching external experts, a local or national academic department, a journal and/or use previously published appraisals, such as are found on the Cochrane Schizophrenia Journal Club (Table 9.1 and Box 9.3).

Where the primary aim is the impact on clinical practice, hold longer sessions or run the club over cycles of several weeks, so that formulating a question from a clinical dilemma, searching the literature, appraising the chosen paper and thinking about its applicability can all be given time. Help with search strategies should be sought from a librarian wherever possible.

Consider also the social role. Clubs that address social needs of participants are more likely to be well attended and persist for longer. Skilled facilitators who provide continuity and create a welcoming, stimulating learning environment are an important component in a successful club. Fully online clubs are less likely to persist and clubs that have a synchronous element find it easier to promote social interaction. Facilitators now need skills in engaging remote participants. Often this will involve input from technically adept colleagues but it is also worth thinking about how to support faculty in acquiring skills in online education.

Trainees value opportunities to meet with more experienced colleagues, so the club needs to attract senior staff: think about how to enhance the attractiveness of the club for them.

Online learning brings challenges but, as ever, also opportunities. Adopting a willingness to experiment and embracing the playful aspects of technology may reinvigorate journal clubs and shape the next generation of psychiatrists in their use of EBM.

References

Alguire PC (1998) A review of journal clubs in postgraduate medical education. *Journal of General Internal Medicine*, 13: 347–53.

Cave MT, Clandinn DJ (2007) Revisiting the journal club. *Medical Teacher*, 29: 365–70.

Coomarasamy A, Khan KS (2004) What is the evidence that postgraduate teaching in evidence-based medicine changes anything? *BMJ*, 329: 1017.

Daniel M, Gordon M, Patricio M, et al. (2021) An update on developments in medical education in response to the COVID-19 pandemic: a BEME scoping review: BEME Guide No. 64. *Medical Teacher*, 43: 253–71.

Deenadaylalan Y, Grimmer-Somers K, Prior M, et al. (2008) How to run an effective journal club: a systematic review. *Journal of Evaluation in Clinical Practice*, 14: 898–911.

Ebbert JO, Montori VM, Schultz HJ (2001) The journal club in postgraduate medical education: a systematic review. *Medical Teacher*, 23: 455–61.

Franquet E, Parker J, Donohoe K (2016) Question-writing journal-club is an alternative learning method for the residents. *Journal of Nuclear Medicine*, 57(supplement 2), 1252.

Gilbody S (1996) Evidence-based medicine: an improved format for journal clubs. *Psychiatric Bulletin*, 20: 673–5.

Glasziou P (2007) Jottings. *BMJ Evidence Based Medicine*, 12: 66.

Gordon M, Patricio M, Horne L et al. (2020) Developments in medical education in response to the COVID-19 pandemic: a rapid BEME systematic review: BEME Guide No. 63. *Medical Teacher*, 42: 1202–15.

Gottlieb M, King A, Byyny R, et al. (2018) journal club in residency education: an evidence-based guide to best practices from the

Council of Emergency Medicine Residency Directors. *Western Journal of Emergency Medicine: Integrating Emergency Care with Population Health*, 19: 746–55.

Groopman J (2005) *The Anatomy of Hope: How People Prevail in the Face of Illness*. Random House Trade Paperbacks.

Harrison J (2007) The work patterns of consultant psychiatrists. Revisiting . . . How consultants manage their time. *Advances in Psychiatric Treatment*, 13: 470–5.

Heilligman PM, Wollitze, OW (1987) A survey of journal clubs in US family practice residencies. *Journal of Medical Education*, 62: 928–31.

Honey PH, Baker, JA (2011) Exploring the impact of journal clubs: a systematic review. *Nurse Education Today*, 31: 825–31.

Horsley T, Hyde C, Santesso N, et al. (2011) Teaching critical appraisal skills in healthcare settings. *Cochrane Database of Systematic Reviews*, 11: CD001270.

Lin M, Sherbino J (2015). Creating a virtual journal club: a community of practice using multiple social media strategies. *Journal of Graduate Medical Education*, 7: 481–2.

Linzer M (1987) The journal club and medical education: over one hundred years of unrecorded history. *Postgraduate Medical Education*, 63: 475–8.

Mark I, Sonbol M, Abbasian C (2020) Running a journal club in 2020: reflections and challenges. *BJPsych Bulletin*, 25: 1–4.

McGlacken-Byrne SM, O'Rahelly M, Cantillon P, et al. (2020) Journal club: old tricks and fresh approaches. *Archives of Disease in Childhood: Education and Practice*, 105: 236–41.

Nabavi N, Geers, BDW (2020) Re: Covid-19: the medical students responding to the pandemic. *BMJ*, 369: m2160.

Nikolaou V (2016). Statistical analysis: A practical guide for psychiatrists. *BJPsych Advances*, **22**: 251–9.

Roberts MJ, Perera M, Lawrentschuk N, et al. (2015) Globalization of continuing professional development by journal clubs via microblogging: a systematic review. *Journal of Medical Internet Research* **17**: e103.

Rosenberg W, Donald A (1995) Evidence-based medicine: an approach to clinical problem solving. *BMJ*, **310**: 1122–6.

Royal College of Psychiatrists (2011) MRCPsych Paper B critical review – evidence-based practice syllabic content. Available at: www.rcpsych.ac.uk/docs/default-source/training/examinations/exams-paper-b-critical-review-syllabus-may2011.pdf?sfvrsn=8d07f1a5_2.

Royal College of Psychiatrists (2015) Continuing professional development: guidance for psychiatrists. OP98: Occasional Paper 98. Available at: www.rcpsych.ac.uk/docs/default-source/members/cpd/members-cpd-op98.pdf?sfvrsn=1de40c5f_4.

Royal College of Psychiatrists (2021) Eligibility criteria and regulations for MRCPsych written papers and Clinical Assessment of Skills and Competencies (CASC). Available at: www.rcpsych.ac.uk/docs/default-source/training/examinations/exams-eligibility-criteria-and-regulations—january-2022.pdf?sfvrsn=83f28e63_44.

Sackett DL (1997) Seminars in perinatology. *Evidence-Based Medicine*, **21**: 3–4.

Stallings A, Borja-Hart N, Fass J (2011) Strategies for reinventing journal club. *American Journal of Health-System Pharmacy*, **68**: 14–16.

Swift G, Crotty F, Moran M, et al. (2001) Inviting a statistician to join an evidence-based journal club. *Psychiatric Bulletin*, **25**: 397–9.

Taylor R, Warner J (2000) National survey of training needs for evidence-based practices. *Psychiatric Bulletin*, **24**: 272–3.

Thakurdesai A, Ghosh A, Menon V, et al. (2018) Electronic journal clubs for capacity building: a case study in psychiatry as a model for medical disciplines in developing countries. *Asian Journal of Psychiatry*, **34**: 93–7.

Warner JP, King M (1997) Evidence-based medicine and the journal club: a cross-sectional survey of participants' views. *Psychiatric Bulletin*, **21**: 532–4.

Western Cape HPSR Journal Club Team (2020) "Not just a journal club – it's where the magic happens': knowledge mobilization through co-production for health system development in the Western Cape Province, South Africa. *International Journal of Health Policy and Management*; doi: https://dx.doi.org/10.34172/ijhpm.2020.128.

Yager J, Linn LS, Winstead DK, et al. (1991) Characteristics of journal clubs in psychiatric training. *Academic Psychiatry*, **15**: 18–32.

Chapter

10

Workshops: An Important Element in Medical Education

Allys Guérandel, Brían Ó Ruairc
and Hiberet Tessema Belay

Introduction

Medical conferences such as those held by the American Psychiatric Association, the Royal College of Psychiatrists, the College of Psychiatrists of Ireland and many other international medical academic bodies include workshops in their programmes. They are also included in the academic teaching programmes aimed at undergraduates, postgraduates and continued professional development. Teaching methods such as workshops, which actively require the learner to participate, are widely accepted to achieve a deeper level of learning. Educational research recognizes student engagement as valuable and as having a significant impact on their learning (Mandernach 2015). However, it is only when workshops are correctly planned and appropriately used that these interactive learning environments foster sound pedagogic principles and result in effective learning. Guidelines for conducting workshops are available and guidelines specific to psychiatry can also be found (Tiberius and Silver 2001), but for workshops to be effective it is important to understand the concepts of adult learning, the learning targets and the principles and process of delivering a workshop.

What is a workshop? Although both sound pedagogic principles and available evidence support the use of interactive teaching and learning approaches, the format is often variable and the terms small-group teaching, tutorial, seminar, group discussion, problem-based-learning group and workshop are used indiscriminately. In common, such formats imply the engagement of students interacting among themselves and with the teacher and, regardless of the format taken, sessions most often take place in small groups or, if in a large group, the group is divided into smaller subgroups. In tutorials, students are set a task; in seminars, students research a topic and make a presentation for group discussion of its content (Jaques 2000); and in problem-based learning, students follow a specific process to discuss appropriate problems in a group, to increase knowledge and understanding (Wood 2003). In workshops, however, students are encouraged to engage in active experiential learning using planned learning activities focused on the desired learning outcome.

The term workshop has various definitions when applied to learning, and we have chosen one that sits closely to the broadly accepted concept of work- shops in education (Brooks-Harris and Stock-Ward 1999: p. 6):

> A workshop is a short-term learning experience that encourages active, experiential learning and uses a variety of learning activities to meet the needs of diverse learners.

How Do Adults Learn?

Principles from Knowles's work in adult learning inform us that, to be most successful, learning must be interactive; the material presented must be practical, contextual and applicable (Knowles 2012). Presenting learning materials in chunks of approximately 20 minutes is in keeping with the belief that learners have a limited attention span. Some new evidence has emerged that the length of the attention span may perhaps vary and relates to how motivated and engaged students are (Bunce 2010).

This, however, does not take away from presenting materials in relevant chunks to facilitate engagement and encourage active learning. These principles are likely to influence the overall design of the workshops (Knowles 2012). Workshops should therefore be designed to be varied and broken up into activities lasting approximately 20 minutes at a time to optimize learning (Bowen 1998).

To utilize experiential learning theories, teaching methodologies that encourage and support learner engagement and foster interaction are required. Engagement is positively related to a host of desired outcomes, including high grades, student satisfaction and persistence in learning. For this reason, such activities as student–faculty interaction, peer-to-peer collaboration and active learning are thought to be important in both face-to-face and online learning environments (Chen et al. 2011). This involves didactic approaches such as replacing a speaker lecturing to passive learners with discussions, role play and other such interactive teaching and learning methods.

The evidence for the benefit of interactive teaching and learning styles is found not only in learning theories such as the ones described above but also in research. The literature on medical education informs us that teaching methods that require the learner to participate actively achieve a deeper level of learning. A Cochrane systematic review comparing conferences, lectures, workshops, seminars, symposia and courses on their effectiveness in medical education showed that interactive teaching methods are more effective than didactic lecture-based teaching (Forsetlund 2009). The review also recommends that every effort be made to incorporate interactive learning into standard didactic lessons.

Changes in Medical Education

As mentioned, in recent years our evidence-based understanding of adult learning has informed new practices in medical education. This has led to a move towards a learner-centred approach. Alongside these advances in education, the boom in social media and, more importantly, the emergence of the current internet-savvy medical students and trainees have also led to changes in the practices of medical education. Lectures can be podcasted, clips of medical procedures can be viewed on video-sharing websites such as YouTube, and virtual patients can be assessed and managed online, all at the convenience of the learner.

There is a call for medical educators to incorporate technology and innovation in medical education (Mehta et al. 2013). In problem-based learning, an emphasis is given to active learning with constructive facilitation. Similarly, the flipped classroom model urges educators to 'flip' the traditional classroom into an interactive learning environment and advocates the use of online portals to support learning (Tucker 2012). The flipped classroom entails the giving of materials to students ahead of the allocated classroom time. Such materials can include recorded videos or lecture notes on a topic. After students engage with the content they are then brought in for small-group tutorials or online webinars where they can discuss applying the knowledge they have acquired to clinical situations or review any difficulties they had with the content.

The new paradigm in medical education calls on medical educators to 'just imagine' medical education's renaissance through a massive central collaborative online learning environment and redirecting of valuable faculty time to interactive activities such as workshops for discussion and problem solving, rather than traditional didactic lectures (Mehta et al. 2013). While embracing technology and incorporating it as a virtual learning support environment, educators urge the use of the 'freed' face-to-face time for more interaction and student engagement (Tucker 2012). In recent times, incorporating technology into teaching delivery has accelerated. The potential for face-to-face teaching opportunities have reduced in frequency and length, and resources to promote interactivity and student engagement in online activity has developed in parallel and may even have become more prevalent. Online teaching delivery, however, brings its own issues. For example, online delivery lacks a humane dimension that can potentiate social isolation (Liu et al. 2016) and this needs to be addressed when planning to use online teaching delivery.

Why Choose Workshops?

Workshops with well-defined learning outcomes, utilizing principles of experiential learning fit well with current trends in medical education, aligning with interactive teaching principles. They can be a powerful and effective medium for teaching and potentiating a deeper level of learning. With appropriate pre-planning and design they are a time-efficient way of meeting desired learning outcomes. They are great for brainstorming and building relationships by providing learners with invaluable structured face-to-face contact. They can be delivered in a consistent fashion by different facilitators at a single teaching site or at multi-site teaching centres. They can help remove any ambiguity about individual tutors' approaches to the use of face-to-face time and cater to different facilitation styles. Properly designed, they are a cost-efficient method of producing active involvement of learners compared with individual training activities (Tiberius and Silver 2001).

Workshops can be used to deliver teaching for a variety of educational topics and set-ups. They can be used in undergraduate, postgraduate and continuing medical education, as well as at various professional or personal development forums. They are often designed for people working together or in the same field.

Workshops have the added advantage that they can be delivered online via facilities such as virtual classrooms or other independent online meeting providers. These resources have a built-in facility to create smaller breakout groups and provide interactivity via raising hands, instant messaging. etc., which resembles what happens in a in-person workshops, while at the same time incorporating interfaces that the current generation of students are comfortable and familiar with. Often, students are slow to turn their camera or microphone on; however, if moved into smaller breakout groups they are more likely to do so and this leads to an increase in discussion, participation and practise of a skill. Organizing the teaching delivery and including such breakout moments foster interactive small-group tasks. Multiple-choice questions (MCQs) or online polls are often available in the virtual classroom, and planning their use judiciously during teaching delivery can also be used to engage students or to identify learning points that need further clarification.

It is well established that online learning can lead to a sense of isolation but by using these functions and fostering student-to-tutor or student-to-student interaction online that burden can be reduced. The importance of having a sense of belonging is very important and can be addressed by developing a sense of collegiality (Eachampati and Ramnarayan 2020; Fawns et al. 2020). Peer social support can be facilitated by making the virtual classroom available to students to meet each other outside of teaching times for discussion. Equally, having access to a tutor as a personal point of contact is another way to facilitate online collegiality.

What guides one in choosing when to use workshops lies in what one hopes to emphasize for the educational meeting, for example problem solving, skill building, increasing knowledge, systemic change or personal awareness/self-improvement (Brooks-Harris and Stock-Ward 1999). Workshops that problem-solve facilitate systemic change and increased personal awareness/self-improvement; they are therefore favoured in forums providing for continuing medical education or the workplace.

Example of a Workshop in Practice

University College Dublin's medical school currently has approximately 250 students in their final year of medical training. The psychiatry module is delivered over six weeks, four times, in the final year, with a group of about 60 at a time. Face-to-face teaching time is being reconfigured from didactic lectures to interactive workshops. To date, the following topics are delivered as workshops: psychopathology; the Mental Health Act; eating disorders; psychopharmacology; liaison psychiatry and medically unexplained symptoms; alcohol use and misuse; psychotic disorders; and mood disorders. The workshops fit well with the other interactive teaching deliveries used in the module. Outcomes for the workshops are aligned to the overall module learning outcomes and to the assessment methods, which include a continuous clinical assessment, an MCQ paper, a reflective essay and an objective structured clinical examination (OSCE). We will draw from this example to go through the three main stages involved in developing a workshop, which we think are essential to achieving an effective teaching and learning experience.

Stage 1: Pre-planning

Regardless of the topic or the emphasis of the workshop, adequate pre-planning is mandatory. When designing a workshop, one should be clear as to its objectives and structure learning activities in line with these. It is sometimes necessary to do a needs assessment for learners before deciding on objectives. In the pre-planning stage consideration should be given to who the participants/learners of the workshop will be, their current level of understanding of the topic and the needs the workshop is aiming to meet. In our workshops this understanding is clearly identified well in advance, as well as the venues and times allocated.

Access to technologies such as laptops, tablets and projectors is ensured, where available. Students and tutors have access to the university portal system, Blackboard; this is used extensively throughout module delivery.

It is important to be aware that workshops in medical schools need to be short, generally one to two hours, as face-to-face teaching time is limited. In our module, most workshops are one-hour long, but for more complex topics, such as psychopharmacology, modules lasting two hours are often required. Remember that the execution of an exercise in a workshop often takes longer than anticipated during pre-planning, therefore it is wise to allow additional time (Tiberius and Silver 2001).

Box 10.1 Key elements of workshop pre-planning

Learning objectives
Clearly define the learning objectives

Time allocation
Fix the duration: usually limited to one–two hours in medical schools; allow enough time for each activity
Content should be divided in to chunks of activity

Venue
Ensure the room is big enough
Ensure access to the technology needed for both educators and students (e.g., the internet, a projector) if being used

Resources
Facilitator/tutor
Training of the facilitator
Comfort of the facilitator with relevant technology

In our workshops, the ratio of tutor to students is about 1:30, but the students are divided into small groups of three or four to perform tasks/activities.

Box 10.1 sums up the key elements of workshop pre-planning.

Stage 2: Planning and Workshop Structure

Every workshop should have an introduction, interactive learning activities and a conclusion. In planning our workshops, the focus was on ensuring that the learning objectives of the session were clearly identified in advance and were also obvious for the tutors to understand. It is crucial when planning learning activities that these are matched to set objectives. Care should be taken that the workshop does not drift away from these objectives and remains cohesive as it navigates through the learning activities and comes to a planned conclusion. Although the style of delivery is often informal and fosters discussion it is important that workshops are well structured. While recent circumstances have accelerated the need for the use of online teaching it is very important to keep to good principles of medical education and the knowledge that integration of online education should be done in a planned manner (Kern et al. 1998).

Access to technology is variable and due consideration should be given both to the resources available to teachers but more importantly what resources students have access to without imposing a financial burden on them. It is also important to note that difficulties can arise due to poor access to the Internet in some places, and this can be a barrier to the use of technology in education.

The introduction should give a concise objective of the workshop and clearly state the expected learning outcomes. A brief outline of the structure of the workshop to follow should then given. Visual means such as PowerPoint presentations or digital photography can be used creatively to illustrate the introduction. In our course, clear introductions set up the student to understand exactly what is expected from the workshop.

The crux of the workshop falls in the middle section, where learning activities take place. We designed workshops using Kolb's experiential learning theory, and we chose learning activities to meet the four phases of the learning cycle: concrete experiences, reflective observation, abstract conceptualization and active experimentation (Kolb and Kolb 2005).

For the chosen activities to be effective they must be relevant and presentation of the material should be varied and engaging. It is important to encourage learners to relate the workshop content to their reality. Enough time to discuss and reflect on the activities is built in.

Allowing time to conclude the workshop is also very important. Facilitators usually bring a workshop to an end by allowing time for summing up, drawing conclusions, and reviewing outcomes and feedback.

Getting the plan right is crucial to a successful workshop. The sequence and timing of the activities and discussions must match the allocated time, resources and budget. The more detailed the plan, the more effective the workshop will be.

Box 10.2 sums up the key elements of workshop planning and structure.

The workshops in the psychiatry module have been designed to emphasize the development of clinical skills and to increase knowledge. In a skill-building workshop, the content focus is on students practising a specific set of clinical skills; for example, eliciting psychotic symptoms or using the Alcohol Use Disorders Identification Test (AUDIT).

Each workshop is carefully planned to have an introduction. Learning activities are listed and timed. Each activity allows time for reflection and there is time at the end of the

---

Box 10.2 Key elements of workshop planning and structure

Introduction
Set out the plan/structure
State the learning objectives: tell the students what they should learn from the workshop
Tell them how they will learn it

Learning activities
Focus on Kolb's four stages
Make appropriate use of technology available
Check the experience of the tutor

Conclusion
Focus on repeating the learning objectives
Ensure understanding of all participating students

Feedback
Prepare a questionnaire for students and tutors to assess the workshop

workshop for summing up. For our module, a manual has been produced detailing the plan, content and activities of all the workshops delivered. This ensures standardization of delivery across teaching and also facilitates the training of tutors, who change every one or two years.

The content of one of the workshops in the module is detailed below.

Workshop on Alcohol Use and Misuse

The content of this workshop, which teaches students about alcohol use and misuse, was developed to follow Kolb's experiential learning theory, with each of its four phases targeted by specific teaching activities.

Reflecting on experience. Students are asked to discuss the topic in subgroups and write down harmful consequences of the misuse of alcohol in various areas, as well as completing a quiz.

Assimilating and conceptualization. Students' responses are gathered by the facilitator and listed on a flip chart for visual effect. PowerPoint slides on adverse effects of alcohol are shown. A video illustrating harmful use of alcohol is shown for purpose of assimilation and conceptualization.

These steps allow the learners to reflect and review their knowledge, correcting inconsistencies in their previous understanding of the topic, leading to abstract conceptualization. The next steps facilitate full understanding.

Experimenting and practising. Students are shown a visual image on PowerPoint and are asked to calculate the number of units of alcohol displayed on the slide. They are asked to use the AUDIT tool in pairs and practise screening patients for alcohol misuse.

Planning for application. Students are asked to write down what they will do when next seeing a patient with suspected alcohol misuse.

Completion of these four phases is viewed as being significant for effective learning to occur.

In our example we used Kolb's experiential learning theory which has been widely influential in adult learning theory but is not without criticism. As we move towards more online teaching delivery the principles of the ARCS model of motivational design may also be considered (Keller 2010). This design promotes learner-centred teaching. It aims to help develop learning experiences to create and sustain student motivation in learning new content. This model prioritizes four key factors for the learning environment: attention, relevance, confidence and satisfaction. For example, to capture the students' attention, content is presented in short texts, using images and short clear messages, which is the format that students are familiar with in this age of digital communication. Tutors discussing their lived experience of clinical cases that they encounter at work bring relevance, potentiating the clinical context. Providing feedback and support on the completion of tasks are ways of helping the students build confidence. Satisfaction can be fostered by marking the completion of a workshop, this can be done using MCQs or by giving digital badges that can be uploaded to a personal portfolio for a module.

Stage 3: Delivery

Facilitators are obviously crucial to a workshop. For our course, we use a mix of experienced tutors as well as younger doctors to deliver the material. They do not have to be subject experts: it is more important that they are enthusiastic, able to engage learners and start

Box 10.3 Potential workshop learning activities

Video clips

Quizzes

Flip charts

Role-play exercises

Skills practice

Online discussion group

Online whiteboards

discussions, and have core knowledge of the topic of the workshop. They need to make the group of learners feel comfortable and use humour and ice-breakers appropriately. Facilitators need to bring the learners to the forefront of the learning experience and support them in being active participants in completing their individual cycle of learning. This is a shift in the role of educators from teacher to facilitator (Brooks-Harris and Stock-Ward 1999). There is a vast array of software and interactive platforms that can be used to support the planning and delivery of workshops. They range from Blackboard and Brightspace to Socrative and Mentimeter. As seen in Box 10.3, videos, quizzes and online forums are just some of the numerous technologies that can be used to support the interactivity of a workshop. With all these options available it is best not to give into techno-centrism, but rather to take into consideration the technological capability of both the learners and the facilitators and then choose the appropriate technology to support the learning tasks.

Stage 4: Feedback

Evaluation is the last step. Often, the summing up of the workshop allows for informal discussion on feedback. This is essential to ensure the quality of further delivery of the workshop, but also for the facilitators and their own professional development as educators. At the end of each running of our course, feedback is collected informally by facilitators, and also formally from all stakeholders, including students, facilitators and academic staff, via a questionnaire.

Students taking the psychiatry module were asked to rate the relevance of the workshops to the topic using a five-point Likert scale (0, strongly disagree; 5, strongly agree). The responses of 246 students are shown in graph form in Fig. 10.1. It is clear that a majority of the students surveyed agreed that the workshops were relevant to the teaching of the topics covered.

The students were also asked to compare and rate lectures, workshops and small-group case-based discussions in terms of how they best aided their learning of various topics. These are the three teaching methods used in set face-to-face time. From the results (Fig. 10.2) it is clear that students prefer to learn in interactive settings rather than the more traditional lecture settings. Students were also given an opportunity to write their own individual feedback on the workshops, which also provided some interesting comments (Fig. 10.3).

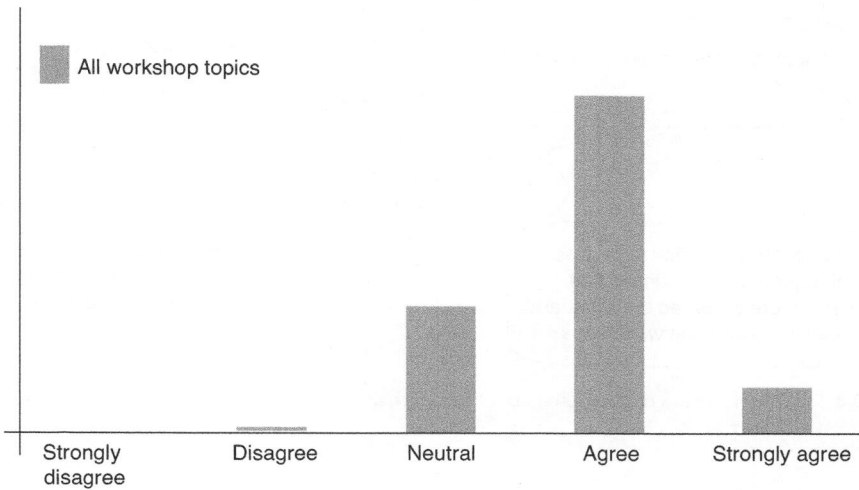

Fig. 10.1 Students' ratings of the relevance of the workshops to the topic covered in the psychiatry module at University College Dublin's medical school.

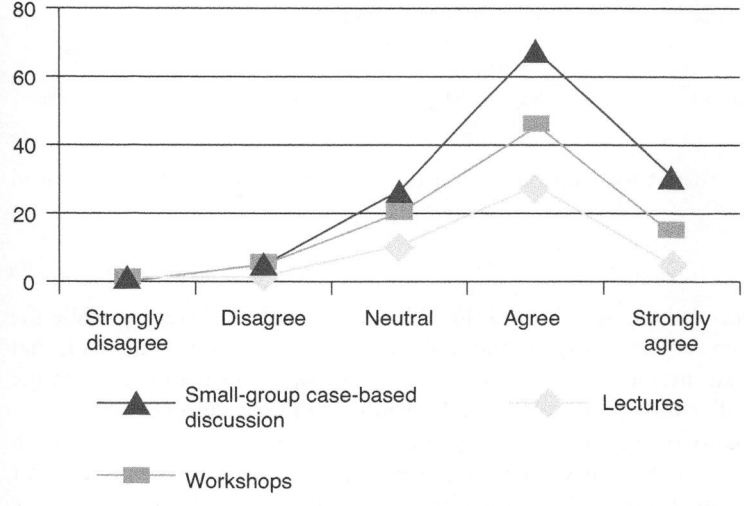

Fig. 10.2 Students' ratings of whether small-group case-based discussion, workshops and lectures were good aids to their learning in the psychiatry module at University College Dublin's medical school.

Workshop facilitators were also surveyed anonymously for their feedback on the use of workshops (Fig. 10.4). All our facilitators had at least a minimum of 6 months' previous teaching experience. Three-quarters reported that they had a clear understanding of the differences between workshops and other small-group teaching methods. All our facilitators unanimously responded that they were comfortable using workshops for teaching. They also responded that using workshops as a teaching method made it easier to facilitate learning in the chosen topic and made teaching sessions interactive. They all also felt that learning objectives were appropriately met through the use of workshops.

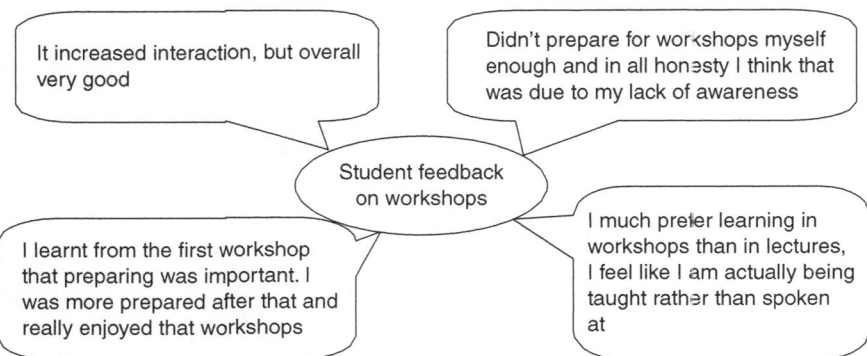

Fig. 10.3 Students' feedback on the workshops of the psychiatry module at University College Dublin's medical school.

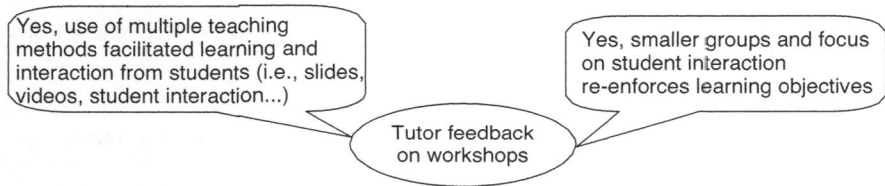

Fig. 10.4 Tutors' feedback on delivering the workshops of the psychiatry module at University College Dublin's medical school.

All tutors also reported that it was fun delivering the workshops and that they enjoyed delivering them.

Conclusion

Most students still expect to be taught in traditional lectures, passively listening while the lecturer speaks on a given subject. However, the feedback from some of our students is that they prefer learning in an interactive setting such as a workshop. They are engaged in the learning process and Kolb's theory on experiential learning is more accurately followed.

Although workshops are recognized in medical education as facilitating a deep approach to learning, and in our example the students reported a preference for workshops over didactic lectures, workshops are not without their limitations. To be effective they need to be well prepared and the principles and steps discussed here must be followed. Tutors have to be trained to be facilitators. Many are used to delivering didactic lectures and it can take time to normalize using workshops instead.

Finally, not all students take to being taught through workshops: indeed, from the feedback received, our students preferred small-group case-based teaching to workshops. However, what is clear is that most students prefer interactive teaching to traditional didactic lectures and sometimes they just need to be given time to adjust to a new dynamic in the teacher–student relationship. Many students straight out of school struggle initially, having always been taught by teachers sitting at the front of a classroom; graduate-entry students adapt more quickly as they have usually come across workshops before.

When participating in a workshop, either as a facilitator or as a learner, one should anticipate the interactivity and learner-centred approach taken in their delivery. Facilitators have to see their role as enabling learners to engage with the taught material and with each other in a positive way. Equally, learners will maximize the benefit of attending a workshop by preparing appropriately for it and then engaging with the activities and each other.

References

Bowen JL (1998) Models that work: the nuts and bolts of faculty development for general internal medicine, family medicine and general paediatrics. Ambulatory Paediatric Association. Available at: www.ambpeds.org/education/nutsandbolts/pdfs/modelsthatwork.pdf.

Brooks-Harris JE, Stock-Ward SR (1999) *Workshops: Designing and Facilitating Experiential Learning*. SAGE Publications.

Bunce D, Flens E, Neiles K (2010) How long can students pay attention in class? A study of student attention using clickers. *Journal of Chemical Education*, **87**: 1438–43.

Chen PD, Gonyea R, Kuh G (2011). Learning at a distance: engaged or not? Innovate, 4; doi: https://nsuworks.nova.edu/innovate/vol4/iss3/3.

Eachempati O, Ramnarayan K (2020). Ten maxims for out of class learning to outclass the academic challenges of COVID-19. *MedEd Publish*, **9**: 89; doi: 10.15694/mep.2020.000089.1.

Fawns T, Jones D, Aitken G (2020) Challenging assumptions about "moving online" in response to COVID-19, and some practical advice. *MedEdPublish* 9: 83; doi: 10.15694/mep.2020.000083.1.

Forsetlund L, Bjørndal A, Rashidian A, et al. (2009) Continuing education meetings and workshops: effects on professional practice and health care outcomes. *Cochrane Database of Systematic Reviews*, **2**: CD003030; doi: https://doi.org/10.1002/14651858.CD003030.pub2.

Jaques D (2000) *Learning in Groups: A Handbook for Improving Group Work*, 3rd ed. Routledge.

Keller JM (2010) *The ARCS of Motivational Design*. Springer.

Kern D, Thomas P, Howard D, Bass E (1998). *Curriculum Development for Medical Education*. John Hopkins University Press.

Knowles MS, Holton EF, Swanson RA (2012) *The Adult Learner: The Definitive Classic in Adult Education and Human Resource Development*, 6th ed. Butterworth–Heinemann.

Kolb AY, Kolb D (2005) Learning styles and learning spaces: enhancing experiential learning in higher education. *Academy of Management Learning and Education*, **4**: 193–212.

Liu Q, Peng W, Zhang F, et al. (2016) The effectiveness of blended learning in health professions: systematic review and meta-analysis. *Journal of Medical Internet Research*, **18**: e2; doi: 10.2196/jmir.4807.

Mandernach J (2015) Assessment of student engagement in higher education: a synthesis of literature and assessment tools, *International Journal of Learning, Teaching and Educational Research*, **12**: 1–14.

Mehta NB, Hull AL, Young JB, et al. (2013) Just imagine: new paradigms for medical education. *Academic Medicine*, **88**: 1418–23.

Tiberius R, Silver I (2001) *Guidelines for Conducting Workshops and Seminars that Actively Engage Participants*. Department of Psychiatry, University of Toronto.

Tucker B (2012) The flipped classroom online instruction at home frees class time for learning. *Education Next*, **12**: 82–3.

Wood DF (2003) Problem based learning. *BMJ*, **326**: 328.

Delivering a Good Lecture

Brendan D. Kelly

Introduction

The traditional lecture has proven to be a remarkable survivor in the fickle world of medical teaching and learning. The traditional, 50-minute, didactic lecture is continually under attack, with critics arguing that its format is inflexible, audiences lose interest and there is insufficient interaction, if any, in most lectures. But while the lecture certainly violates many of the sacred tenets of contemporary education, it has nonetheless survived and even thrived in a world of incessant educational innovation and countless online teaching initiatives. Why?

Why is the traditional lecture still so popular? How has it survived? And how can we use the enduring appeal of the lecture format to best advantage in modern medical education and postgraduate training?

The past three decades have seen an increasing amount of research address these questions and provide an improved evidence base for teaching methods in the health sciences. It is, perhaps, best to start with some general findings about the value and place of the lecture format, before moving on to specific techniques for planning and delivering good lectures.

Thirty years ago, Butler (1992) reported the results of a study of teaching methods and the lecture format among 126 occupational therapy students in the journal *Medical Teacher*. Butler found that students perceived the traditional didactic lecture as the least effective teaching method, but that involving students actively within the lecture enhanced the format and was regarded as a more effective teaching and learning tool. In other words, the problem with lectures was the idea of one voice dominating for 50 minutes, rather than any problem intrinsic to the lecture format itself. This could be remedied by enhancing learner participation within the lecture, without abandoning the basic lecture format. This simple adjustment improves the educational value of lectures considerably and allows the lecturer to respond to the learning needs of students immediately.

This was, however, just one study, albeit a compelling one. Thirty years later, is there now systematic evidence that the lecture format itself, if used imaginatively, is as good as other teaching formats, such as seminar-based teaching? And in a world with so many teaching formats, does the lecture still hold any special value?

In 2020, Zeng and colleagues (2020) performed a meta-analysis of randomized controlled trials to explore the effects of seminar teaching methods compared to lecture-based learning for medical students. Their analysis included 16 randomized controlled trials with a total sample size of 1,122 medical students. These authors found that seminar teaching methods significantly improved knowledge and skills; that the effects of seminar teaching methods in practice courses were better than in theory courses; and that there appeared to be no difference in teaching basic concepts for students taught by seminars compared to lecture-based teaching.

Consistent with Butler's conclusions, this meta-analysis supports a role for lectures in medical education and training, especially for teaching basic concepts, once there is interaction with students, rather than a single voice dominating the entire lecture. Unsurprisingly, seminar-based teaching appears particularly suited to practice-based learning, which is a central element of medical education and postgraduate training. Clearly, a blend of teaching methods is needed, with lectures forming part of the mix.

Smits and colleagues (2003) reach a similar conclusion in their study of problem-based learning versus lecture-based learning in postgraduate medical education. This group performed a randomized controlled trial, with a mean follow-up of 14 months, involving 118 doctors training as occupational health physicians in the Netherlands. They compared problem-based learning with a traditional lecture-based approach and found that knowledge increased equally in both groups directly after the programs, and decreased equally at follow-up. While performance indicator scores increased in both groups, and significantly more so in the problem-based group, the problem-based group was less satisfied with the course.

Against this background, it is clear that the lecture format still has specific roles within medical education. It is effective and acceptable to students, once it is used correctly and for appropriate purposes. This chapter explores specific ways to optimize the lecture format in order to prepare a good lecture, deliver it well, learn from the experience and so inform future teaching and learning. While the lecture will never be the sole teaching method in any course, it has specific roles to play in medical education and postgraduate training once we use the format correctly and with care.

Preparing the Lecture

The first step in preparing a lecture is to identify objectives or learning outcomes for the teaching session. To do this, it is important to understand your audience, be they undergraduate medical students, postgraduate psychiatry trainees, colleagues, allied health professionals, patients, families, voluntary groups, the general public or any other group. Given the diversity of possible audiences, the lecturer needs to understand both what the audience wants or needs to know and what the lecturer wants or needs to convey. These requirements do not always match up precisely so it is good to be clear which requirements are being met. Ideally, the title of the lecture will help ensure that key objectives are shared between the audience and the lecturer.

There is good evidence that setting out three learning objectives ahead of time both clarifies the lecturer's thoughts and helps students to focus on what matters. Butler (1992), in her study of teaching methods among occupational therapy students, found that setting clear objectives for each lecture well ahead of time helped students to check their notes, prepare for the teaching session and focus revision on key learning points. The fact that these objectives were provided in handout format at the start of the course also meant that they were useful if students missed a lecture, lost their notes or were confused about particular points.

Chapman (2018) recommends clarifying the precise goals of the teaching session when developing educational materials for the lecture. She suggests starting with less complex educational objectives and proceeding to more complex ones. Chapman also points out that more is not necessarily better. It is useful to focus on a small number of clear, achievable learning objectives rather than a large number of poorly defined ones that are difficult to describe let alone achieve within a lecture. It is likely that many students will be distracted, tired or otherwise inattentive, so a small number of clear, direct, comprehensible objectives are best.

Once the objectives of the lecture are clear, decide on the presentation format. There are many possibilities here. You can just talk (with no audio-visual aids), simply have a structured discussion with the students, use a presentation programme (such as Microsoft PowerPoint or Prezi) or develop a blended approach. The key is to decide what you are going to do beforehand and think it through fully. Few people have the ability to command an audience's attention with speech alone for 50 minutes, so most people opt to use some visual aids. If you decide to use slides (e.g., PowerPoint), do not let the slides distract from the key objectives of your lecture. Keep the number of slides small, focus on pictures rather than words, and familiarize yourself with your slides beforehand.

Above all, be sure to avoid the three key errors with PowerPoint (a) having too many slides (while there is no absolute limit, the fewer the better); (b) not knowing your slides, with the result that you simply read your slides aloud (slides are a support, not a script); and (c) having too much information on slides. If you need to say that 'this is a very busy slide', that slide should not be in your presentation. Address this issue before your lecture, rather than apologizing during it.

Despite many years of experience with PowerPoint, many PowerPoint presentations are still too long, too complicated and, as a result, entirely unhelpful. This is a pity. PowerPoint is not the enemy. Most problems with PowerPoint presentations stem not from the programme itself, but from how it is used by presenters.

Harden (2008) argues that, all too often, PowerPoint leads to the elevation of form over content, as bullet points, animation and other features of the programme are used in a way that distracts students from the key points of the lecture, rather than underlining them. It is not enough simply to repeat the information on the slides or to show words and graphs, there also needs to be discussion around important points, added information and inter action with students in order to bring learning to life.

Harden (2008) recommends that, when planning a lecture, we forget about PowerPoint to begin with and focus instead on the target audience, the message we wish to convey, the strategies we can use and various other features of the presentation. He suggests looking at simple ways to improve PowerPoint techniques, such as avoiding pre-set templates, which are available within PowerPoint and are also offered by meeting organizers, who often generate PowerPoint templates with the organizer's branding on every slide. These tem plates homogenize presentations and should be avoided when possible. If absolutely neces sary, put the organizer's branding on your opening and closing slides, but do not carry it on every slide, as this is immensely repetitive and distracting for audiences (Chapman 2018).

Finally, Harden (2008) advises us to break out of the mould of standard PowerPoint presentations and focus on the story we are telling, rather than the slides we are showing. Lectures are about communication and understanding, not ranting our way through dozens of slides on a screen.

Your opening slide should have the title of your presentation, your name and, possibly, your email address. Chapman (2018) offers further advice about constructing slides, noting that black text on a white background or white text on a black background both work well

It is useful to stick to two or three colours per slide and remember that some audience members might be colour blind. Text should be chunky and readable (with fonts such as Arial, Calibri or Verdana) and font sizes should be large (40 for titles; 28 to 36 for content). Avoid clutter and distractors which obstruct the passage of information from the slide to the student's brain. Simple is best, less is more.

PowerPoint is not the only presentation programme you can use. Prezi is another option; it was launched in 2009 and had over 35 million users by 2015 (https://prezi.com/). This software is straightforward to use and has the key benefit of allowing lecturers to organize and view their presentation as a whole. Lecturers can also develop ideas and produce 'mind maps' as they might do on an old-style blackboard. Duffy and colleagues (2015) studied the benefits of Prezi among final-year medical and physiotherapy students and reported that almost all students (99%) found Prezi to be a more engaging experience than other styles of lecture and a majority (89%) found the overview or 'mind map' provided by Prezi to be helpful.

Overall, preparation is the key to a good lecture. Focus on clear, direct objectives; decide your presentation format beforehand, and do not let the features of presentation software distract you and your audience from the central purpose of the lecture: to share knowledge and increase understanding.

Delivering the Lecture

Many people feel anxious speaking in front of a group. There are several ways to address this issue, centred on practicing your lecture, engaging your audience and maintaining a good degree of flexibility as you speak: not everything goes according to plan. It is good to maintain an awareness of your use of technology throughout your lecture, as you do not want sophisticated technology to distract your audience from the content you seek to convey.

First, practice your lecture. Run through your main points ahead of time so that it is easier to deliver the lecture to the audience when the time comes. Include your three learning objectives on your opening slide in order to focus your thoughts on the key messages you want to share. Do not try to remember specific sentences or specific wordings, because you will not recall them precisely. Trying to recall specific sentences will simply trip you up. Instead, go over your main points again and again beforehand, and be as conversational as possible in the lecture itself, rather than repeating a written script.

Second, be very familiar with your slides (if you are using slides). This means that you will know which slide is coming up next and you can introduce it before it appears on the screen. If you muddle up the order of the slides, do not panic. Just tell the audience that you have muddled up the order of the slides and will do your best to talk through them anyway. The audience will understand and most will be delighted with this very human interaction. Small errors, when handled confidently, can become a highpoint and help regain everyone's attention.

Third, think of the lecture as a conversation. Ask the students some questions early on. This breaks the ice between lecturer and audience, and helps everyone to relax. Interaction is the key to reducing anxiety. While many people are nervous about public speaking, most are comfortable with a conversation. Always support what your audience members say, even if you do not share their viewpoint. Respond generously, especially when you disagree: 'Yes, I see what you are saying, it makes perfect sense. On the other hand, of course, it could be argued that . . .' Avoid telling audience members that they are wrong, even if you feel that they are. Emphasize the merits in their points and then make your own points in return. You want to encourage engagement, not deter it.

Fourth, tell stories. Easton (2016) performed a qualitative study of how medical lecturers use narratives by observing medical lectures and then performing one-to-one interviews with lecturers and focus groups with medical students. He found that lecturers use a variety of narratives on a range of different themes, including clinical cases, patient experiences and narratives about their own professional careers. These stories provide relevant context, act as a 'hook' to engage students and serve as memory aids. Easton's findings are consistent with the broader literature which suggests that narrative is a useful tool for learning in medicine. This approach might be especially relevant to promoting humanistic aspects of medical practice, such as professional identity and empathy. Narratives certainly help to maintain an audience's attention and increase their engagement with the lecture as you deliver it.

Fifth, do not deliberately set out to use humour. Use humour only if an opportunity presents itself naturally and spontaneously. Carefully planned humour rarely works in a teaching setting because humour is highly dependent on timing, atmosphere and the nature of your relationship with the audience. All of these factors are difficult or impossible to predict. Humour also depends on the existence of common ground, knowledge or experience, and you might not always know if you have these in common with your audience (Monks et al. 2018). Therefore, humour should be used sparingly, if at all.

Despite these caveats, if a moment for humour presents itself during the lecture and you are comfortable enough to make a joke, humour can greatly improve the atmosphere and re-engage people whose minds have wandered. It is important that you do not offend any audience members with your remarks; so, the only reasonable object for humour is yourself. Feel entirely free to make jokes or humorous remarks about your own incompetence on the sports field (for example), your idiotic mistakes in the past or your inability to perform simple household tasks with which everyone is familiar. Do not joke about anyone else; if you decide to use humour, make sure that you are the object of it.

Sixth, take a pause in the middle of the lecture to break the atmosphere and ask the audience how they are doing (Butler 1992). For example, you could say: 'I've been talking for 20 minutes now and I need to take a breath. Does anyone have any questions, queries or comments at this point? There will be more time for questions at the end, but I'm happy to pause for some questions or comments now, too.' This is a nice technique that helps get everyone back on track and gives you an opportunity to assess what you have covered so far and what you have left to do.

Seventh, maintain an awareness of the role that technology is playing in your lecture as you deliver it. Is the presentation programme working? If there are technical problems at the start, resolve these briskly. Always bring a print-out of your slides to the lecture with you so that, if you cannot resolve technical problems after five minutes, you can simply speak from notes. Audiences are usually (paradoxically) relieved when a slide presentation definitively does not work and the presenter is able to speak without slides.

The same applies to more elaborate presentation techniques. Embedding videos in presentations, for example, can be helpful for learning clinical skills, once the videos are relevant and focused (Sarıhan et al. 2016). Electronic voting, too, is sometimes used to encourage interaction, although this can prove difficult to prepare (Duggan et al. 2007). As with all technology, however, it is important to remain aware of the effect of these technologies as you deliver your lecture. Stop using them if they do not work, prove distracting or shift focus from substantive content of your lecture to the technology. Lectures are about learning, not mastering the latest interactive technology.

Finishing the Lecture

How you finish your lecture is just as important as how you begin it and what you say during it. Many people deliver good information during a lecture, but then fail to draw their points together on their final slides, talk for too long or fade into an unfocused mumble at the end, rather than finishing crisply and cleanly. It is worth thinking about how you will finish your lecture so as to provide the audience with clear take-home messages and, ideally, a few minutes to draw their thoughts together before they move on to their next lecture or other activity. Several techniques can help.

As you approach the end of your lecture, return to the three learning objectives that you planned ahead of time and outlined at the start of the lecture (Butler 1992). Put these points on a slide and summarize what you have said about them. This gives a useful arc to the lecture as an educational experience and will remind you of anything important that you forgot to say during the lecture itself.

There is strong evidence to support the usefulness of this approach. Lautrette and colleagues (2020) performed a randomized controlled study of the impact of take-home messages in slide presentations on the retention of messages and knowledge by trainee doctors. This group found a strong positive association between writing take-home messages on a slide, retention of take-home messages and doctors' knowledge. Clearly, re-emphasizing key messages is an effective teaching technique.

In terms of rhetorical strategy, it is important to bring your lecture to a crisp close. Do not simply fade out or end up mumbling as you run out of things to say. When you reach the end, announce clearly that you are finished: 'That is all I have to say today. Thank you for listening. I am happy to answer any questions or hear any comments you might have.' This indicates that you have finished the formal part of your lecture and re-directs attention back to the audience for the discussion.

During the discussion, have a final slide prepared to keep on the screen as you answer questions. This slide should be the same as your opening slide and have the title of your presentation, your name and, possibly, your email address. This reinforces who you are and what the lecture was about. It also provides another 'hook' for the new knowledge that the audience has (hopefully) gained from your lecture.

Answer questions generously, directly and briefly. A generous answer always begins with the word 'Yes', regardless of the question. 'Yes' makes everyone feel better. You might need to subtly roll back from the 'Yes' in your subsequent comments, but always start with a 'Yes'. Avoid 'No'. It is important to be generous towards the questioner's viewpoint even if they do not share your perspective. After all, they might be right and you might be wrong.

A direct answer is one that provides a clear response or openly admits a lack of knowledge. 'I don't know' is a good answer, especially if you can follow it up with one or two facts that indicate that you know a little bit about the topic, even if you do not have a definitive answer. Do not pretend you know the answer when you do not. Feel free to speculate briefly, but label this clearly as speculation. Audiences instinctively know when you do not know what you are talking about.

Keep your answers brief. The more questions you can field in the time allotted, the more interactive your lecture will be. Audiences love to ask questions so try to give the opportunity to as many audience members as possible. The best way to do this is not by extending the time for questions and answers, but by keeping your answers brief.

Sometimes, audience members make statements rather than ask questions. Even if an audience member makes a statement that is wrong, try to phrase your response in the positive: 'Yes, I can see where you are coming from and why you reached that conclusion. On the other hand, though, there is evidence that ...' Alternatively: 'Yes, many people hold that view and I can certainly see why. There are, however, other ways of looking at it ...'.

Finally, some audience members will take the opportunity at the end of a lecture to engage in lengthy lectures themselves rather than asking questions, sometimes speaking for so long that other audience members become restless and frustrated. This is a difficult situation, but do not become flustered. Encourage the audience member to finish up so that others have an opportunity to pose questions or make comments. You could, for example, say: 'Thank you for that, but I am keen to give other audience members an opportunity to speak ...'.

If this does not work, you have no choice but simply to let the difficult questioner talk themselves out. The more you interrupt, the more they will talk. Do not feel the need to intervene aggressively. If you simply remain entirely silent, most people are deeply unnerved by this and stop talking quite quickly. Also, be consoled by the fact that the more unreasonable the questioner becomes, the more reasonable you look in the eyes of the rest of the audience.

Conclusion

The lecture is a much maligned but valuable teaching format. Used correctly, a lecture can prove an excellent learning experience for lecturer and audience alike. The keys lie in being clear about your objectives; avoiding distracting technology; sticking to time; finishing crisply; and moving briskly through the questions and answers. Try to turn the lecture into a conversation with the audience and be generous towards their views, which might be different to your own. Above all, remember that audiences are exquisitely sensitive to pomposity and humbug; avoid both by making yourself the object of your jokes.

References

Butler JA (1992) Use of teaching methods within the lecture format. *Medical Teacher*, **14**: 11–25.

Chapman T (2018) Waking up your lecture. *Pediatric Radiology*, **48**: 1388–92.

Duffy RM, Guerandel A, Casey P, Malone K, Kelly BD (2015) Experiences of using Prezi in psychiatry teaching. *Academic Psychiatry*, **39**: 615–19.

Duggan PM, Palmer E, Devitt P (2007) Electronic voting to encourage interactive lectures: a randomised trial. *BMC Medical Education*, 7: 25.

Easton G (2016) How medical teachers use narratives in lectures: a qualitative study. *BMC Medical Education*, **16**: 3.

Harden RM (2008) Death by PowerPoint: the need for a 'fidget index'. *Medical Teacher*, 30: 833–5.

Lautrette A, Boyer A, Gruson D, et al. (2020) Impact of take-home messages written into slide presentations delivered during lectures on the retention of messages and the residents' knowledge: a randomized controlled study. *BMC Medical Education*, 20: 180.

Monks A, Geher G, Johnson J, et al. (2018) Top tips on how to make your lectures interesting. *Times Higher Education*, 18 October. Available at: www.timeshighereducation.com/features/top-tips-how-make-your-lectures-interesting.

Sarıhan A, Oray NC, Güllüpınar B, et al. (2016) The comparison of the efficiency of traditional lectures to video-supported lectures within the training of the emergency medicine residents. *Turkish Journal of Emergency Medicine*, **16**: 107–11.

Smits PB, de Buisonjé CD, Verbeek JH, et al. (2003) Problem-based learning versus lecture-based learning in postgraduate medical education. *Scandinavian Journal of Work, Environment and Health*, **29**: 280–7.

Zeng HL, Chen DX, Li Q, Wang XY (2020) Effects of seminar teaching method versus lecture-based learning in medical education: a meta-analysis of randomized controlled trials. *Medical Teacher*, **42**: 1343–9.

Chapter

12

Giving and Receiving Feedback in Psychiatric Education

Nick Brown

Introduction

Medical education has changed considerably from models based mainly on knowledge acquisition and duration of training towards the achievement of predefined learning outcomes (Krackov and Pohl 2011). In such a competency-based approach to education effective feedback has become an integral and important constituent of teaching and learning.

In the learning process, feedback is a process of sharing observations, concerns and suggestions with another person. Feedback helps to maximize learning and development by raising an individual's awareness of their areas of strength and relative weakness or need as well as outlining the actions required to improve performance.

Detailed and prompt feedback coupled with clear opportunities to improve enables individuals to achieve previously agreed milestones such as curriculum outcomes (Krackov and Pohl 2011) or continuing professional development (CPD) objectives.

Feedback comes in many shapes and forms. In the past it was said that the primary purpose of feedback should be not to judge but to present information (Hyman 1980). However, the advent of workplace-based assessments (WPBAs) (Norcini and Burch 2007) has changed matters somewhat. For WPBAs to be an effective form of feedback that includes honest and accurate judgement is essential (Veloski et al. 2006). It is difficult if not impossible to see how doctors in training can improve their skills and behaviours without practising them and receiving feedback on their performance.

Giving accurate feedback is an activity that is sometimes omitted or not done well (Day and Brown 2000; Adcroft 2011), but it is a skill that can be learned. The observation that after some 10 years or more of WPBAs the perception of trainees about feedback remains little altered (Cheston et al. 2020) makes the need to consider feedback and how to make it effective an important continuing issue.

Background

Any cyclical system controls itself by monitoring performance results: this is feedback. Where only numbers are used, for example an examination score, very simple summative feedback is achieved but little information that could lead to improvement is passed. The individual does not necessarily learn what they have done well and what was done less well. However, if detailed and useful information is provided as feedback and this influences change, the feedback has been effective and learning has taken place. Feedback is part of the learning cycle and should therefore be considered integral to any learning experience.

Most people have a desire to know how well they are performing. The implicit expectation of success is fundamental to motivation and effort (Atkinson 1957) and can lead to enhanced performance. Feedback should concentrate on both the good and the not so good aspects of performance. Medical students' need for and use of performance feedback has been a theme throughout the literature on medical education (Hewson and Little 1998; Bing-You and Trowbridge 2009).

The potential benefits of feedback are manifold within personal development and include:

improved self-awareness;
enhanced performance;
affording the opportunity to change behavior;
better relationships;
improved teamwork;
confirmation of strengths; and
highlighting areas for development.

The realization of these benefits is, however, dependent on the active participation of the learner in accepting the feedback (Algiraigi 2014), internalizing it and taking action using the learning cycle (Kolb and Fry 1975). Successful feedback starts with a degree of self-awareness and active participation. These properties together may constitute insight and contribute to successful lifelong learning (Brown et al. 2014). For feedback to be effective the individual must be able and willing to reflect on what was positive in their performance and what could be improved in the future. Historically, constructive and effective feedback has been shown to improve learning outcomes, including better assessment marks, in school children and university students (Black and William 1998) and to improve competence in medical trainees (Rolfe and McPherson 1995). More recently, studies have, for example, focused on changes in medical professionalism (Parikh et al. 2001; Lerchenfeldt et al. 2019) and consultation skills (Hunukumbure et al. 2017; Dohms et al. 2020) through learning accompanied by feedback.

Unfortunately, in practice, sometimes only the negative aspects of performance are commented on. This may reduce the repetition of certain mistakes and behaviours but it can also make the trainee feel inadequate. Nevertheless, there are some who argue that their most powerful and formative learning experiences resulted from negative criticism and that praise merely overprotects the trainee and does not show them where they are making errors (Boehler et al. 2006).

Perceptions and Dissatisfactions around Feedback

Despite medical trainees' request for high-quality feedback, together with evidence that it is beneficial to future performance and its identified importance within the trainer's role (Chur-Hansen and McLean 2006), both the literature and personal experience suggest that it is often lacking in practice. Several studies have highlighted medical trainees' dissatisfaction with the quality of the feedback they receive, both at undergraduate and postgraduate level. There appears to be a long-standing discrepancy between the way trainees and trainers perceive feedback (Gil et al. 1984). In the past, trainees have reported that feedback is given infrequently and/or ineffectively whereas teachers themselves believe that they provide frequent and adequate feedback (Hewson and Little 1998).

Trainees have highlighted the need for feedback to be relevant to their expected level of performance and competency (Moorehead et al. 2004). This is particularly pertinent to contemporary models of competency-based training curricula. In their review of the literature on medical education, McIlwrick et al. (2006) concluded that the 'best-intended feedback may be unhelpful if it is: (1) not descriptive or specific enough, (2) not age appropriate, or (3) mistaken for assessment'.

Recent findings regarding continuing misperceptions of feedback (Kogan et al. 2012) and dissatisfaction with the accuracy of feedback on WPBAs are concerning (Cheston et al. 2020).

Principles and Characteristics of Effective Feedback

A number of principles govern constructive feedback (Box 12.1). A further simple model is offered using the mnemonic CORBS (Box 12.2, Hawkins and Shohet 1989) The most fundamental factors are that feedback is for the learner's or trainee's benefit and that it should be offered rather than imposed on most occasions; remember, though, that there will also be situations where feedback will be at the behest of the trainer, for example, in the case of problems in performance or where feedback is a compulsory requirement of the training curriculum or programme.

The amount of information should be tailored to need, and the individual must not be overloaded. It should be checked with the individual; for example 'How did you feel that went?' rather than 'That went . . . '. Feedback should always refer to actions or behaviours rather than to the individual's personality, for example 'You are always late for clinic – can we look at this?' (behaviour) rather than 'You are a lazy doctor' (personality).

Box 12.1 Ten basic requirements of feedback

Feedback should meet seven fundamental requirements, thus it should be:
1. For the learner's (trainee's) benefit
2. Timely (and regular), not delayed
3. Specific, not general
4. Descriptive based on direct observation, not evaluative
5. Accurate – good feedback obviously requires accurate observation and assessment
6. Not embarrassing
7. Impersonal
8. Constructive not destructive
9. Relevant
10. It must always end with an action plan for improvement (Krackov 2009)!

Box 12.2 The CORBS model of constructive feedback

Clear: Give information clearly and concisely

Owned: Offer feedback as your perception, not the ultimate truth

Regular: Feedback is offered as soon as possible after each event

Balanced: Offer a reasonable balance of negative and positive feedback

Specific: Feedback must be based on observed behaviour.

Good-quality feedback involves a dialogue between trainer and trainee. If conversation and honest dialogue are fostered, a situation will arise where feedback is actively sought and adult learning flourishes. Strong efforts should be made to facilitate learners' perception of feedback as an opportunity of learning, almost like one-to-one coaching. Offering feedback rather than forcing it, using dialogue rather than monologue, giving the learner a leading role in their feedback and choosing the right setting are all helpful points for the proper perception of feedback. A feedback session should be two-way; the learner plays a critical role in assessing his/her own performance (Krackov 2011) and the teacher should be genuinely receptive to feedback from trainees. Feedback should, where possible and appropriate, include multiple sources, for example, from patients and other healthcare professionals, and include the learner's self-perception.

Trainers must consider the level of the trainee because there is evidence that learner's perceptions of feedback change through stages of development (Murdoch-Eaton and Sargeant 2012). It appears that at more junior stages learners adopt a more passive approach that simply informs about progress in meeting (or otherwise) standards or curriculum outcomes whereas at more senior stages a style that guides and enables adjustments to learning and practice is desired (Murdoch-Eaton and Sargeant 2012).

Barriers to Effective Feedback

There are several potential barriers to giving effective feedback, and awareness of these can be a first step to overcoming them. The key problems are:

- Fear of upsetting the trainee or damaging the relationship between trainer and trainee; trainers may feel uncomfortable, particularly when highlighting areas of deficiency (Gil et al. 1984).
- Fear of doing harm rather than good.
- Resistance or defensiveness in the trainee: poor handling of feedback by the trainer, for example, feedback that is insensitively given is more likely to be ignored; equally, a trainee who finds it difficult to accept feedback is more likely to disregard it.
- Feedback that is too generalized and not related to specific facts or observations.
- Feedback that fails to give guidance on how the trainee can change or improve.
- The trainee's lack of respect for the source of the feedback. When trainees are surveyed, they opine that trust and respect for teachers are factors that would make them more receptive to feedback (Bing-You et al. 1997; Hesketh and Laidlaw 2002).

The last point reinforces the need to establish feedback within the context of a relationship based on honesty and mutual respect, which leads in turn to consideration of the organizational or educational culture in which feedback is offered at the right time for trainer and trainee.

Creating the Environment for Effective Feedback: Changing the Culture

In order to help teachers give effective feedback, increase the acceptance of feedback and enable improvement in performance, it is vital to consider the environment or culture in which the feedback is occurring (Ramani and Krackov 2012); a recent review reinforces the notion that addressing the culture of feedback is critical to improvement in the process (Kornegay et al. 2017). A positive learning climate is essential (Hewson and Little 1998).

The learning environment should be one in which teachers and learners are working together to help the individual learner achieve the expected outcomes.

The field of learner preparedness for engaging with and working with feedback is underdeveloped but has been suggested as a factor in any lack of impact of feedback on personal development (Algiraigri 2014). Algiraigri (2014) suggests ten tips for learners (see Box 12.3).

Although giving feedback is an integral part of the role of the trainer and educational supervisor, trainers may feel uncomfortable about the task, particularly when highlighting areas of deficiency in a student's performance (Gil et al. 1984). Trainers and clinical teachers should be encouraged to reflect upon their skills including skills in giving feedback constructively (Box 12.4, Hardavella et al. 2017); regular workshops for teacher development to improve feedback skills that can be acquired and refined through repeated practice should be a feature of every training school or programme.

Box 12.3 Ten tips for receiving feedback (Algiraigri 2014)

- **Self-assessment:** Try to assess yourself better, break tasks down and consider each item and how you performed
- **Do I really need feedback?:** Regardless of where we are in our career, we all need feedback. Consider blind spots perhaps by using the 'Johari Window'
- **Your teacher:** Do you connect?
- **Little or no feedback?:** Ask for feedback
- **Positive feedback:** Thank your supervisor/teacher and take your performance up a level
- **Your emotion:** It is normal to receive constructive feedback, be a good listener
- **Your turn! What happens next?:** Be part of a constructive action plan
- **Generational differences:** These may influence approach, be aware of them
- **If general or non-specific feedback is received:** Probe and ask questions to find out what exactly is the point

---

Box 12.4 Tips for teachers and supervisors offering feedback (Hardavella et al. 2017)

- Plan in advance
- Try to give feedback promptly, as soon after the event as possible
- Think about what you want to achieve
- Start gently, be specific
- Encourage self-reflection
- Make eye contact, be aware of nonverbal clues
- Remember emotions are deduced through facial expression – smile
- Use you voice and tone in a natural way
- Avoid looking strict, by sitting with your arms crossed, or as if you don't care, by sitting slumped. An open posture helps an open conversation
- Keep calm
- Avoid distractions – think about your situation. Where are you in relation to your workscreen? Those emails and messages can wait. The person in front of you will notice when you glance at your screen!
- Reflect afterwards – what went well? What can you improve? How was this trainee and/or this session unique?

Feedback during Workplace-Based Assessment

The principles above and models below are particularly relevant in the setting of WPBAs. To place an individual WPBA in context and give appropriate feedback on the trainee's performance it is essential to be certain in one's mind of its purpose: for example, is it an assessment of a general area of the curriculum such as communication skills or does it have a specific objective such as a risk assessment by the trainee? Be clear about what is observed. Which curriculum learning outcome or objective is being addressed?

The observer should always take contemporaneous notes during the performance; this will improve the accuracy of the observation and consequently the quality of the feedback offered. If a problem is present, it is axiomatic that it must be clearly defined, communicated and agreed. Otherwise no plan for improvement can begin.

It is of concern that WPBAs do not appear to be well perceived as measuring performance of improving quality of training (Menon et al. 2012, Gilberthorpe et al. 2016). Perhaps part of the key to this lies in the survey finding that only 51% of WPBAs delivered an outcome in terms of an achievable action plan (Gilbertorpe et al. 2016)

Models for Giving Effective Feedback

Training trainers and trainees using a set format for feedback can help overcome many of the problems highlighted above as well as standardize the way in which feedback is given. Some of the most common strategies for delivering effective feedback are outlined below. Each may have a place; different situations or personalities may demand use of a different model in practice.

Pendleton's Rules

Pendleton's rules (Box 12.5), which were developed in UK general practice training, allow both trainee and trainer to comment on how well an activity was performed (Pendleton et al. 1984). The interview follows a format in which the trainee and the trainer state first what they thought was done well, and then what they thought could be improved and how this might be achieved. The rules have been criticized for artificially separating the good and poorer parts of performance and for spending too long appraising the positive aspects, leaving little time for suggestions for change.

Box 12.5 Pendleton's rules

- The trainee performs an activity, for example, carrying out a risk assessment
- The trainee says what they thought they did well, for example, 'I think I established a good rapport with the patient'
- The trainer comments on what was done well, for example, 'You were empathic towards the patient and they appeared relaxed talking to you'
- The trainee identifies what was not done so well and how they could improve, for example, 'The history I obtained was disjointed. I could use a more structured approach next time'
- The trainer comments on the aspects to be improved and offers suggestions in a constructive manner, for example, 'It took a long time to establish the circumstances surrounding the overdose. Next time you could try using more closed questions to clarify the situation'

The Feedback Sandwich

Many people are uncomfortable giving negative feedback. The feedback sandwich (Box 12.6) allows a criticism to be 'sandwiched' between two items of praise. It is particularly useful at the start of a new trainer–trainee relationship. The trainer begins by commenting on a positive area of an activity and praises the trainee on this. The 'meat' of the sandwich is the criticism; this should be constructive and provide suggestions on what could be changed. The trainer then ends the feedback with another positive comment on the trainee's performance.

Silverman's SET–GO

Also known as the Calgary–Cambridge method (Silverman et al. 1997), Silverman's SET–GO (Box 12.7) involves descriptive feedback during which the trainee comments on what they experienced while carrying out a task. The task is often videotaped, which allows the trainee to reflect and comment on what they see when reviewing the tape. The trainee discusses with the trainer what they were thinking during the task and acknowledges any difficulties. An aim or goal is clarified and ways of achieving this are discussed. This method can be particularly useful in teaching sessions where a peer group review the trainee's tape.

Box 12.6 The feedback sandwich

- First, the trainer gives a positive comment, for example, 'I liked the way you reflected on how the patient was feeling at that time'
- Then the trainer comments on an area that needs change and advises how to achieve this change, for example, 'The patient was still crying when you moved on from the family history. Perhaps next time it would help to wait a little longer and give the patient more space to express him/herself'
- The trainer finishes with another positive comment, for example, 'I liked the way you included the patient in decisions about the management of the problem'

Box 12.7 Silverman's SET–GO

- **What the trainee saw:** This should be descriptive, specific and non-judgemental, for example, 'The patient became very upset and tearful when I talked about the diagnosis of bipolar affective disorder'
- **What else they saw:** This again must be descriptive, for example, 'I allowed the patient to calm down before continuing'
- **What the trainee thought at the time:** Reflection, acknowledgement and problem solving, for example, 'I was aware the news was distressing the patient and was concerned that he wouldn't remember a lot about our conversation. I could have given him written information'
- **Clarify the goal:** For example, discussing a diagnosis with a patient
- **Explore offers of how to achieve the goal:** For example, clarifying what the patient believes is wrong and what they understand by the diagnosis given, and discussing the treatment options

The Six-Step (Problem-Solving) Method

This stepwise approach to delivering feedback is particularly effective when it is necessary to reach agreement on what has gone wrong with the trainee's performance and where the problem lies (Box 12.8) (Chambers and Wall 1999).

Feedback as a Gift

Feedback as a gift is a semi-formal and simplified amalgam of the Pendleton and Silverman models (Box 12.9).

The Chicago Model

The six-step Chicago model (Box 12.10) (Brukner et al. 1999) is similar to other methods but has the great advantage of starting with a recapitulation of the aims and objectives that the trainee is supposed to be addressing.

Box 12.8 The six-step (problemsolving) method

When a problem in the trainee's performance is identified, the six steps are:

(1) problem presented (to the trainee by the trainer)
(2) problem discussed
(3) problem agreed
(4) solution proposed
(5) solution discussed
(6) solution agreed

For the method to work it is essential that the trainer:

• is able to connect – establish a rapport with the trainee
• has identified a clear outcome in advance, that is, the trainee must agree that there is a problem and the agreement should not be diluted or obscured by external factors such as the trainee's counter-arguments

---

Box 12.9 Feedback as a gift

The trainer comments on:

• something good that the trainee needs to keep doing, for example, 'I liked the way you asked the patient what she wanted to achieve from the session'
• something that distracts the trainee from their strengths, for example, 'I feel that the patient was not clear about what was expected from her for the next session'
• something that is a weakness, with a suggestion for improvement, for example, 'Towards the end of the session you could summarise what has been discussed and clarify any unclear areas'

Other Models

It is worth noting at this point that the literature from the wider world of healthcare professional and business/occupational personal development is full of easy-to-use models (Box 12.11), which you may wish to consider either in educational work or in dealing with difficulty more widely in your role as a senior healthcare professional.

Box 12.10 The Chicago model

The six steps that the trainer takes are to:

(1) Review the trainee's aims and objectives
(2) Give interim feedback of a positive nature
(3) Ask the trainee to give their own appraisal of their performance
(4) Give feedback focusing on behaviour rather than on personality (what happened, not the trainer's opinions or what the trainer thinks might have happened or been about to happen – this is particularly important in WPBAs)
(5) Give specific examples to illustrate (aided greatly by taking notes during observation)
(6) Suggest specific strategies for improvement

Box 12.11 Other feedback models

Situation–Behaviour–Impact (SBI) feedback model
- **Situation:** Describe the situation. Be specific about when and where it occurred
- **Behaviour:** Describe the observable behavior, do not assume that you know what the other person was thinking
- **Impact:** Describe what you thought or felt in reaction to the behavior

The BOOST feedback model
- **Balanced:** In context with the past, for example, previous events or experience
- **Observed:** What you actually saw or heard
- **Objective:** Requires a change in behavior
- **Specific:** Real examples (when, where, what)
- **Timely:** Feedback offered close to any actual events

The DESICA feedback model
- **Describe** the issue
- **Express** how the behavior makes you or others feel
- **Specific examples** of when the behavior is noticed
- **Implications** on service including stakeholders
- **Consequences** of not changing the behavior
- **Agreed actions** to resolve the issue

Feedback on Written Work

It is important to remember that clinical performance includes written work. A psychiatrist needs to be able to write coherent, legible and understandable notes, letters and reports (Pullen and Loudon 2006). Very similar principles to all of the above apply but with an important caveat that comments should not be so specific that the learner simply seeks to implement what appear to be instructions and mimic their teacher rather than developing their own style (Willingham 1990).

Dealing with Difficulty

Telling a trainee that they are doing well is very satisfying. However, telling a trainee that there are problems with their performance can be very difficult. It is not always easy to give feedback that separates the performance from the individual. Making apparently intrusive comments can be awkward and individual trainees will respond in different ways. Setting the scene should be done carefully and thoughtfully. Think about how the trainee has responded to feedback before; explain what is going to happen. Giving the trainee space in which to express themselves and their feelings is essential. They should not be interrupted or confronted at such times, even if their response is aggressive, defensive or tearful. When they are in control of themselves they should be asked how they would describe what they are doing and what they would see as a positive way forward.

Practical issues may need to be addressed, such as not allowing the trainee to perform a particular task until the trainer has had the opportunity to give them detailed feedback followed by a reassessment. But the main points that trainers should bear in mind when addressing problems with performance are to:

- address the issue(s) or problem(s) immediately, do not put it off;
- find out or have to hand the facts;
- share the problem;
- explain the problem;
- give support; and
- document what the trainee says and does.

Feedback Using Other Communication Instruments

Sometimes it is necessary or appropriate to give feedback in ways that are not face-to-face.

Telephone- or Video-Call Feedback

Telephone feedback without video is difficult for trainer and trainees as there are no non-verbal cues; therefore, it is necessary to be extremely sensitive to changes in voice or hesitations that may suggest doubt or disagreement. Voices sound different over the telephone and many statements that are delivered comfortably face-to-face sound aggressive or rude down the phone line. Some calls, particularly international calls, may introduce a dimension of delay and echo into an already difficult situation. The use of video calling may overcome some of these hurdles, providing both parties are comfortable with the technology and the quality of connection is good. If feedback has to be given by telephone or video call, the trainer should keep a short written record of the conversation for future reference and in case of misunderstandings.

Written Feedback

Written feedback may be needed even when the trainee is seen regularly. The correspondence must be clear, concise and supportive. It can be more difficult to express thoughts in the written rather than the spoken word and cultural differences in the use of language may lead to misunderstandings. If in doubt, trainers should ask a colleague to see how the letter 'reads' to them.

Email Feedback

Email can be used for quick, relatively informal communications. However, the very lack of social niceties that is common in emails may give rise to misinterpretation and it may again be wise to check content with a colleague. The send button should never be pressed without due thought!

Text and Messaging Feedback

Text either through SMS or other messaging systems provides a very quick and convenient form of communication. Literature is emerging that suggests there may be a significant role for instant messaging applications (IMAs) in medical education, with evidence of a positive outcome on educational attainment, particularly when used with defined local networks (Raiman et al. 2017; Coleman and O'Connor 2019). These networks of teachers and students appear to generate high frequencies of participation and foster feedback between teachers and learners and also between learners as peers.

Videoconferencing, Teleconferencing and Feedback

The challenges of COVID-19 have brought the use of technology to the fore in almost all aspects of medical education, and already a body of literature is appearing (Hilburg et al. 2020; Emanuel 2020; Rose 2020). The use of conferencing technologies in giving and receiving feedback has not received much attention thus far but a study on the use of videoconferencing in medical students (Zhou et al. 2019) suggests that feedback sessions may be performed successfully using web-based programmes, although particular attention needed to be paid to the students' ability to fully participate and the need to avoid group problems such as shaming. Recent experience suggests that using one of the above models for feedback, perhaps with modification, will aid success. For example, in a Zoom session with say six students (all trained in giving feedback), a modified Pendleton model in which the observed students say what they believe they can improve on is followed by their peers and a tutor giving suggestions for improvement. At the end of the session the student receives all information (positive and negative) from all participants in a written format (M. R. Rhodes 2021, personal communication).

Continuing Professional Development or Continuing Medical Education

CPD has long been recognized as essential to medicine and, in 2000, the General Medical Council (General Medical Council 2000) began the path to the current system of revalidation. Revalidation incorporates the need for continuing learning, which in turns begs the question of feedback guiding the individual's learning programme. The need for attention to learning requirements is highlighted by the potential for poor performance to occur across all domains of clinical practice (O'Leary et al. 2010). There is a link here to the issues of self-awareness and insight and the need for all doctors to be active in seeking feedback on their performance throughout their career from a variety of trusted sources, including patients, colleagues and other members of the healthcare team (Brown et al. 2014).

Conclusion

Interactive feedback is indispensable in aiding the education and professional development of clinical medical students and doctors in all stages of their careers. It provides any learner with information on their performance, which can be used to inform a plan to improve that performance.

In the UK, trainees in psychiatry have always viewed feedback as desirable (Day and Brown 2000) and it is now even more important after the adoption of WPBAs. The greatest value of the latter as an educational tool is their formative assessment of the real performance of doctors at their service base. They allow areas of performance to be observed and clear, accurate, regular feedback to be offered that appropriately adjusts the trainee's learning objectives and plan.

In giving good feedback the supervisor or trainer is helping the trainee to change: feedback is a powerful instrument which, if used wisely and well, will further a trainee's personal and professional development. The ability to give feedback is a core skill for trainers. This underlines the need to include training in feedback skills in basic 'training for trainers' – a view that was reinforced by the Royal College of Psychiatrists, which commissioned an early CPD online module on the subject (Oakley and Oyebode 2008, reviewed in 2015). The General Medical Council has continued to support the identification and support of educators with a range of skills including the ability to give and receive feedback (General Medical Council 2012, 2016).

Providing and receiving feedback can sometimes be challenging. The consolidation of the use of competency-based models of education throughout the medical career and the introduction of WPBAs mandate that all doctors including psychiatrists must become proficient in giving, seeking and receiving feedback. That there were over 800 review articles on feedback in medical education published in the decade up to 2017 only serves to underline the importance of the subject (Bing-You et al. 2017).

Training can increase the comfort and skill of the teacher in offering the feedback and also the learner, including importantly the lifelong learner (Brown et al. 2014), in receiving and acting upon timely, specific and quality feedback.

Acknowledgements

For information, the original paper on which this chapter is based was: Brown N, Cooke L (2009) Giving effective feedback to psychiatric trainees. *Advances in Psychiatric Treatment*, 15: 123–8. The author gratefully acknowledges the contribution of Dr Louise Cook, who was involved in writing the original article.

References

Adcroft A (2011) The mythology of feedback. *Higher Education Research and Development*, 30: 405–19.

Algiraigri AH (2014) Ten tips for receiving feedback effectively in clinical practice. *Medical Education*, 19: 25141.

Atkinson JW (1957) Motivational determinants of risk taking behaviour. *Psychology Review*, **64**: 365.

Bing You RG, Trowbridge RL (2009) Why medical educators may be failing at feedback. *JAMA*, **302**: 1330–1.

Bing You RG, Paterson J, Levine MA (1997) Feedback falling on deaf ears: Residents' receptivity to feedback tempered by sender credibility. *Medical Teacher*, **19**: 40–4.

Bing-You R, Hayes V, Varaklis K, et al. (2017) Feedback for learners in medical education: what is known? A scoping review. *Academic Medicine*, **92**: 1346–54.

Black P, William D (1998) Assessment and classroom teaching. *Assessment in Education*, **5**: 7–73.

Boehler ML, Rogers DA, Schwind CJ, et al. (2006) An investigation of medical students' reactions to feedback: a randomised controlled trial. *Medical Education*, **40**: 746–9.

Brown N, McAvoy P, Joffé M (2014) Defining insight: a challenge that matters. *The Clinical Teacher* **11**: 170–3.

Brukner H, Altkorn DL, Cook S, et al. (1999) Giving effective feedback to medical students: a workshop for faculty and house staff. *Medical Teacher*, **21**: 161–5.

Chambers R, Wall D (1999) *Teaching Made Easy: A Manual for Health Professionals*. Radcliffe Publishing.

Cheston H, Graham D, Johnson G, Woodland P. (2022) Changes in UK medical trainees' perceptions of workplace-based assessments across 10 years: results from two cross-sectional studies. *Postgraduate Medical Journal*, **98**: 269–75.

Chur-Hansen A, McLean S (2006) On being a supervisor: the importance of feedback and how to give it. *Australasian Psychiatry*, **14**: 67–71.

Coleman E, O'Connor E (2019) The role of WhatsApp® in medical education: a scoping review and instructional design model. *BMC Medical Education*, **19**: 279.

Day E, Brown N (2000) The role of the educational supervisor. A questionnaire survey. *Psychiatric Bulletin*, **24**: 216–18.

Dohms MC, Collares CF, Tibério IC (2020) Video-based feedback using real consultations for a formative assessment in communication skills. *BMC Medical Education*, **20**: 57; doi: https://doi.org/10.1186/s12909-020-1955-6.

Emanuel EJ (2020) The inevitable reimagining of medical education. *JAMA*, **323**: 1127–1128

General Medical Council (2000) *Revalidating Doctors: Ensuring Standards, Securing the Future: A Consultation Document*. General Medical Council.

General Medical Council (2012) Recognising and approving trainers: the implementation plan. Available at: www.gmc-uk.org/education/10264.asp.

General Medical Council (2016) *Promoting Excellence: Standards for Medical Education and Training*. General Medical Council.

Gil DH, Heins M, Jones PB (1984) Perceptions of medical school faculty members and students on clinical clerkship feedback. *Journal of Medical Education*, **259**: 856–64.

Gilberthorpe T, Sarfo MD, Lawrence-Smith G (2016) Ticking the boxes: a survey of workplace-based assessments. *BJPsych Bulletin*, **40**: 89–92.

Hardavella G, Aamli-Gaagnat A, Saad N, Rousalova I, Sreter KB (2017) How to give and receive feedback effectively. *Breathe (Sheffield)*, **13**: 327–33.

Hawkins P, Shohet R (1989) *Supervision in the Helping Professions: An Individual, Group and Organizational Approach*. Open University Press.

Hesketh EA, Laidlaw JM (2002) Developing the teaching instinct: feedback. *Medical Teacher*, **24**: 245–8.

Hewson MG, Little ML (1998) Giving feedback in medical education: verification of recommended techniques. *Journal of General Internal Medicine*, **113**: 111–18.

Hilburg R, Patel N, Ambruso S, Biewald MA, Farouk SS (2020) Medical education during the coronavirus disease 2019 pandemic: learning from a distance. *Advances in Chronic Kidney Disease*, **27**: 412–7.

Hunukumbure AD, Smith SF, Das S (2017) Holistic feedback approach with video and peer discussion under teacher supervision. *BMC Medical Education*, **17**: 179.

Hyman RT (1980) *Improving Discussion Leadership*. Teachers College Press.

Kogan JR, Conforti LN, Bernabeo EC, et al. (2012) Faculty staff perceptions of feedback to residents after direct observation of clinical skills. *Medical Education*, 46: 201–15.

Kolb DA, Fry RE (1975) Towards an applied theory of experiential learning. In Cooper CL (ed.). *Theories of Group Processes*. Wiley, pp. 33–58.

Kornegay JG, Kraut A, Manthey D, et al. (2017) Feedback in medical education: a critical appraisal. *AEM Education and Training*, 1: 98–109.

Krackov SK (2009) Giving feedback. In Dent JA, Harden RM (eds.), *A Practical Guide for Medical Teachers*, 3rd ed. Churchill Livingstone Elsevier, pp. 357–67.

Krackov SK (2011) Expanding the horizon for feedback. *Medical Teacher*, 33: 873–4.

Krackov SK, Pohl H (2011) Building expertise using the deliberate-practice curriculum planning model. *Medical Teacher*, 33: 570–5.

Lerchenfeldt S, Mi M, Eng M (2019) The utilization of peer feedback during collaborative learning in undergraduate medical education: a systematic review. *BMC Medical Education*, 19: 321.

McIlwrick J, Nair B, Montgomery G (2006) 'How am I doing?': many problems but few solutions related to feedback delivery in undergraduate psychiatry education. *Academic Psychiatry*, 30: 130–5.

Menon S, Winston M, Sullivan G. (2012) Workplace-based assessment: attitudes and perceptions among consultant trainers and comparison with those of trainees. *Psychiatric Bulletin*, 36: 16–24.

Moorehead R, Maguire P, Thoo SL (2004) Giving feedback to learners in the practice. *Australian Family Physician*, 33: 691–5.

Murdoch-Eaton D, Sargeant J. (2012) Maturational differences in undergraduate medical students' perceptions about feedback. *Medical Education*, 46: 711–21.

Norcini J. Burch V. (2007) Workplace-based assessment as an educational tool: AMEE Guide No. 31. *Medical Teacher*, 29: 855–71.

Oakley C, Oyebode F (2008) Giving feedback to trainees (online CPD module). Royal College of Psychiatrists. Available at: https://elearninghub .rcpsych.ac.uk/.

O'Leary D, McAvoy P, Wilson J (2010). Performance concerns in psychiatrists referred to the National Clinical Assessment Service. *The Psychiatrist*, 34: 371–5.

Parikh A, Mcreelis K, Hodges B (2001) Student feedback in problem based learning: a survey of 103 final year students across five Ontario medical schools. *Medical Education*, 35: 632–6.

Pendleton D, Schofield T, Tate P, et al. (1984) *The Consultation: An Approach to Teaching and Learning*. Oxford Medical Publications.

Pullen I, Loudon J (2006). Improving standards in clinical record-keeping. *Advances in Psychiatric Treatment*, 12: 280–6.

Raiman L, Antbring R, Mahmood A (2017) WhatsApp messenger as a tool to supplement medical education for medical students on clinical attachment. *BMC Medical Education*, 17: 7.

Ramani S, Krackov SK (2012) Twelve tips for giving feedback effectively in the clinical environment. *Medical Teacher*, 34: 787–91.

Rolfe I, McPherson J (1995) Formative assessment: how am I doing? *Lancet*, 345: 837–9.

Rose S (2020) Medical student education in the time of Covid-19. *JAMA*, 323: 2131–2.

Silverman J, Draper J, Kurtz S (1997) The Calgary–Cambridge approach to communication skills teaching II: the SET–GO method of descriptive feedback. *Education for General Practice*, 8: 16–23.

Veloski J, Boex JR, Grassberger J, Evans A, Wofson DB (2006) Systematic review of the literature on assessment, feedback, and physicians' clinical performance: BBEME Guide No. 7. *Medical Teacher*, 28: 118–28.

Willingham DB (1990) Effective feedback on written assignments, *Teaching of Psychology*, 17: 10–13.

Zhou Z, Mims T, Dugan A, et al. (2019) Randomized evaluation of videoconference meetings for medical students' mid-clerkship feedback sessions. *Western Journal of Emergency Medicine*, 20: 163–9.

The Postgraduate Curriculum and Assessment Programme in Psychiatry: The Underlying Principles

Gareth Holsgrove, Amit Malik and Dinesh Bhugra

Introduction

Assessment is a key part of the educational process. It directs learning and significantly influences the learners' behaviour. Not only can assessment form the basis for planning educational programmes, it can also enable learners and their teachers and mentors to check progress and attainment. However, the process of assessment has potential pitfalls, which are mainly due to the content and methods of assessment, the expertise of the assessors and the outcomes of assessment in respect to feedback and career progression. Issues connected with appeal procedures and feedback must form an integral part of the process so that both trainees and trainers/assessors can learn from it. Another key problem is the burden of assessment and the extent to which this impairs, rather than supports, good learning practices and takes time away from actual learning.

In this chapter, we summarize some characteristics of good practice in designing and carrying out assessments, and the way in which the assessment programme in psychiatry related to the curriculum, and the learners' journey through it, when significant changes were made just over a decade ago. However, it is helpful to set the context in which assessment in medicine was developing even further back in history than this. For example, at the beginning of the twentieth century, 'assessment' usually meant little more than formal examinations. Assessments in the workplace (which might previously have been carried out only occasionally and informally) are now widely used in medical education. In this chapter, we also look at the relationship of examinations and workplace-based assessments (WPBAs) to the curriculum. We outline their contribution to the overall assessment programme and explain how information from both sources can be integrated to monitor progress.

Recent Developments in Medical Education

The past 20 years have seen significant developments in medical education in the UK and elsewhere. In the UK, these began mainly with changes in undergraduate education and came about with the introduction of new curricula following the recommendations in *Tomorrow's Doctors*, published in 1993 by the General Medical Council (GMC 1993), and their implementation, which was facilitated by Kenneth Calman's Undergraduate Medical Curriculum Implementation Support Scheme (UMCISS). With the inception of the Postgraduate Medical Education and Training Board (PMETB) in 2003 (although it became fully functional only in 2005), many similar changes were introduced into postgraduate training. Prior to this, the GMC had regulated the undergraduate curricula, whilst postgraduate curricula (insofar as they existed at all) were in the domain of the medical Royal Colleges. However, in 2010 the PMETB became incorporated into the GMC, which then regulated both undergraduate and postgraduate training and assessments.

The PMETB, in order to support their changes in requirements and regulation regarding postgraduate medical curricula, published documents that set the standards for curricula and assessments (Southgate and Grant 2004; Grant et al. 2005). The standards themselves are summarized in Box 13.1.

Box 13.1 Summary of PMETB standards (PMETB 2008)

Curriculum purpose and development
Standard 1: The purpose of the curriculum must be stated, including linkages to previous and subsequent stages of the trainees' training and education. The appropriateness of the stated curriculum to the stage of learning and to the specialty in question must be described.

The assessment system must be fit for purpose
Standard 2: The overall purpose of the assessment system must be documented and in the public domain.

Content of the curriculum
Standard 3: The curriculum must set out the general, professional and specialty-specific content to be mastered, including:

- the acquisition of knowledge, skills and attitudes demonstrated through behaviours, and expertise;
- the recommendations on the sequencing of learning and experience should be provided, if appropriate; and
- the general professional content should include a statement about how *Good Medical Practice* is to be addressed.

The content of the assessment will be based on curricula for postgraduate training, which themselves are referenced to *Good Medical Practice*
Standard 4: Assessments must systematically sample the entire content, appropriate to the stage of training, with reference to the common and important clinical problems that the trainee will encounter in the workplace and to the wider base of knowledge, skills and attitudes demonstrated through behaviours that doctors require.

Managing curriculum implementation
Standard 5: Indication should be given of how curriculum implementation will be managed and assured locally and within approved programmes.

Model of learning
Standard 6: The curriculum must describe the model of learning appropriate to the specialty and stage of training.

Learning experiences
Standard 7: Recommended learning experiences must be described which allow a diversity of methods covering, at a minimum:

- learning from practice;
- opportunities for concentrated practice in skills and procedures;

- learning with peers;
- learning in formal situations inside and outside the department;
- personal study; and
- specific trainer/supervisor inputs.

Assessment system methods
Standard 8: The choice of assessment method(s) should be appropriate to the content and purpose of that element of the curriculum.

Supervision of the trainee
Standard 9: Mechanisms for supervision of the trainee should be set out.

Role of the assessor
Standard 10: Assessors/examiners will be recruited against criteria for performing the tasks they undertake.

Assessment feedback to the trainees
Standard 11: Assessments must provide relevant feedback to the trainees.

Standards for classification of trainees' performance/competence
Standard 12: The methods used to set standards for classification of trainees' performance/competence must be transparent and in the public domain.

Documentation will be standardized and accessible nationally
Standard 13: Documentation will record the results and consequences of assessments and the trainee's progress through the assessment system.

Curriculum review and updating
Standard 14: Plans for curriculum review, including curriculum evaluation and monitoring, must be set out.

Resources
Standard 15: Resources and infrastructure will be available to support trainee learning and assessment at all levels (national, deanery and local education provider).

Lay and patient involvement
Standard 16: There will be lay and patient input in the development and implementation of assessments.

Equality and diversity
Standard 17: The curriculum should state its compliance with equal opportunities and anti-discriminatory practice.

It became clear that all assessments needed to relate directly to the curriculum and that the assessment programme was integral to the curriculum. The PMETB expected post-graduate medical education bodies to produce curricula for its approval in which the assessment programme was fully integrated. To meet this obligation, the Royal College of Psychiatrists developed an entirely new Core and General Curriculum.

Mapping Assessments to the Curriculum
Mapping the assessment programme to the curriculum, which in turn is mapped to *Good Medical Practice* (GMC 2006), was a good way to satisfy PMETB Standard 4. Therefore, the

Core and General module of the new curriculum was constructed using headings from *Good Medical Practice*. This model then served as a template upon which almost all of the specialty and subspecialty modules were subsequently structured.

The Curriculum Framework

In the 1990s, there had been a number of national initiatives in the western hemisphere to define the roles (general categories of competencies) expected of doctors. Notable among these are the general competencies defined by the Accreditation Council for Graduate Medical Education (ACGME) in the USA, the Royal College of Surgeons and Physicians in Canada's CanMEDS model and the GMC's *Good Medical Practice* guidance in the UK. These three models all set out the broad roles within which various specialties needed to define competencies.

In the UK, the PMETB required that all medical Royal Colleges should map their curriculum framework to the *Good Medical Practice* domains set out by the GMC. For the sake of clarity and simplicity, the Royal College of Psychiatrists' curriculum for specialist training was based directly on the *Good Medical Practice* framework. However, *Good Medical Practice* was quite complicated and not really intended as the foundation for designing a curriculum, but rather as a guidance document, so mapping directly to this framework involved some problems. In the original version of *Good Medical Practice* there were four main domains and the content was organized in a hierarchical structure within each domain. Below the domain level is the subdomain, followed by major competency, aspect and, finally, supporting competencies.

Most of the major competencies have a number of aspects, and the supporting competencies for each aspect are set out under the headings of 'Knowledge', 'Skills' and 'Attitudes'. Table 13.1 shows just one branch from the first of the *Good Medical Practice* domains ('Good clinical care') down to one of the supporting competencies, listed as 'Knowledge'.

The Core and General module ran throughout the six years of specialist training in psychiatry (at the time this was ST1–ST6, which has now changed to CT1–3 (core training) and ST4–6 (specialist training)). It was necessary to indicate the developing competencies throughout training because, in most instances, a specialty registrar in ST1 would be performing at a lower level of expertise than one approaching the end of their training. The College Curriculum Group decided to do this by placing the developing competencies in three categories ('Under supervision', 'Competent' and 'Mastery') and to use a colour code to indicate the stage of training in which different levels of performance should be achieved: red indicated specialist training stage 1 (ST1); gold, ST2 and ST3; violet, ST4 and ST5; and green, ST6.

Developing an Assessment Programme

In developing an assessment programme that follows modern principles and is integrated into the curriculum, a variety of issues needed to be considered such as the purpose and psychometric properties of assessments, their blueprinting and their utility (Wass et al. 2001). We consider each of these in the next three sections.

Purpose of Assessments

Each assessment should be considered in the context of its assessment programme, and the PMETB required that the purpose of an assessment be explicit (Southgate and Grant 2004).

Table 13.1 Mapping curriculum competencies to aspects of *Good Medical Practice* domains

Curriculum hierarchy	Competency
Domain from *Good Medical Practice*	Providing good clinical care
Subdomain from *Good Medical Practice*	Providing a good standard of practice and care
Major competency	Undertaking clinical assessment of patients with mental health problems
Aspect of major competency	Consultation
Supporting competency (knowledge)	Psychiatrists apply knowledge of specific techniques and methods that facilitate effective and empathic communication between the psychiatrist, patient, carers, colleagues and the wider healthcare system, including: acknowledgement of diversity relating to age, gender, race, culture, disability, spirituality and sexuality

Assessments should be educational and formative (i.e., providing educational feedback) (Wass et al. 2001), particularly since we know that assessment is the most important driver of learning (Newble and Jaeger 1983).

However, within a programme such as specialist medical training, assessments also need to have a summative or pass–fail function. The same assessment tool can often be used for both a summative and a formative purpose, but it is very important that this should be made clear at the outset (Crossley et al. 2002a).

In the College curriculum, WPBAs have a predominantly formative function (discussed in greater detail below). The Member of the Royal College of Psychiatrists (MRCPsych) examination, of course, forms the backbone of the summative assessments in postgraduate psychiatric training. The MRCPsych examination will remain mandatory for trainees to progress, complete their training and obtain their certificate of completion of training (CCT).

Blueprinting

As we have noted, assessment is the most powerful driver of learning in medical education. To a considerable extent, this is probably because trainees feel burdened by their workload and focus on learning only what is assessed. Therefore, it is reasonable to require that assessments validate the outcomes set by the curriculum. To achieve this, test content should be planned with reference to the learning objectives (the College uses the more recent Intended Learning Outcomes framework now) – a process known as blueprinting (Wass et al. 2001). A blueprint is a matrix in which the test designer determines how many items/tasks are to be assessed for each subject or category. Then, all the outcomes to be measured are explicitly stated in the blueprint, thus allowing an assessment programme to be developed that contains and utilizes appropriate types of assessment method in the varying clinical settings (Crossley et al. 2002a). Inadequate blueprinting of assessments raises concerns about the validity of an assessment programme. The intricate relationship between the various aspects of clinical competence and the characteristics of different assessment instruments means that multiple forms of tests should be used, particularly for high-stakes summative assessments.

Although not explicitly stated in the PMETB principles and standards documents (Southgate and Grant 2004; Grant et al. 2005), there was a clear expectation that the assessment programme will feature WPBAs as well as formal, national examinations.

However, the assessment programme was designed in such a way that much of the curriculum could be assessed both in the workplace and in the MRCPsych examination. Table 13.2 shows the assessment matrix for 'Consultation', for which the place in the curriculum hierarchy was illustrated in Table 13.1. The assessment matrix shows that consultation skills can be assessed in the workplace using assessment of clinical expertise (ACE), case-based discussion (CbD), case presentation (CP) and the mini-assessed clinical encounter (mini-ACE). It can also be assessed in the MRCPsych in the objective structured clinical examination (OSCE).

Utility of Assessments

Utility has been defined as a multiplicative function of reliability, validity, educational impact, acceptability and cost, with different weights attributed to each (van der Vleuten 1996). As most of these elements cannot be quantified, this is a purely conceptual model and not a psychometric index. However, it does highlight the trade-offs involved in assessments, which are always necessary because perfect utility is a Utopian concept (van der Vleuten 1996). In reality, those responsible for the assessments must give different weights to the different component variables of utility, depending on the context and the purpose of the assessment (van der Vleuten and Schuwirth 2005). In this model, the relationship between all of the variables has deliberately been kept multiplicative so that if one of the elements is zero then the utility will be zero. Let us consider each variable.

Reliability

Reliability is the technical term that describes the extent to which the results of an assessment reflect all possible measurements of the same construct (Crossley et al. 2002b). It is the property of assessment data that refers to how much the results of an assessment can be reproduced (van der Vleuten and Schuwirth 2005). It is important because all stakeholders involved must have confidence in its results. To achieve this, the results must be accurate and reproducible and are therefore likely to be reliable.

The internal consistency of an assessment is usually expressed as a coefficient (Cronbach's α) with values ranging from 0 to 1. This is just one of the estimations of error, but it includes aspects of other error sources and can be calculated using SPSS software (a standard platform of the assessment analyst). This makes Cronbach's α convenient, and it has proved very useful for many years to developers of tests; it still remains the most common contemporary measure. An α value of 0.8 is regarded as the minimum acceptable value, but this acceptability really depends on the purpose of the examination (van der Vleuten and Schuwirth 2005). Generally speaking, the higher the stakes in an examination, the greater the reliability should be, and for some years $\alpha = 0.90$ has been regarded as the gold standard for high-stakes examinations. In practical terms, however, because of their formative/summative characteristics and (if they are appropriately designed

Table 13.2 Assessment of consultation skills

	Workplace-based assessment methods									MRCPsych assessment		
	Assessment of clinical expertise (ACE)	Assessment of teaching (AoT)	Case-based discussion (CbD)	Case presentation (CP)	Direct observation of procedural skills (DOPS)	Journal club presentation (JCP)	Mini-assessed clinical encounter (mini-ACE)	Mini-peer assessment tool (mini-PAT)	Team assessment of behaviour (TAB)	Multiple choice questions (MCQs)	Extended matching questions (EMQs)	Objective structured clinical examination (OSCE)
	X	X	X	X			X					X

and utilized) high validity, a reliability coefficient below 0.8 would often be acceptable for WPBAs. This is an example of the utility trade-offs mentioned in the preceding section.

Moreover, work by Schuwirth and van der Vleuten, who are in the vanguard of assessment in medical education, challenged our assumptions on assessments and the interpretation of the results. They questioned the value of relying solely on strict psycho-metric tools such as reliability and validity to interpret modern assessment methods such as WPBAs (van der Vleuten and Schuwirth 2006).

However, it was recognized that achieving good reliability in assessments in medical education poses two particular challenges. Crossley and colleagues discuss these in more detail, pointing out that the professional role of a doctor comprises complex behaviour and is highly dependent on the characteristics of the problem at hand (Crossley et al. 2002b). The classical approach to statistical support for assessments, which includes the calculation of Cronbach's α, calculates the components of reliability one by one, and the most important of these components are summarized below. However, in recent years an extension of classical theory has become more prominent and Lee Cronbach himself has endorsed it (Cronbach 2004).

Crossley and colleagues (2002b) introduce this *generalizability theory* particularly well. Essentially, the theory quantifies all the sources of error simultaneously. These sources include errors within and between the assessed and the assessors, as well as the random errors that occur in all assessments. Moreover, and of special interest to test developers, it utilizes mathematical modelling to predict the generalizability coefficient (G) from a number of different simulations (such as changing the number and duration of assessments or using different numbers of assessors) based on pilot data.

The number of variables involved allows us to see that the reliability of WPBAs is subject to many challenges. These might include the following.

Interrater Reliability

This refers to the extent that different assessors observing the same thing will make similar (or dissimilar) assessments. Some authorities claim that interrater reliability is the single most important component of reliability where direct ratings are used (as opposed, for example, to computer-marking in MCQs). Poor interrater reliability is a common and potentially serious problem in assessments – particularly in some oral and essay-type examinations. However, interrater reliability can be improved, often to a considerable extent, by assessor training and by using structured assessment instruments. The crucial factor in assessing a doctor's competence is adequate sampling of their performance across different patients by different examiners. This has been found to have a greater impact on reliability than standardization (van der Vleuten and Schuwirth 2005). Therefore, the most straightforward way to increase interrater reliability is to use a reasonably large number of observers and patients/cases.

Case Specificity

This is also known as domain or content specificity, and the reliability of assessment outcomes is more dependent on what is being assessed rather than on how (van der Vleuten 1996), particularly if a number of cases are assessed by different assessors. This implies that a trainee may perform differently when assessed for the same competency in different clinical contexts or with different cases, thus affecting the reliability of clinical assessment. Just as with interrater reliability, the simplest way to overcome this problem is to increase the number of cases used to assess a competency; but this too is handicapped by feasibility and cost. Also, it is important to use predominantly cases of medium difficulty for the group of trainees being assessed (Downing and Haladyna 2004) because these tend to be the best discriminators between those who have reached the required standard and those who have not.

Intrarater Reliability

This recognizes that the same trainee, when assessed for the same competency in the same clinical context and by the same assessor, can perform differently on different occasions. This could be due to a variety of factors intrinsic to the trainee, the assessor or external factors. The reliability issues in this situation can, once again, be addressed by using multiple assessments that form the basis of the overall assessment of a competency. In other words, we can think of an assessment programme as a mosaic, gradually building up a picture of progress and attainment, rather than the single snapshot over a short timescale that tends to occur in the examination hall.

These issues of reliability, along with systemic bias (e.g., gender, ethnicity, age), are important factors that affect reliability in assessment scores. Yet their effects can be reduced by a number of strategies.

Validity

Validity is a complex matter, with many aspects. Put simply, it is a measure of how thoroughly, accurately and appropriately a test measures what it purports to measure (Brown and Doshi 2006). Messick (1995) defines validity as 'the degree to which empirical evidence and theoretical rationales support the adequacy and appropriateness of inferences and actions based on test scores or other models of assessment'.

Reliability, of course, is a prerequisite for validity (since if an assessment is not reliable it cannot be valid) and high reliability allows for a greater measure of validity. However, this does not mean that high reliability alone is sufficient to demonstrate validity (Streiner and Norman 2003). On the other hand, it is of course pointless to design a reliable assessment that has no validity.

Although a complicated issue, validity has traditionally been classified into five aspects: face, content, construct, criterion and, more recently, consequential validity. Criterion validity is further divided into predictive and concurrent validity. We can summarize validity to mean that we are reliably assessing the right things in the right way, using the right people, and are having a positive effect on learning, behaviour, professional development and outcome.

There have been criticisms of some of the technical aspects of validity. For example, Streiner and Norman (2003) discuss the concept of face validity ('Does a test appear to assess what it claims to?'). In response to these challenges, the College is aiming to collect evidence of the validity of their assessment programme from a wide variety of sources and to use appropriate blueprinting of the curriculum's assessments to support the content validity of the assessment framework.

Predictive validity studies using longitudinal data (e.g., WPBAs predicting clinical and/ or examination performance) are invaluable when establishing the long-term credibility of the assessment framework. Focus groups, qualitative studies and survey questionnaires also need to be considered in order to assess the consequential validity (educational impact) of the assessment framework.

Feasibility

This is a particular issue with WPBAs and it needs to be evaluated in respect of the various clinical settings and the number of assessors. More contemporarily, it must be evaluated with different types of assessors (e.g., senior doctors, other healthcare workers, patients, carers, simulated patients).

There are major and specific concerns regarding the feasibility of WPBAs, including such practical matters as assessor and trainee fatigue, yet it is also recognized that certain trainees, in some specific areas of their work, require more assessment than others. To minimize potential disruption, a framework should be developed to give guidance on how much assessment is enough to ensure confidence in the outcome of the training (the delivery and assessment process). Not only is there a danger of having too many assessments, it is also important that time is provided for assessments to take place. Above all, it has to be accepted that this is a huge cultural change in the delivery and assessment of postgraduate medical education and its overall assimilation into the in-service training system will take time to be properly implemented and researched.

In any system, logistical issues need to be considered such as assessor training, automating the processing and reporting results. and good local administration strategies are essential.

Acceptability

For the assessment programme to be successful, the framework must be acceptable to all concerned – particularly the assessors and the trainees. For example, assessors might not properly administer a potentially highly valid and reliable assessment instrument if they were not convinced of its educational value. Neither were they likely to correctly use assessment instruments that significantly limited their freedom to employ their professional judgement.

First, the assessors needed to understand information about the relevance of a particular domain and the ability of the assessment tool to assess it effectively as part of the overall assessment framework. Second, it was important for the test designers to listen to the feedback from the assessors and take this into account. This required that the acceptability of the assessment instruments and the curriculum framework was evaluated on an ongoing basis; that the key concerns, principal benefits, reliability and validity were identified; and that this information was properly disseminated and acted upon.

Educational Impact

The educational impact of assessment is technically known as consequential validity.

Trainees who already feel burdened (maybe over-burdened) by the pressures of clinical work – being on-call, attending courses, participating in audits, giving presentations – are almost certain to concentrate their learning efforts on what is being assessed. Therefore, assessment can be a powerful driver of learning. In fact, 'assessment is usually the most powerful factor in the entire curriculum, because it determines the real curriculum, the one which the students follow, rather than the one which the faculty may intend or believe that they follow' (Holsgrove 1997a: p. 182).

There are a variety of ways in which assessment can influence learning. These include the content (blueprinting), the format, the feedback, the scheduling (van der Vleuten 1996) and the consequences of failure (van der Vleuten and Schuwirth 2006). Not only are students likely to learn topics that are assessed, they are more likely to learn and practice well those topics that are assessed more thoroughly or frequently, or to which the most importance is attached. For these same reasons, assessments can also have unexpected and unintended negative effects – for example, by focusing on trivia while ignoring the essentials.

To make the best use of assessment, it is best practice to use multiple formats of assessment within an assessment programme. It is important that each format is validated for a particular purpose. For example, MCQs have been traditionally used to test knowledge (typically, straightforward factual recall) but, when based on a clinical scenario, they can also be used to test clinical reasoning and the application of knowledge.

Cost-effectiveness

This is an important point because good assessments are expensive to develop, deliver and quality assure. Assessor training takes time and money – and medical education in the UK is usually short of both. Therefore, it is important that adequate funds are identified at the beginning for development, implementation and quality assurance of the assessment programme. However, besides the development and quality assurance costs there are hidden costs such as the assessor's time, trainee's time and administrative costs. These should all be identified and made explicit.

There is also a broader question of who pays for assessments – trainees, trusts, deaneries, etc. In the curriculum project described here, the College bore the initial costs of developing many of the assessment instruments for both WPBAs and the MRCPsych examinations. This includes piloting them and developing the electronic portal for WPBAs.

The Royal College of Psychiatrists' Assessment Programme

The College's assessment programme has been designed to determine or contribute to a number of different functions, all concerned with progression of a trainee towards achieving specialist registration as a psychiatrist.

Purposes of the Assessment Programme

At the most basic, but extremely important, level, the assessment programme provides information to help the trainee and trainer to identify areas of strength and those aspects where further input and support are required. These latter aspects are mainly identified through WPBAs, and this is why it is so important for trainees to undertake WPBAs early in each phase of training

The programme of WPBAs was envisaged not only to lead to eligibility to sit the MRCPsych examinations, but also help the trainees to prepare to succeed when reaching these important professional milestones. Both the WPBAs and the MRCPsych examination were to contribute to the annual review of competency progression (ARCP) process, which will determine whether trainees can proceed to the next stage of their training.

Workplace-Based Assessments

Ten WPBA methods were identified and became the subject of literature reviews and practical experience in the pilot studies. These methods are discussed in detail in *Workplace-Based Assessments in Psychiatry* (Bhugra 2007) and the pilot studies are also reported in the same book (Brittlebank 2007). The function of WPBAs in the College curriculum was designed to be predominantly (but not exclusively) formative, to assist with planning educational programmes and to provide the feedback on progress and attainment that is essential to both trainees and their supervisors. However, there are also certain requirements for successfully completing WPBAs before progressing to the next stage of training or being eligible to take the MRCPsych.

The MRCPsych Examination

The MRCPsych examination, the backbone of summative assessment in the curriculum, has been redesigned several times since this paper was first written. The content of the examination is determined by the curriculum, of course, and the examination methods have been selected according to three principles:

- they must supplement the WPBAs in sampling across the whole curriculum;
- they must have the high degree of reliability (accuracy and internal consistency) that contemporary best practice demands;
- they should be predominantly computer-marked to reduce the administrative workload (which for the 'old' MRCPsych examination was massive), to improve reliability by reducing the potential effects of different examiners awarding different marks for a similar standard of work and to enable marks to be agreed and notified to candidates quickly after the examination.

The new examination (in 2009) comprised four elements (three written papers and one clinical practical) and used just three examination methods. These methods were well established and thoroughly validated and have been discussed elsewhere (e.g., Holsgrove 1997b, c, d). The three written papers (Papers 1, 2 and 3) used a combination of MCQs using the single-best-answer format, and extended matching questions (EMQs; also called extended matching items – EMIs). On successfully passing all three written papers, candidates were permitted to sit the fourth part, the extended objective structured clinical examination (OSCE).

Subsequent Developments

Since the PMETB approval for its curriculum and assessment programme was given almost two decades ago there have of course been further developments.

The MRCPsych examination was amended in 2015 to two written papers, A and B, and a practical examination, the Clinical Assessment of Skills and Competencies (CASC). The curricula have been reformulated in the last two years to incorporate the GMC professional capabilities framework which began to be introduced in 2017 (www.gmc-uk.org/education/standards-guidance-and-curricula/standards-and-outcomes/generic-professional-capabilities-framework). This new curriculum is being introduced at the time of publication. Further changes to the examination were made as a result of the pandemic and these are reviewed by Greening et al. in Chapter 2.

The MRCPsych examination will undoubtedly continue to be fine-tuned on the basis of piloting, examiner experience and psychometric analysis. Therefore the College curriculum and its programme of WPBAs and the MRCPsych examinations will continue to be seen as work in progress.

Acknowledgements

The authors acknowledge financial support from the Department of Health via the National Institute for Health Research (NIHR) Specialist Biomedical Research Centre for Mental Health award to the South London and Maudsley NHS Foundation Trust and the Institute of Psychiatry at King's College London.

References

Bhugra D, Malik A, Brown N (eds.) (2007) *Workplace-Based Assessments in Psychiatry.* RCPsych Publications.

Brittlebank A (2007) Piloting workplace-based assessment in psychiatry. In D Bhugra, A Malik, N Brown (eds.), *Workplace-Based Assessments in Psychiatry.* RCPsych Publications, pp 96–108.

Brown N, Doshi M (2006) Assessing professional and clinical competence: the way forward. *Advances in Psychiatric Treatment,* **12**: 81–91.

Cronbach L (2004) My current thoughts on coefficient alpha and successor procedures. *Educational and Psychological Measurement,* **64**: 391–418.

Crossley J, Humphris G, Jolly B (2002a) Assessing health professionals. *Medical Education,* **36**: 800–4.

Crossley J, Davies H, Humphris G, et al. (2002b) Generalisability: a key to unlock professional assessment. *Medical Education,* **36**: 972–8.

Downing SM (2003) Validity: on the meaningful interpretation of assessment data. *Medical Education,* **37**: 1–8.

Downing SM, Haladyna TM (2004) Validity threats: overcoming interference with proposed interpretations of assessment data. *Medical Education,* **38**: 327–33.

GMC(1993) *Tomorrow's Doctors.* General Medical Council.

GMC (2006) *Good Medical Practice.* General Medical Council.

Grant J, Fox S, Kumar N, et al. (2005) *Standards for Curricula.* Postgraduate Medical Education and Training Board.

Holsgrove G (1997a) The purpose of assessing medical students. In C Whitehouse, M Roland, P Campion (eds.), *Teaching Medicine in the Community: A Guide for Undergraduate Education.* Oxford University Press, pp. 179–82.

Holsgrove G (1997b) Principles of assessment. In C Whitehouse, M Roland, P Campion (eds.), *Teaching Medicine in the Community: A Guide for Undergraduate Education.* Oxford University Press, pp. 183–5.

Holsgrove G (1997c) Assessing knowledge. In C Whitehouse, M Roland, P Campion (eds.), *Teaching Medicine in the Community: A Guide for Undergraduate Education.* Oxford University Press, pp. 186–94.

Holsgrove G (1997d) Assessing clinical skills. In C Whitehouse, M Roland, P Campion (eds.), *Teaching Medicine in the Community: A Guide for Undergraduate Education.* Oxford University Press, pp. 195–7.

Messick S (1995) Standards of validity and the validity of standards in performance assessment. *Educational Measure: Issues Practice,* **14**: 5–8.

Newble DI, Jaeger K (1983) The effect of assessments and examinations on the learning of medical students. *Medical Education,* **17**: 165–71.

PMETB (2006) *Quality Assurance, Quality Management and Assessment System Guidance (Revised).* Postgraduate Medical Education and Training Board. Available at: www.pmetb.org.uk/fileadmin/user/QA/Assessment/QAQMASG_New.pdf.

PMETB (2008) *Standards for Curricula and Assessment Systems*. Postgraduate Medical Education and Training Board.

Southgate L, Grant J (2004) *Principles for an Assessment System for Postgraduate Medical Training*. Postgraduate Medical Education and Training Board.

Streiner DL, Norman GR (2003) *Health Measurement Scales*, 3rd edn. Oxford University Press.

van der Vleuten CP (1996) The assessment of professional competence: developments, research and practical implications.

Advances. *Health Sciences Education*, 1: 41–67.

van der Vleuten CP, Schuwirth LW (2005) Assessing professional competence: from methods to programmes. *Medical Education*, **39**: 309–17.

van der Vleuten CP, Schuwirth LW (2006) *How to Design a Useful Test: The Principles of Assessment. Understanding Medical Education*. Association for the Study of Medical Education.

Wass V, van der Vleuten CP, Shatzer J, et al. (2001) Assessment of clinical competence. *Lancet*, **357**: 945–9.

Supervision of Psychiatric Trainees

David Cottrell

Introduction

Doctors in training do their learning 'on the job'. Supervision in the workplace has a key role in ensuring patient safety and promoting professional development as part of this learning process. These twin elements are critical to understanding good supervision. If trainees are learning in their workplace, there must be systems in place to ensure they do not make mistakes that affect patient safety, but at the same time support them in learning new skills.

This chapter discusses the supervision of trainee psychiatrists and is based on an article first published in 1999 (Cottrell 1999). It is gratifying to note the many significant and positive changes in the organization of supervision that have taken place since that date. In 1999, the Royal College of Psychiatrists had responsibility for approving training schemes and specified that each trainee should have a 'protected hour per week' with his or her educational supervisor. This time should belong 'exclusively' to the trainee and be 'for the benefit of the trainee'. Training consultants, as they were then known, were expected to be 'readily available' to trainees, and to provide a 'regular, weekly, timetabled supervision session'.

Whilst supervision was clearly perceived as a key activity, there was a marked lack of clarity as to what constituted good and effective supervision and few opportunities for learning how to supervise. Today, we have clear standards for what constitutes adequate supervision and structures in place to ensure that it is delivered as intended. The General Medical Council (GMC) rather than the College now has responsibility for standards setting and regulation of supervision, and there is a new section in this chapter briefly summarizing how the governance and regulation of supervision now works.

The evidence for the effectiveness of supervision, the characteristics of good supervision and the implications of this evidence for UK practice have been well summarized (Kilminster et al. 2007; Kilminster and Cottrell 2013). There is good evidence that supervision has a positive effect on patient safety and that good supervision is dependent on characteristics such as the quality of the supervisory relationship, frequent constructive feedback, direct supervision with trainee and trainer working together so that the trainee can be directly observed and structured supervision with regular, timetabled meetings and agreed learning objectives.

There is also general agreement about the purposes and functions of supervision (Box 14.1).

Nevertheless, despite this increasing consensus, trainees and trainers still struggle with how to create supervisory relationships that deliver these dual goals of patient safety and professional development.

> **Box 14.1** The functions and purposes of supervision (Health Education England 2019)
>
> **Good Supervision has three main functions:**
>
> - **Normative:** Ensuring that the supervisee can provide high-quality patient care
> - **Formative:** Learning in the workplace occurs through good supervision, with high-quality timely feedback to the supervisee from a senior professional fundamental to this learning
> - **Restorative:** Good supervision enhances the wellbeing of the supervisee
>
> **The purpose of supervision is to:**
>
> - Enable the progression of healthcare professionals along a training and/or professional development pathway with respect to acquisition of knowledge, clinical skills and competencies
> - Enhance general (clinical) and professional skills and attitudes
> - Ensure both good patient experience and safety

Governance and Regulation of Supervision

With greater recognition of the critical role of supervision has come greater regulation and quality assurance. The GMC now sets the standards and requirements for the delivery of all stages of medical education and training in the UK. Its publication *Promoting Excellence: Standards for Medical Education and Training.* (GMC 2015) sets out standards for supervision under five themes:

- learning environment and culture;
- educational governance and leadership;
- supporting learners;
- supporting educators; and
- developing and implementing curricula and assessments.

Briefly, these themes require that the environment must be safe for patients, supportive for learners and educators and support and value education; that there is measurement of educational outcomes and systems in place for quality improvement; that learners receive both educational and pastoral support; that educators are selected, trained and supported; and that assessments are implemented that enable demonstration of learning outcomes having been met.

In England, and local education and training boards (LETBs, the 13 regional structures in the health education and training system of the National Health Service (NHS) in England) and their constituent postgraduate deaneries work with local educational providers (LEPs, i.e., places where doctors in training work such as NHS trusts, primary care settings etc.) to ensure these GMC standards are met.

The GMC distinguishes between clinical supervisors who oversee trainees in a placement on a day-to-day basis and educational supervisors who are responsible for overseeing a trainee's progress over a period of time and across placements. Health Education England suggests a third category of workplace supervisor, who takes responsibility on any particular shift where the clinical supervisor is not present and who may be any competent member of the clinical team (Health Education England, 2019).

Box 14.2 GMC criteria for trainer recognition

1. Ensuring safe and effective patient care through training
2. Establishing and maintaining an environment for learning
3. Teaching and facilitating learning
4. Enhancing learning through assessment
5. Supporting and monitoring educational progress
6. Guiding personal and professional development
7. Continuing professional development as an educator

Training programme directors take responsibility for leading and coordinating the training of specialty trainees within a specialty training programme. In the important task of recognizing and approving trainers, the GMC uses criteria drawn from the Academy of Medical Educators' 2014 guidance on Professional standards for medical, dental and veterinary educators (Academy of Medical Educators 2014); see Box 14.2.

Effective Supervisors

Evidence suggests that effective supervisors have good interpersonal skills, are seen as clinically competent and engage in 'helpful' supervisory behaviours such as giving direct guidance on clinical work, linking theory and practice, engaging in joint problem solving, providing positive and constructive feedback, being reassuring and providing a role model (Kilminster et al. 2007). The evidence also supports the need for supervision to be organized and managed.

Psychiatric trainees are adult learners and bring with them to their training a wide range of past experience, learning abilities and styles. The motivation of adult learners is often stronger and their learning more purposeful than in earlier years. They want to learn in order to pursue a particular self-chosen outcome, and therefore require meaning and relevance in what is taught. They want active involvement in the learning process and usually expect clear goals and objectives and require feedback and time for reflection. Training against this background has to manage a constant tension between a respect for the autonomy of trainees as mature adults and the need for the trainer to specify particular learning objectives as part of the requirements for the successful completion of training. Some knowledge of educational theory with respect to styles and processes of learning is helpful for supervisors. Educational theories of supervision are often rooted in cognitive and social learning theories and so are likely to be familiar to psychiatrists.

Appraisal and assessment are also key skills for the effective supervisor but can sometimes be misunderstood. Traditionally, appraisal has been seen as being primarily for educational purposes, is usually confidential and is designed to assist the progress of the learner. It is focused on the trainee and his or her needs and is designed to make training and learning more efficient and effective.

Assessment is concerned with career regulation and the measurement of the trainee against pre-agreed standards. It leads to decisions about career progress and therefore is not confidential. Managing the tension between these two conflicting demands can be difficult and requires all of the skills of effective supervisors described above.

Structure and Content of Supervision

Much of what has gone before would be applicable to trainees in any medical specialty. But from here on, the focus is on psychiatry supervision and the weekly supervision by the clinical supervisor in psychiatric placements. Direct supervision in such settings is less common. In surgical training, for example, direct observation and supervision of practical procedures is essential to ensure safe practice whilst skills are learnt. Psychiatric supervision of clinical work can be direct but most often involves face-to-face discussion of cases after the event.

Supervision will always be different for each trainer/trainee pair, at different stages of training, and will differ from one session to the next according to the needs of training. The suggestions about the structure and content of supervision which follow are drawn from my own experience of being supervised and being a supervisor, but also from the published literature on good supervision, including surveys of trainer and trainee views about supervision.

Structure

Whilst all supervision experiences will differ, they cannot be effective without a clear structure and explicit aims and objectives. Six key elements of the supervisory structure are discussed below.

(i) Ground Rules

It is essential that ground rules should be agreed for supervision in the early stages of the supervisory relationship. These should clarify what it is appropriate to discuss, what the trainer and trainee expect of each other and what to do if urgent problems require discussion between supervision sessions. The boundaries of confidentiality must be established at the outset. It is essential that supervision sessions cover areas of difficulty for the trainee. This is more likely to happen if trainees know which aspects of their discussions will be confidential and used for appraisal purposes, and which will contribute to formal assessment reports. There must be clarity about, for example, what might be shared with an educational supervisor, or about the fact that the clinical supervisor may wish to examine the trainees medical note keeping. Supervisors need to remember that their supervision may be discussed by the trainee with the educational supervisor or training programme director.

However, trainees and trainers need to be aware that no confidentiality agreements are absolute. From time to time the trainer may become aware of behaviour or performance which has to be shared with others, irrespective of the trainee's wishes, for example behaviour likely to cause significant harm to patients. In these situations, it is good practice for trainees to be told exactly what the concerns are, and with whom they are being shared, before any third party is involved. It can be helpful if a written contract is drawn up specifying what has been agreed concerning timing, ground rules and content of supervision. This will make dealing with any subsequent difficulties in the supervision process much easier.

(ii) Timing

One hour of individual supervision per week is usually seen as the irreducible minimum. This should happen at a regular time and in a fixed place each week. The time should be protected as far as is possible from interruptions by bleeps, telephone calls and the demands of colleagues and patients. The creation of such a predictable space for supervision helps to contain trainee anxieties and is likely to reduce demands from trainees for additional supervision time. If a trainee knows that supervision will be available at a particular time, the need for advice, help and support can usually be delayed until that time. However, arrangements need to be in place concerning how trainees can access support in a crisis and cannot wait until the next supervision session

Although supervision should usually be on an individual basis, there are occasions when other models may be useful. If a trainer is supervising two trainees at the same grade, there may be occasions when joint supervision, with the opportunities this affords for sharing experiences, may be appropriate. If this does occur, sessions would need to be longer than the usual one hour per week. There would also have to be agreed mechanisms for either of the trainees to see the trainer individually if the need arose. Joint supervision is probably not helpful for supervising two trainees at different levels of training except for occasional sessions with specific objectives, for example discussing the supervision of a specialty trainee by a specialty registrar.

(iii) Flexibility

Trainees will vary in past experience and, therefore, in current training needs. Clinical supervisors and placements will differ with respect to the training opportunities that they can offer. The first one or two supervision sessions in a placement should, therefore, include a review of the trainee's prior training with a view to identifying gaps in experience and matching these to training opportunities in the forthcoming placement.

Thereafter, supervision sessions should be trainee-led as far as is possible. Trainees should be encouraged to come to supervision with an agenda of topics that they wish to be discussed. The supervisor should monitor the content of supervision over time and ensure that there is a good balance of the various subjects that need to be discussed (see below). The exact frequency of discussion of any one case or topic, and the depth of that discussion, will depend on the particular trainee's experience.

(iv) Learning Outcomes and Their Assessment

Agreed curricula, set by the College, will dictate clear learning objectives and outcomes for trainees and the stage of career at which these should be met. If trainees are to achieve all the learning outcomes within the time available and be awarded a certificate of completion of training (CCT), then training needs to be organized and managed. The annual review of competency progression (ARCP) is a requirement for all doctors in training. It is a summative assessment that checks the trainee meets the requirements necessary to progress to the next stage of training and for GMC revalidation, and it also ensures patient safety.

The most recent ARCP will inform the learning outcomes set at the beginning of a new placement. Trainees will arrive in placement with specific training needs identified for that placement and it is essential that these are discussed at the beginning of the placement, and agreement reached that the placement can provide the opportunities needed to meet these learning needs. It is not enough for trainers to just offer trainees experience of the generality of what happens in the placement. Instead, particular aspects of that placement will need to be singled out to meet training needs, and other areas not used for training at all.

Trainees are then expected to keep their e-portfolios up to date with a record of their training experience during the placement. Supervisors are expected to carry out a series of workplace-based assessments (WPBAs) during the placement. These are intended to focus on performance and be evidence-based (with evidence triangulated where possible). A wide range of these assessments (case-based discussions, journal-club presentations) have been incorporated into the training portfolios for psychiatric trainees. WPBAs are largely formative and form a basis for giving constructive feedback, and they can be very useful discussion topics in supervision sessions. However, a certain number are taken into account in the ARCP and so also have a summative function. In addition, a set number of WPBAs need to have been completed in order to enter for the College examinations. WPBAs are discussed in greater detail in Chapters 3, 12 and 13.

(v) Record-Keeping

Trainees should maintain and bring to supervision an up-to-date list of their current cases and the case notes of any patient that they wish to discuss, as well as the means to access logbooks and e-portfolios. They should also keep notes of any decisions reached in supervision and, if these concern patient care, record these in the patients' notes.

Clinical supervisors should also keep their own list of the trainee's cases to assist them in helping the trainee to monitor their workload and should always know how many ongoing cases their trainee has at any one time. Trainers should also make notes about cases which are discussed so that they can: (a) monitor whether any cases have not been discussed for too long; and (b) remind themselves of previous discussions when cases are reviewed again. In the fortunately rare event of serious concerns about a particular trainee, or about standards of patient care, the existence of accurate and contemporaneous records is essential.

(vi) Liaison with the Educational Supervisor and Programme Director

It is important for the trainee and clinical supervisor trainer to be clear about the boundaries of supervision. It is usually impossible for any one consultant trainer to provide supervision to meet all of a trainee's needs. Who provides training and supervision is less important than the fact that there is a clearly organized system which takes all trainees' needs into account and does not allow important areas to be neglected because everyone thinks that area is someone else's responsibility.

Clinical supervisors should review all of the areas described below with their trainee and ensure that if they are not providing supervision, others are. There needs to be clarity and agreement about what the intended learning outcomes are for the current placement, what has been achieved already and what can be left for subsequent placements. Liaison with the educational supervisor and training programme director about the totality of supervision and training will be essential. Difficulties within the supervision relationship should be resolved internally as far as is possible. However, every training programme should ensure that there is a way for trainees who are having difficulties in supervision to have access to outside help when needed. This might be via the educational supervisor, the training programme director or perhaps another consultant designated specifically for this purpose.

Content of Supervision

This is the most difficult aspect of supervision to specify. If the structures outlined above are in place, trainers and trainees should have a good idea of what needs to be discussed in supervision. The exact content will vary according to the needs of the trainee, the skills of the supervisor and the opportunities within the placement. It should include the following broad topics.

(i) Clinical Management

- Setting and regular review of learning outcomes and priorities.
- A review of e-portfolio and discussion of workplace based assessments.
- Theoretical and practical management of cases. In particular, helping trainees to integrate theoretical and research knowledge into clinical practice. This should include an examination of a random selection of medical records to ensure that the trainee is competent in the essential task of keeping good records.
- Management of case loads.
- In-depth supervision of particular cases.
- Consideration of trainee career stage. With very senior trainees who are soon to be awarded their CCT, it may be helpful to agree that supervision will be relatively 'light-touch' for some cases, whilst still agreeing that advice will always be available if needed. This recognizes the seniority of the trainee and affords an opportunity for them to manage cases without regular supervision, a situation they will soon experience when they attain consultant status.
- Supervision for specific therapeutic modalities, for example, cognitive behavioural therapy.

(ii) Teaching and Research

- Teaching skills training.
- Discussion of the learning and supervision process – an important component of supervision is reflection, by trainer and trainee, on the process of supervision itself, and consideration of whether the supervision is meeting the needs of the trainee.
- Appraisal skills and the supervision of others.
- Research methodology teaching and research project supervision.

(iii) Management and Administration

- Management skills training and provision of knowledge regarding medical politics and National Health Service structures. It can be particularly helpful for the supervisor to share, when appropriate, details of management tasks that they are engaged in, and to invite trainees to 'shadow' them at management meetings.
- Issues concerned with the functioning of and working with multidisciplinary teams.

(iv) Pastoral Care

- Personal guidance and support. In particular, the supervisor has an obligation to bring up personal issues if he or she thinks they are affecting their trainee's capacity to work.
- Career guidance.

Finding Further Support

Although it will not be possible, or appropriate, for all trainers to offer supervision in all of the above areas personally, most supervisors should be able to provide some supervision or know a colleague who could help with a particular issue. Local courses may provide some training in teaching skills, but the consultant supervisor may still be able to provide supervision of a particular teaching engagement during a placement. Similarly, many schemes provide separate research supervisors for trainees, but this should not stop consultants pointing out and discussing relevant research in relation to clinical work.

Additional Training Experiences

In addition to the minimum, one hour per week of supervision, there are a number of other activities which contribute to the supervision process. Trainers should endeavour to provide some or all of the following during placements, depending upon the nature of the placement and the needs of the trainee:

- Opportunities for the trainee to observe the consultant working in a variety of different settings, including attendance at meetings or conferences with the consultant where appropriate.
- Observation, by the supervisor, of one session with a particular case, perhaps chosen by the trainee, as a way of providing more detailed supervision of complex cases. This might include live supervision of the trainee either individually or as part of a family therapy team, where appropriate.
- Joint work with the trainee.
- Opportunities for all of the above with other members of the team who have different skills to the consultant supervisor.

Emotional Aspects of Supervision

As a child psychiatrist who has researched into supervision, I have been struck by how most of the academic literature focuses on cognitive models of learning and professional development. These are critical to understanding supervisory processes, as highlighted above. However, I suspect they are necessary but not sufficient for effective supervision. Learning has been described as a form of 'becoming' and is more than just the acquisition of new facts and skills. Treading carefully, for fear of sounding patronizing to the adult learners who are supervised, I think there are potentially helpful parallels with parenting and child rearing.

Good parenting involves helping a young person acquire a wide range of behavioural skills with the aim of enabling them to move from relative dependence on the parent to achieve independence. This of course includes intellectual stimulation and providing the right kind of learning experiences to promote cognitive development. But it also includes the provision of warmth, affection and approval, the modelling of values and behaviour appropriate to the family's culture, continuity of care within a caring relationship and the graded opportunity and encouragement to acquire autonomy. It also includes monitoring, vigilance and protection from harm.

We have ample evidence that children who grow up in warm, caring and supportive relationships and who are praised for their achievements do well in life. Why should this not also be true of supervision?

We also have good evidence that those who have been well parented tend to make better parents. I am sure the same is true of supervision. The experience of being well supervised makes one a better supervisor. Fortunately for those who have not had this experience, supervision is still a skill that can be learnt.

One important implication of thinking about the links between parenting and supervision is the need to consider abuse. Children can be abused emotionally, physically or sexually and through neglect. Abuse is facilitated by the power imbalance between parent and child. Sadly, that same power imbalance in supervision can lead to all these forms of abuse within the supervisory relationship. All those involved with training of junior doctors and other healthcare students and professionals need to be alert to this possibility and know how to respond. Trainees and students must have information on how they can safely report any concerns about abuse and the reassurance that any reports will be taken seriously and acted on.

Conclusion

Supervision is one of the key mechanisms by which we train juniors doctors and enable them to become consultants. Over the last 20 years, much more interest has been taken in ensuring that supervisors are properly trained, and trainees are properly supervised. Research into supervision has highlighted characteristics of effective supervisors and supervision and this research can be used to help construct effective supervisory relationships. Nevertheless, at the heart of effective supervision there is still a largely individual relationship between two people working together to learn about and reflect on good psychiatric practice in order to deliver better care to patients. All parties in this endeavour need to be valued and supported in order to reach this important goal. Supervisors would do well to remember that part of helping their trainees to learn is to provide a warm and caring environment in which learning and good practice will thrive.

References

Academy of Medical Educators (2014) *Professional Standards*, 3rd ed. Academy of Medical Educators.

Cottrell D (1999) Supervision. *Advances in Psychiatric Treatment*, 5: 83–8.

GMC(2015) *Promoting Excellence: Standards for Medical Education and Training*. General Medical Council.

Health Education England (2019) *Enhancing Supervision for Postgraduate Doctors in Training*. Health Education England.

Available at: www.hee.nhs.uk/sites/default/files/documents/SupervisionReport_%20FINAL1.pdf.

Kilminster S, Cottrell D (2013) Educational supervision. In Walsh K (ed.). *Oxford Textbook of Medical Education*. Oxford University Press, ch. 22.

Kilminster S, Cottrell D, Grant J, Jolly B (2007) AMEE Guide No. 27: effective educational and clinical supervision. *Medical Teacher*, 29: 2–19.

15 Psychiatry in the Foundation Programme: An Overview for Supervisors

Holly Smith and Arthita Das

Introduction

The Foundation Programme (Box 15.1) was instituted in 2005 and brought together the preregistration house officer grade and the first year of the senior house officer grade (UK Foundation Programme Office 2015). This created an integrated two-year programme, governed by a single curriculum produced by the Academy of Medical Royal Colleges (2016). The majority of students completing undergraduate medical training in the UK will enter the Foundation Programme directly after leaving medical school.

The Foundation Programme is coordinated nationally by the UK Foundation Programme Office, which is commissioned by the four UK national health departments: Health Education England (HEE), National Health Service (NHS) Education for Scotland (NES), the Northern Ireland Medical and Dental Training Agency (NIMDTA) and the Wales Deanery. These four bodies are responsible for ensuring that the Foundation Programme is delivered across the UK in accordance with the standards set by the General Medical Council (GMC). Foundation schools are the structures through which each of the education authorities (HEE/NES/NIMDTA/Wales Deanery) delivers foundation training. Training is provided by local education providers (LEPs) through primary, secondary and academic placements (UK Foundation Programme Office 2021). Outside of the UK, the Foundation Programme has been replicated in Malta. The Maltese programme was launched in 2009 and it uses the same curriculum and provides the same educational and training opportunities (Foundation Programme Malta 2021). As far as we are aware, the Foundation Programme is not being used elsewhere. However, in other countries, such as Australia and the USA, graduates undertake an internship during which they are supervised until they gain full registration (Wilson and Feyer 2015).

Foundation training consists of a series of placements over two years in a wide variety of specialty areas, including psychiatry. Each placement lasts a minimum of four months and a maximum of six months. Foundation doctors complete a 'Preparing for Professional Practice Programme' or shadowing period before starting their placements (Miles et al. 2015).

Recent Changes to the Foundation Programme

Developing and maintaining a skilled workforce is one the greatest challenges for the NHS (NHS England 2019). To start to address this challenge, the UK government created 1500 new medical school places and five new medical schools across England between 2016 and 2019. Five hundred new medical places were allocated in 2018, with another 1000 places in 2019/20. There will be a concomitant expansion of the Foundation Programme to accommodate the newly graduated medical students (although not exactly matched in numbers), planned between 2023 and 2025.

Box 15.1 Essential functions of the Foundation Programme (from HEE 2019)

- To welcome future doctors to the healthcare workforce, and offer support for continued self-development and professional self-development.
- To provide a safe space environment in which to learn and care, allowing the transition from student to doctor and an increasing level of responsibility as the programme progresses.
- To allow development of clinical skills through the delivery of patient care under supervision, [with the foundation trainee] taking increasing responsibility for guiding others as the programme progresses.
- While training, to allow doctors to learn to play an increasingly important role in service delivery, including gaining experience in the provision of out-of-hours care.
- To offer an exposure to the breadth of medicine and an introduction to the delivery of compassionate, effective care across a range of clinical environments based on an understanding of patient and service needs. Within the programme, foundation doctors should be offered additional opportunities to develop specific skills such as research, management and quality improvement.
- To be able to demonstrate the professionalism expected of doctors, for those they care for, the healthcare system in which they work and the requirements of the regulator.
- To develop an interest in pastoral care, moving from self-care to the support of other foundation doctors where appropriate.
- To develop the ability to learn while working, ensuring self-directed learning through the seeking out and giving of feedback where appropriate.
- To future proof the doctor, by instilling a lifelong commitment to learning and improving practice.
- To establish a professional careers portfolio which will allow the doctor to demonstrate up-to-date clinical practice.
- [To facilitate the] independence and preparedness to progress through the foundation programme and into specialty training.

As well as increasing the size of the workforce, there was also the intention to develop the skills of the medical workforce – both specialist (with an increase in the number of psychiatrists) and generalist (improving training in mental health for all doctors).

Three reports were published contemporaneously, all pertaining to the Foundation Programme and particularly the delivery of mental health within the Foundation Programme. In 2019, the Health Education England (HEE) review of the Foundation Programme, 'Supported from the start; ready for the future' was published (HEE 2019). The Royal College of Psychiatrists commissioned a qualitative study focussing on trainees' experience of Foundation posts in psychiatry. They made recommendations based on this study and the full research paper was published in 2021 (Stott et al. 2021). The updated Foundation Curriculum by the Academy of Medical Royal Colleges was due for publication in 2020. However, this was delayed due to the impact of Covid-19 on the healthcare system, and it was published in 2021 (UK Foundation Programme Office 2021).

The HEE review sets out recommendations; Box 15.2 lists the most relevant of these. There are multiple transitions, not just at entry but throughout the Foundation Programme. Recommendations (7) and (8) make specific reference to psychiatry, with Recommendation

Box 15.2 Some of the recommendations of the HEE Foundation Programme Review 2019 (from HEE 2019)

1. The transition for, and preparation of, those entering foundation training must be improved to better prepare foundation doctors for the next stages of their development.
7. HEE will preferentially distribute the 1500 foundation doctor training places in the geographies where the NHS most needs them, in alignment with regional plans to support population healthcare needs and local specialty recruitment.
8. During 2019/20 and 2020/21, HEE will introduce and evaluate a number of Foundation Priority Programmes, specifically designed to attract and retain trainees in: remote, rural and coastal geographies, under-doctored geographies and shortage specialties, aligned to the Long-Term Plan with psychiatry as the initial priority.
10. HEE will work with foundation schools to identify opportunities to enhance support to doctors with specific needs including wider use of supportive placements.
11. Foundation schools will support greater flexibility in foundation training, including expanding access to Less Than Full Time Training (LTFT) and allowing access to a greater variety of working patterns and percentages of full time.
12. LEPs must ensure that foundation supervisors are valued and have appropriate training and skills and specific time allocated for their roles.
13. Senior trainees should be encouraged to take on the role of mentors. Trusts should develop this based on successful local 'good practice' schemes. To support this, HEE, working with the Academy of Medical Royal Colleges, will develop plans for a sustainable model for the role of senior trainees as mentors, including how such a role could be incorporated as a training opportunity for senior trainees.
14. HEE will engage with key stakeholders to assess how foundation doctors can be given time in the working week for professional self-development ('self-development' time).

(8) being translated into the Psychiatry Foundation Fellowship Programme. Self-development time (Recommendation 14) is detailed later in this chapter.

Supporting Transitions from Undergraduate Training to Postgraduate Practice

Surveys show that new graduates can experience significant anxiety at the transition from undergraduate training to postgraduate practice and can feel ill-prepared for the foundation year 1 (FY1) role. This is especially problematic for FY1 trainees whose first post is in a psychiatry placement. These posts are often (although not always) geographically separate from acute LEPs, leading to trainees feeling isolated from their peers and unable to access the peer support, which is important in helping to ameliorate their anxiety and stress (HEE 2019). These trainees also expressed concerns that their skills in acute medical and surgical care diminished or did not develop at the same pace as their peers, leaving them at a disadvantage when starting their second post in an acute hospital.

There are a number of ways in which mental health placements and supervisors can support trainees :

- Many mental health trusts have reciprocal arrangements with local acute trusts where FY1 trainees participate in the medical on-call rota. This enables them to continue to develop acute care skills, as well as maintaining contact with peers.

- Ensuring attendance at FY1 weekly teaching (organized and hosted by the acute LEP), again providing them with ongoing learning as well as informal contact and support with their peers.
- Use of e-learning and simulation packages to provide learning and development of skills.
- Arranging informal 'shadowing' prior to the transition from the first to the second post. Although this is mandatory for all FY1 trainees starting in August, a second period of shadowing can help to ease the transition into a new LEP.

What Does This Mean for Psychiatrists?

The principal implication of these changes for the medical workforce in psychiatry is a large and rapid increase in the number of foundation placements in psychiatry. Many more consultants will become supervisors of foundation doctors. Other non-consultant-grade psychiatrists will encounter foundation doctors in their teams and many will also be involved in their training. Many psychiatrists will not have had experience of working with foundation doctors before. Psychiatrists are used to providing core and specialist training; with foundation doctors they will need to provide more generalist training, which meets the requirements of the Foundation Programme curriculum. A key aim of the Foundation Programme in psychiatry is that doctors will be able to develop generic, transferrable skills that will be useful in their future careers, regardless of the specialty.

What Do Psychiatrists Need to Know About Foundation Doctors?

What Is the Difference between FY1 and FY2?

Foundation year 1 enables medical graduates to begin to take supervised responsibility for patient care and consolidate the skills they have learned at medical school. Satisfactory completion of FY1 allows the relevant university (or their designated representative in a foundation school) to recommend to the GMC that the foundation doctor can be granted full registration (GMC n.d.). It is worth noting that this may change in the future, as the 'Shape of Training' review led by Professor David Greenaway (Shape of Training 2013) has recommended that full registration should move to the point of graduation from medical school.

When they first start, most FY1 doctors will be very inexperienced and will require a substantial amount of support from their supervisors and the wider multidisciplinary team (MDT). This will change as the year goes on and they move into FY2, as they will start to develop skills, knowledge and confidence in their clinical work. FY2 trremain under clinical supervision, but take on increasing responsibility for patient care. They begin to make management decisions, develop their core generic skills and contribute more to the education/training of the wider healthcare workforce. At the end of FY2, doctors should have started to demonstrate clinical effectiveness, leadership and decision-making respon-sibilities (Goodyear et al. 2014). Satisfactory completion of FY2 will lead to the award of a Foundation Programme certificate of completion (FPCC), which indicates that the foundation doctor is ready to enter a core, specialty or general practice training programme (UK Foundation Programme Office 2021).

What Is the Difference between Foundation Training and Psychiatric Specialty Training?

It is important to remember that foundation doctors are not learning to be psychiatrists, unlike core and specialty psychiatry trainees. The aim of the Foundation Programme is to give foundation doctors a meaningful experience of psychiatry and to allow them to achieve the Foundation Programme competencies. However, if foundation doctors have an interest in psychiatry, they can be supported in accessing additional learning opportunities.

All trainees play a key role in the delivery of NHS care and it is important that foundation doctors 'learn by doing', as they will learn more effectively when they are responsible for their actions (Swanwick and Buckley 2014). FY1 doctors are new medical graduates and will be inexperienced compared with core psychiatry trainees. Therefore, they need to be well supervised to allow them to develop as doctors while ensuring patient safety.

What Are the Boundaries of Responsibility for Foundation Doctors?

Although technically FY1 doctors can prescribe anywhere, including in the community, the Royal College of Psychiatrists recommends that those in psychiatry placements should only prescribe in an in-patient setting. However, local exceptions to this may occur if adequate safeguards are in place (Boyle and Perry 2015). Although FY1 doctors may work out of hours, they should not be assigned to work on the same rotas as core trainees, and special arrangements should be made to ensure that they are adequately supported and supervised. In practice, this means that there must be a senior colleague on site. This colleague could be a senior nurse, as long as they have the necessary knowledge and skills to advise the foundation doctor appropriately (Boyle and Perry 2015).

How Can Supervisors Ensure That Their Posts Are of High Quality?

High-quality training in new and existing foundation posts requires careful planning and execution in order to maintain patient safety, inspire trainees and preserve enthusiasm. There are many ways in which psychiatrists can develop high-quality placements for foundation doctors. The Royal College of Psychiatrists has curated and published examples of best practice: innovative posts, bespoke teaching programmes, Balint groups and inspiring taster days (Royal College of Psychiatrists 2017).

Shadowing and Induction

Before beginning their first placement, FY1 doctors should undertake a shadowing period of at least four days' duration (which includes induction) overseen by their clinical supervisor.

All new foundation doctors should normally have sat a prescribing safety assessment (PSA) before commencing the programme. UK medical students should have been given the opportunity to sit the PSA during their degree course. Appointees from non-UK medical schools will be offered the opportunity to sit the PSA before or during their shadowing period where possible. Foundation doctors who have not passed the PSA before starting the programme are offered support and are required to sit/re-sit the assessment. All foundation doctors are required to pass the PSA within the two years immediately preceding the date on which they are signed off as having completed their FY1 year (GMC 2020).

Foundation doctors should have an induction from their foundation school and their employer/LEP. To ensure patient safety, all rotations should also initiate foundation doctors through a formal induction to the department and place of work.

Consultants should discuss the level of training and competency of the new incoming doctor with members of the MDT, managing expectations and clarifying the duties and responsibilities of foundation doctors. Team members should be told explicitly what is and what is not expected of a foundation doctor: for example, FY1 doctors should not undertake unsupervised section 136 Mental Health Act assessments and they do not have powers of detention.

Supervisors should organize a workplace induction process and timetable which ensures that the foundation doctor is introduced to all team members and is familiarized with the working environment (and health and safety procedures). The supervisor should give the foundation doctor an overview of key issues in psychiatry such as the Mental Health Act, the Mental Capacity Act and risk and safeguarding, which can be expanded on in supervision sessions.

The MDT should be involved in the foundation doctor's induction and placement. Members of the team will be able to support the doctor's training, for example through conducting joint assessments with the doctor, undertaking supervised learning events (SLEs) and giving feedback on their progress.

Teaching

Supervisors should consider the specific learning needs of foundation doctors and try to align teaching opportunities with their curriculum. All foundation doctors are required to attend their mandatory foundation teaching programme; this usually takes place at the acute trust and forms part of doctors' annual review of competence progression (ARCP) requirement.

Supervisors may also consider supporting foundation doctors to attend local educational activities for psychiatry trainees, such as journal clubs, case conferences or Member of the Royal College of Psychiatrists (MRCPsych) examination teaching sessions. For example, a foundation doctor could be supported to attend a teaching session on 'assessing capacity', as this is in their curriculum. LEPs and foundation schools may also consider developing a teaching programme specifically for foundation doctors.

Box 15.3 Induction Checklist for Supervisors

1. **MDT involvement:** Involve the whole team and ensure that they know that a foundation doctor is starting and what the new doctor can/cannot do.
2. **Local induction:** Ensure someone is there to meet with them on their first day, orientate them to the local workplace; that they have a timetable; consider shadowing different members of the team for the first two weeks.
3. **Seeking help/advice:** Foundation doctors should be given written guidance on who to contact and how to contact them (email/phone/working days) both during the day and out of hours, as needed.

Supervision

Each foundation doctor will have a preassigned educational supervisor for the year and one clinical supervisor for each placement. Foundation doctors should aim to meet with each supervisor at the beginning and end of each rotation. In addition, clinical supervisors in psychiatry rotations are expected to deliver weekly one-hour face-to-face supervision. Part of the supervision process should involve a review of the foundation doctor's progress and a review of which competencies they have met from the curriculum. From the outset, clinical supervisors should agree with the foundation doctor the times of these meetings and the consultant or higher trainee who will conduct the meetings in the clinical supervisor's absence. This is particularly important in the first year of the Foundation Programme, as it helps to support doctors in the often-difficult student-to-doctor transition (Steele and Beattie 2013).

Supervised Learning Events and Assessments

Foundation doctors have to complete a number of SLEs and obtain various other assessments for a successful ARCP. SLEs are formative workplace-based assessments that involve an interaction between the trainer and the foundation doctor, leading to immediate qualitative feedback and reflective learning. They replaced workplace-based assessments (WBPAs) in the Foundation Programme from 2012. SLEs may appear superficially similar to WBPAs, but they represent a desire to make the process more formative, although this shift was not universally well understood (Rees et al. 2014). SLEs have three components, which are outlined in Box 15.3:

- directly observed interactions;
- case-based discussions; and
- developing the clinical teacher.

The additional assessments, reports and evidence that foundation doctors must obtain for the ARCP are shown in Box 15.4. In brief, they are:

- a team assessment of behaviour;
- end-of-placement and end-of-year reports; and
- evidence of performance of core procedures.

All SLEs and assessments are designed to monitor foundation doctors' progress and provide a platform for further development. They are all completed in the electronic portfolio (e-portfolio), where further information about each SLE and assessment can be located. It is advised that consultant supervisors become familiar with the e-portfolio system in order to provide optimum support to their trainees. Completion of SLEs should be consultant-led where possible and should be undertaken early in the placement, when the doctor has the most to learn (Academy of Medical Royal Colleges 2016).

Tasters

Clinical exposure can be further complemented by taster days organized locally by supervisors. The Royal College of Psychiatrists suggests that posts should be developed to include five taster days in other subspecialty areas of psychiatry (Boyle and Perry 2015). These days are provided through study leave for FY2 doctors, but the opportunity for FY1 doctors to

---

Box 15.3 The components of SLEs for foundation doctors in FY1 and FY2 (Academy of Medical Royal Colleges 2016)

Directly observed interactions
- Mini-clinical evaluation exercises (mini-CEXs): a mini-CEX is an observed clinical encounter, for example, observing the doctor taking a patient history
- Direct observation of procedural skills (DOPS): the primary aim of a DOPS is to give feedback on the doctor's interaction with a patient while performing a procedure, for example, an ECG or taking bloods; the secondary aim is to demonstrate the progression of procedural skills

Case-based discussions (CBDs)
- A CBD is a structured discussion of a clinical case managed by the doctor; it has a focus on clinical reasoning

Developing the clinical teacher
- This tool aims to assess and develop the doctor's teaching and presentation skills by observing a teaching session

---

Box 15.4 2 Additional formal assessments and evidence required for successful completion of the ARCP for foundation doctors (Academy of Medical Royal Colleges 2016)

Team assessment of behaviour
- A multi-source feedback tool completed by a mix of appraisers recruited by the foundation doctor

Reports
- Clinical supervisor's end of placement report:

  one per placement

- Educational supervisor's reports:

  at the end of the placement

  at the end of the year

Core procedures
- E-portfolio evidence of satisfactory performance of core procedures (e.g., venepuncture, cannulation): FY1 only

---

undertake taster days will depend on local arrangements. Clinical supervisors can maintain quality through the bespoke design of taster days, focusing on the two main objectives: namely, informing career intentions, within and outside psychiatry, and fitting with the foundation doctor's interests (UK Foundation Programme Office 2011). Examples of suitable tasters might include child and adolescent mental health services for a doctor who is interested in paediatrics as a career, or neuropsychiatry for a doctor who is interested in neurology.

In the next section we focus on how foundation placements in psychiatry can offer doctors the opportunity to develop both generic and mental-health-specific skills. These opportunities will also help to ensure that posts are of high quality.

Supporting Foundation Doctors in Achieving the Generic and Specific Mental Health Competencies of the Curriculum

Most competencies can be demonstrated by behaviour in the workplace and training programme and there is emphasis on the importance of experiential learning and reflection.

MDT Working

All supervisors should aspire to give their foundation doctors a high-quality experience of MDT working. Care programme approach meetings are a gold standard of multiprofessional working in mental healthcare, so supervisors should encourage foundation doctors to attend them. Supervisors can organize for foundation doctors to undertake joint assessments with other MDT members to give them an appreciation of the broad range of professions involved and the skills they bring to mental healthcare. Supervisors should support their foundation doctors to attend clinical team meetings and encourage them to contribute. These opportunities for MDT working should allow other team members to make reliable judgements about the foundation doctor's ability and performance. This feedback can be used in their appraisal.

Communication Skills

Supervisors should develop posts that allow foundation doctors to acquire and develop communication skills. This could be done by enabling foundation doctors to work with patients, their families and other professionals in both straightforward and more complex situations. It might involve the foundation doctor explaining a treatment plan to a patient with chronic schizophrenia and an intellectual disability in a way that the patient can understand. It might involve breaking bad news, such as a new diagnosis of dementia, to a patient and their family in a sensitive and supportive manner. It is vital that foundation doctors are able to communicate empathically in this post-Francis era (Francis 2013).

Reflective Ability

The Foundation Programme curriculum encourages doctors to reflect on, and learn from, both their positive and negative experiences in order to demonstrate clinical development (Academy of Medical Royal Colleges 2016). Supervisors can support the development of reflective ability through the one-hour face-to-face weekly supervision. If there is the opportunity, supervisors should encourage their doctors to attend a specific Balint group for foundation doctors. Balint groups enable doctors to gain experience of reflection, listening and supporting others in the group, as well as developing a deeper understanding of their patients (Salinsky 2015).

Interface with Different Specialties and with Other Professionals

In mental health settings, the supervisor can signpost the foundation doctor to cases that will allow them to experience working across health and social care boundaries (Duncan 2015). For example, a foundation doctor could observe a core trainee assess a patient on a psychiatric ward, who has a medical problem that requires discussion with the on-call medical registrar and transfer to the accident and emergency department. This would allow the doctor to develop an understanding of working across mental health and acute trusts. Another example might be inviting a social worker to attend a ward round for a patient about whom there are safeguarding concerns. This would allow the foundation doctor to understand more about working across mental health and social care boundaries.

History Taking, Mental State Examination and Core Medical Skills

The supervisor should ensure that the foundation doctor has the opportunity to develop skills in history taking and mental state examination through teaching, practical experience and reflection (by SLEs and supervision). Supervisors and other team members should signpost foundation doctors to opportunities to acquire core medical skills within their day-to-day clinical work (e.g., physical health assessments of new admissions in an in-patient setting). Local providers may like to consider developing posts that have timetabled sessions in an acute medical setting (e.g., one day a week on-call in a co-located acute trust).

Management of Patients with Long-Term Conditions

The Foundation Programme curriculum outlines how doctors should gain experience of managing patients with long-term conditions (Academy of Medical Royal Colleges 2016). In mental health settings, the supervisor should highlight, through teaching and supervision, the interplay between long-term physical illness, psychological factors and mental disorders. For example, the foundation doctor could undertake a case-based discussion of a patient with chronic schizophrenia and diabetes, who experienced trauma in childhood.

Opportunities to have experience of holistic care in both acute presentations and in long-term conditions are likely to be widely available in all psychiatry placements.

Specific Areas of Core Learning

The list of core topics in psychiatry has expanded significantly from the four previously specified topics (self-harm, acute psychosis, cognitive impairment, psychiatric presentations of physical health illnesses); see Box 15.4. Foundation doctors also need to develop skills in managing clinical scenarios where they may be required to apply knowledge of mental health legislation/treatment to a patient with a physical health presentation (see Box 15.5).

Teaching and Quality Improvement

Supervisors must ensure that foundation doctors have protected time to engage in audit and quality improvement work (Cai et al. 2009). It is recommended that half a day per week is embedded in all foundation psychiatry placement timetables to support this activity (Boyle and Perry 2015).

Supervisors and other team members should seek out opportunities for foundation doctors to teach others. For foundation doctors in psychiatry, this could include teaching

Box 15.4 Core topics in mental health

- Depression
- Mania
- Psychosis
- Anxiety/panic
- Personality disorder
- Delirium
- Chronic cognitive impairment/dementia
- Eating disorders
- Substance misuse
- Somatization disorders including functional syndromes

Box 15.5 Examples of mental health presentations in acute settings

- Assessing capacity and using the Mental Capacity Act
- Mental Health Act 1983 (or equivalent, e.g., Mental Health Scotland Act 2015)
- Relevant ethical framework around difficult decision making (e.g., treating patients with eating disorders or who self-harm)
- Understanding that physical disease can present with psychiatric symptoms (e.g., multiple sclerosis, Cushing's syndrome, hypothyroidism) when ordering and interpreting investigations
- Serious adverse effects of common psychotropic medications
- Communicating with and managing a disturbed or challenging patient
- Explaining a diagnosis to a patient (or carer) who has medically unexplained symptoms or a non-organic cause for their symptoms (e.g., panic disorder presenting as chest pain)

topics that align with their curriculum to medical students who are on psychiatry rotations or teaching a medical topic to the MDT. It may be helpful for the foundation doctor to do this in conjunction with a senior colleague who can provide supervision and feedback. This could also be done as an SLE (developing the clinical teacher).

Recognition and Management of the Acutely Ill Patient

Foundation doctors should be supported by their supervisors to gain experience of recognizing and managing patients who are acutely unwell and those who have self-harmed. Supervisors could organize for foundation doctors to conduct home visits, undertake a taster in liaison psychiatry or observe a Mental Health Act assessment. This would enable foundation doctors to gain experience of conducting risk assessments and considering underlying causes of severe mental disturbance, such as acute confusional states, psychosis and substance use/withdrawal.

Medicolegal Issues

Supervisors should help their foundation doctors to acquire knowledge of medicolegal and ethical issues in healthcare. This could be, for example, through the supervisor's own teaching or through a larger programme, such as MRCPsych teaching. Teams should ensure that foundation doctors are able to gain an understanding of the Mental Capacity Act and experience of using it, for example through observing/participating in the assessment of whether a patient has capacity to consent to treatment on an in-patient ward (Nicholson et al. 2008). Supervisors must ensure that they provide specific teaching and supervision concerning the powers of detention for FY2 doctors who are on-call out of hours and are deputizing for the responsible clinician under the Mental Health Act.

Learning Opportunities

Foundation doctors must be afforded equitable access to learning opportunities in the psychiatry placement. It is a risk that the most routine service delivery tasks such as 'scribing' in medical records during ward rounds are regularly delegated to the foundation doctor by the more senior specialty trainees. Another risk is that the foundation doctor may be forced to shadow more experienced clinicians for the duration of their placement. Teams will need to identify and support a range of experiential learning opportunities for the post, to allow the foundation doctor to grow in confidence and to safely support their wider professional development as a doctor.

Self-Development Time

Self-development time was introduced for all foundation doctors in England as a result of the HEE Foundation Programme Review (HEE 2019). It was piloted across some sites from April 2020 onwards and became mandatory for all foundation (FY1) trainees working in England from August 2021.

FY1 trainees are allocated one hour per week of self-development time, increasing to three hours weekly for FY2 trainees. This time does not have to be given every week and can be amalgamated fortnightly or monthly to enable the trainee to attend a learning activity or event. It is time which should be formally included in the personalized work schedule of a foundation doctor to allow them to carry out non-clinical activities related to their curriculum or career exploration. It is similar to the supporting professional activity time included in consultant contracts.

Self-development time can be used for:

- meetings with supervisor;
- quality improvement work;
- developing career interests (not taster days);
- preparing or designing teaching; and
- some reflection and e-portfolio work (but trainee should not use all their self-development time for their portfolio),

However, it should **not** be used for:

- clinical work;
- mandatory trust e-learning;
- taster days, which are a separate entitlement in addition to self-development time; or
- annual leave, study leave or time owed in lieu.

Experience beyond the Curriculum

Some foundation doctors will wish to acquire competencies beyond the Foundation Programme over the course of their placement. They may already have decided on psychiatry as a career, or they may wish to maximize their learning opportunities. Further learning opportunities could include additional experience in psychotherapy (e.g., participation in a psychotherapy group), emergency psychiatry (e.g., observation or supervised undertaking of Section 136 assessments) and medicolegal aspects of psychiatry. The Good Practice Guide also includes creative examples of other possibilities (Royal College of Psychiatrists 2017).

Conclusion

The implication of the increase in the number of psychiatry posts as a result of changes to the Foundation Programme is that consultant psychiatrists and the wider team will be supervising and training more foundation doctors. There is a need to ensure that these new psychiatry foundation posts are of high quality so that doctors have a positive experience of the specialty.

The qualitative research conducted by the Royal College of Psychiatrists (Stott et al. 2021) confirmed that the quality of posts and psychiatric experience currently is inconsistent. Poor experience will have an impact on foundation doctors' future career choices. It also does not equip the wider medical workforce with the necessary skills and knowledge to deal with patients with mental disorder effectively and compassionately.

This chapter has focused on the role of the psychiatric supervisor and improving the quality of foundation posts in psychiatry. However, only 45 per cent of foundation doctors rotate through a psychiatry post, a proportion which will likely decrease in the future. This still leaves over 50 per cent of doctors graduating from the Foundation Programme without a consistent level of mental health knowledge or skills. There is an urgent need to deliver high-quality education and training for all doctors within the Foundation Programme, if we are to ensure high-quality care for people with mental disorders across all services in the future.

Acknowledgements

For information, the original paper on which this chapter is based was: Perry J, Ryland H, Thoms L, & Boyle A (2017) Psychiatry in the Foundation Programme: an overview for supervisors. *BJPsych Advances*, 23(2), 123–30. doi:10.1192/apt.bp.116.015909. The authors wish to acknowledge with thanks the contributions of Jennifer Perry, Howard Ryland, Lesley Thoms and Ann Boyle to the original paper.

References

Academy of Medical Royal Colleges (2016) *The Foundation Programme Curriculum 2016.* Academy of Medical Royal Colleges.

Boyle A, Perry J (2015) *A Guide to Psychiatry in the Foundation Programme for Supervisors.* Royal College of Psychiatrists.

Cai A, Greenall J, Ding DCD (2009) UK junior doctors' experience of clinical audit in the Foundation Programme. *British Journal of Medical Practitioners,* 2: 42–5.

Duncan E (2015) Liaison psychiatry is a good foundation for junior doctors. *BMJ Careers,* 9 Nov.

Foundation Programme Malta (2021) Welcome to the Foundation Programme – Malta.

Available at: http://fpmalta.com (accessed June 2022).

Francis R (2013) *Report of the Mid Staffordshire NHS Foundation Trust Public Inquiry: vols 1–3*. The Stationery Office.

GMC (n.d.) Full registration for UK graduates moving from F1 to F2. Available at: https://www.gmc-uk.org/registration-and-licensing/join-the-register/registration-applications/application-guides/full-registration-for-uk-graduates-moving-from-f1-to-f2 (accessed June 2022).

GMC (2020) Outcomes for graduates. Available at: www.gmc-uk.org/education/standards-guidance-and-curricula/standards-and-outcomes/outcomes-for-graduates/outcomes-for-graduates.

Goodyear H, Bindal N, Bindal T, et al. (2014) Foundation doctors' experience and views of mentoring. *British Journal of Hospital Medicine*, **74**: 682–6.

HEE (2019) Supported from the start; ready for the future: the Postgraduate Medical Foundation Programme Review. Available at: www.hee.nhs.uk/sites/default/files/documents/FoundationReview%20FINAL%20for%20web.pdf.

Miles S, Kellett J, Leinster SJ (2015) Foundation doctors' induction experiences. *BMC Medical Education*, **15**: 118.

NHS England (2019) Interim people plan. Available at: www.longtermplan.nhs.uk/wp-content/uploads/2019/05/Interim-NHS-People-Plan_June2019.pdf.

Nicholson TRJ, Cutter W, Hotopf M (2008) Assessing mental capacity: the Mental Capacity Act. *BMJ*, **336**: 322–5.

Rees CE, Cleland JA, Dennis A, et al. (2014) Supervised learning events in the Foundation Programme: a UK-wide narrative interview study. *BMJ Open*. Available at: http://dx.doi.org/10.1136/bmjopen-2014-005980.

Royal College of Psychiatrists (2017) Foundation Good Practice Guide (CR202 Mar 2017). Available at: www.rcpsych.ac.uk/improving-care/campaigning-for-better-mental-health-policy/college-reports/2017-college-reports/good-psychiatric-practice-relationships-with-pharmaceutical-and-other-related-organisations-cr202-mar-2017.

Salinsky J (2015) A very short introduction to Balint groups. Available at: http://balint.co.uk/about/introduction/.

Shape of Training (2013) *Securing the Future of Excellent Patient Care: Final Report of the Independent Review Led by Professor David Greenaway*. Shape of Training.

Steele R, Beattie S (2013) Development of foundation year 1 psychiatry posts: implications for practice. *Advances in Psychiatric Treatment*, **19**: 410–9.

Stott J, Haywood J, Crampton P (2021): Early career doctors' experiences of psychiatry placements: a qualitative study. *Medical Teacher*, **43**: 1196–202.

Swanwick T, Buckley G (2014) Introduction: understanding medical education. In Stanwick, T (ed.), *Understanding Medical Education: Evidence, Theory and Practice*. Wiley Blackwell, pp. xv–xviii.

UK Foundation Programme Office (2011) *Specialty Tasters in the Foundation Programme: Guidance for Foundation Schools*. UK Foundation Programme Office.

UK Foundation Programme Office (2015) *Rough Guide to the Foundation Programme*, 4th ed. UK Foundation Programme Office.

UK Foundation Programme Office (2021) New Foundation Programme curriculum. Available at: https://foundationprogramme.nhs.uk/curriculum.

Wilson A, Feyer AM (2015) *Review of Medical Intern Training: Final Report*. Australian Health Ministers' Advisory Council.

Interprofessional Education in Mental Health Services

Daniel Kinnair, Elizabeth Anderson and Kris Roberts

Introduction

Interprofessional education was originally defined by the Centre for the Advancement of Interprofessional Education in 1997 and clearly articulated in 2002 (Barr 2002). There has been international agreement that it 'occurs when two or more professions learn about, from and with each other to enable effective collaboration and improve health outcomes' (World Health Organization 2010: p. 13). This definition implies that students from different professions must come together in the learning process to achieve their intended learning outcomes. In this way, students bring their uniprofessional specific knowledge and skills into interprofessional learning to mirror the complexity of team-based clinical practice.

Interprofessional education has existed in the formal preregistration curriculum for about 15 years, and is affirmed as essential by the General Medical Council in *Outcomes for Graduates* (General Medical Council 2018). As a result, students are emerging from preregistration courses primed to learn in this way. Indeed, the Foundation Programme curriculum expects ongoing training to include preparation for team working (UK Foundation Programme 2016). It is implicit in the psychiatry core training curriculum (Royal College of Psychiatrists 2017) that good interprofessional collaboration is key for those who choose to train in psychiatry. In addition, all doctors in the UK are now required to produce evidence for revalidation, for which one of the domains is communication, partnership and teamwork (General Medical Council 2019).

This chapter explores the continuing paucity of interprofessional education in current postgraduate programmes for doctors and other practitioners preparing to work in mental health teams. We offer solutions based on our extensive experience, which are framed in sound theoretical principles for team-based learning and involve patients as a central component.

Team Working in Mental Health Services

Team working and collaborative practice have always been a key component of patient care in mental health services. This is because patients present with complex mental health needs and interrelated social problems that often require a response from medicine, nursing, psychology, occupational therapy and social work. Traditionally, the doctor has taken a leadership role relating to diagnosis, whereas treatment plans and long-term care – areas in which concepts such as recovery, support and therapy are important – have been

> **Box 16.1** The care programme approach (Department of Health 1990)
>
> The key components of the CPA are:
> - an interagency assessment of the individual's health and social care needs
> - an assessment of risk factors for the individual or others
> - a CPA care plan to address the assessed needs
> - the identification of a care coordinator
> - regular reviews
> - the identification of gaps in service

shared across medicine, nursing, occupational health and psychology. In addition, the social worker places the patient (client) in their social and cultural context. On the whole, these teams have learnt 'on the job' how to work with each other. Community mental health teams (CMHTs) are seen as providing joined-up multi-professional services for individuals with complex care needs and, in the UK, the care programme approach (CPA) was designed to support team working (Department of Health 1990) and collaborative practice (Box 16.1). However, despite efforts within organizations to improve team working there continue to be errors, concerns and national inquiries that highlight poor team working within mental health services (Prins 2004).

The day-to-day practicalities of team working in mental health services remain difficult, and conflicts and challenges arise when professions have different value bases and report to different statutory accountable structures. The concept of values within health and social care includes anything that is 'valued', and might embrace ethics, justice, principles, morals and individuals' personal beliefs. A number of obstacles to good collaborative practice have been identified. These include structural, procedural, financial, professional and status-based factors, not least of which is who takes the lead and has the power (Peck and Dickinson 2008).

A review of partnership working across different teams and organizations in mental healthcare delivery (Glasby 2004b) identified several barriers to good team working and possible solutions. The barriers included:

- professional self-interest, including aspects of autonomy and accountability;
- financial resources and constraints; and
- procedural differences between teams.

No easy solutions to these difficulties were found. There has been an ongoing call for more training to prepare practitioners to work effectively in teams (Whittington 2003).

Team Roles of Psychiatrists

There has been a plethora of documents looking at how psychiatrists should work in teams (Department of Health 2005). The recent UK government reform of the Mental Health Act highlights the need for multidisciplinary working throughout all patient-facing areas (Department of Health and Social Care 2021). Psychiatrists' roles are changing to provide expertise in assessment and treatment and operate on a consultative model. Other team members (e.g., nurse prescribers) are taking on some of the roles more commonly associated with doctors, and doctors within the team are asked to see only the patients with the complex problems. Responsibility for care, which once sat firmly with the psychiatrist, is now shared between team members. Care depends on collaborative work, with each team member sharing their unique skills and abilities.

Current Provision

Interprofessional education has been endorsed for preregistration courses as it prepares undergraduate students for collaborative working (Barr and Low 2012). There are examples of programmes for mental healthcare, although contact is often limited and not all professions are included (Curran et al. 2008). Looking at the educational continuum, there are also some examples of interprofessional education for postgraduate mental health teams, but these initiatives are rare, mostly because of the complexity of aligning postgraduate courses (Barnes et al. 2000; Reeves and Freeth 2006). There is evidence that attendance at postgraduate courses organized as part of continuing professional development is higher among nursing staff than among psychiatrists and psychologists (McCann et al. 2012). There is huge scope for developing more relevant interprofessional education relating to the complexity of mental healthcare for all professionals. In medicine, the need to provide evidence for revalidation might encourage the provision of postgraduate interprofessional education.

Solutions: The Way Forward

Interprofessional education may offer solutions for shaping professional behaviour and for developing effective teams. It focuses on theories of learning centred not on the individual but on learning with others in sociocultural clinical contexts. Its premise lies in adult learning theory, where the process of learning, that is, through experience or reflection, is key (Knowles 1978; Kolb 1984; Wenger 1998). Interprofessional education at its best can set up a complex and challenging social learning environment that mirrors the realities of clinical practice and teaches effective team working (Bleakley 2006). It is also an important vessel for change in reducing mental health stigma among healthcare students (Maranzan 2016). There are obviously socially constructed and mediated power differentials in these mixed student interactions and managing these must be considered (Hean et al. 2013).

Undergraduate Models of Interprofessional Education

In its original version, the Leicester Model of Interprofessional Education was designed and developed with undergraduate students to enable them to appreciate the complexities of health and social care delivery in meeting the needs of disadvantaged inner-city communities (Lennox and Anderson 2007). The model combines practical understanding of team working and collaborative practice using a patient-centred approach (Anderson and Lennox 2009). It uses a learning cycle based on the work of Kolb (Fig. 16.1).

From the student's perspective learning takes place (cyclically) following four consecutive steps:

(1) **Concrete experience**: Experiential learning in which students work with and learn from patients, carers and professionals in day-to-day clinical practice. The students

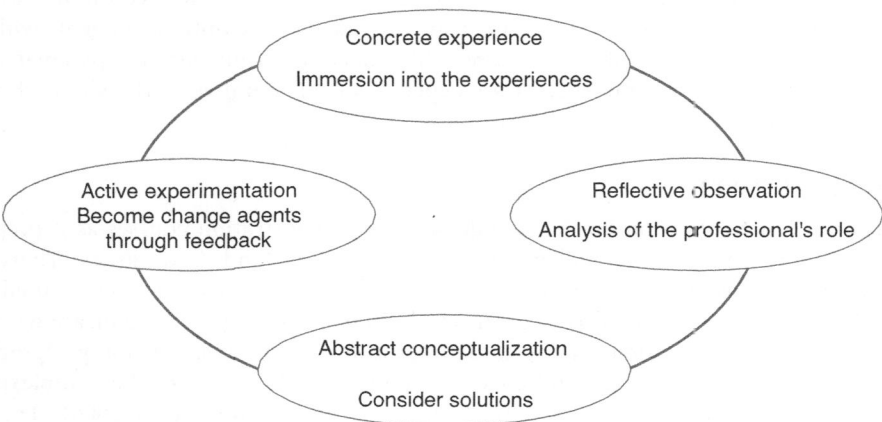

Fig. 16.1 The learning cycle of the Leicester Model of Interprofessional Education (adapted from Kolb 1984).

are immersed in the complexity of team working, and patient/carer perceptions of care are central to and drive the learning.

(2) **Reflective observation**: Students are helped in tutorials to apply theory and policy to their experiences and thus to gain a richer and deeper understanding of patients' and professionals' perspectives of care delivery. In this way, students come to understand professional roles and responsibilities.

(3) **Abstract conceptualization**: Students faced with the complexity of care are helped to reanalyse clinical problems and consider new ways to address and manage care. These new solutions are student generated and can often raise issues not yet considered by the professionals, mostly because students have more time to reflect on what they see.

(4) **Active experimentation**: In the final stage, students feed back to the professional teams changes to practice that they think might improve patient outcomes and that might be introduced into day-to-day procedures.

Shadowing the Professionals

The Leicester Model of Interprofessional Education places patients at the heart of the experience for undergraduate interprofessional groups, and this mirrors team working with patients in practice (Department of Health 2008). The model has been evaluated from the perspective of students, professionals and patients (Anderson and Lennox 2009). The learning template has been adopted in different team-based clinical settings, including mental healthcare (Kinnair et al. 2012). The essence of the model is that students are given clinical responsibilities, becoming shadow teams accountable to the professional team. They analyse and explore the existing professional care plans for patients, and throughout are directly involved in the realities of day-to-day practice. In the mental health adaptation, the students mirror the work of a CMHT and feed back on inter-agency care plans. In this and other adaptations, student teams have identified unmet needs and unsafe practice (Anderson and Thorpe 2010; Lennox and Anderson 2012).

Involving Patients in Interprofessional Education

The involvement of patients has the benefit of putting the teaching in a real-life clinical context. The Department of Health and Social Care requires the involvement of members of the public in education (Department of Health 2003), and, as already mentioned, the Leicester model places patients at the centre of the cycle of experiential learning. Towle et al. (2009) propose six levels of patient involvement, from case studies through to policy development. The level of engagement may be crucial to the patients' experiences or perspectives of the value they place on participating in interprofessional education.

A number of studies have shown the successful inclusion of patients in undergraduate interprofessional education (Cooper and Spencer-Dawe 2006; Anderson et al. 2011). Patients involved in the mental health interprofessional education course in Leicester reported that they could see the purpose and benefit of bringing students from different professional groups together to learn (Kinnair et al. 2012). They recognized that they received care provided by teams and that joined-up care between teams is sometimes difficult. Although patients were initially nervous about participating in the course, the overwhelming feedback was that they enjoyed taking part and felt that their contribution to education was valued. There is also evidence that postgraduate interprofessional education courses can have a positive effect on patient care (Zwarenstein et al. 2005).

Interprofessional Education in Postgraduate Mental Healthcare

Effective interprofessional collaboration has been seen by policy makers as a key mechanism for tackling poor-quality service delivery, improving patient safety and minimizing waste of resources, including clinical time (Department of Health 2001). However, despite repeated suggestions in national policy documents and statements that an interprofessional education approach should be taken in mental healthcare, there is little evidence to demonstrate benefits in postgraduate training, and no national strategy.

There is published evidence to demonstrate the benefits of interprofessional education at the post-graduate level in a pilot project involving CMHTs (Reeves and Freeth 2006). Interprofessional education was offered to two CMHTs, with the aim of improving collaborative working by providing an opportunity for team members to reflect on collaborative practice and the contribution to care made by each profession within the teams. The teams met for three two-hour workshops. The study reported that the workshops did help to clarify roles and were seen by participants as a valuable space to reflect on different professional perspectives.

The idea of different professional perspectives is an important one in health and social care, and particularly in mental healthcare, where successful recovery requires a biopsychosocial approach. Patients with mental health problems may also experience health inequalities dependent on income, housing, environment, powerlessness to effect change and wider notions of unfairness (Duggan et al. 2002). A collaborative approach between different professionals and agencies is needed to tackle these complicated difficulties.

From Silo to Interprofessional Education

There is an opportunity to improve the quality of mandatory training programmes within UK National Health Service (NHS) trusts. Many of these courses are multi-professional, but not truly interprofessional. Courses in areas such as risk assessment, child protection, working with vulnerable adults and resuscitation skills require good collaborative care in clinical practice, and could benefit from an interprofessional education approach. Within postgraduate medical education, most core and higher trainees are taught in uniprofessional silos, separately from other branches of medicine for the majority of the time. There is an opportunity to develop interprofessional educational events to cross some of the existing barriers. All psychiatrists will work with a wide variety of professional groups, including general practitioners, physicians, social workers and others, and there should be formal learning events to support the development of high-quality multi-agency work.

Taking Forward Interprofessional Education at Postgraduate Level

Planning and implementing interprofessional education necessitates the involvement of faculties from different health and social care schools, within or across universities. This first step of bringing staff together from different services and backgrounds is often difficult and requires a collegiate approach. If patients are to be involved, it will also be necessary to include clinical, practice-based staff to identify, recruit and support them.

If interprofessional education events are to be successful, they should have several important characteristics. They need the shared enthusiasm of the different disciplines involved in the project, not only in the developmental phase, but to sustain and embed it in several different curricula (Reeves 2008). Staff must model good interprofessional practice and communication in their collaboration and facilitation of learning events. And events must stay abreast of changes in policy at a national level and service changes at a local level that can affect staff and collaborative efforts.

Setting Up a Postgraduate Course

Three key steps need to be considered in the development of a postgraduate interprofessional education course. First, train and bring together the course leaders/facilitators so that they can:

- learn more about each other and begin to work interprofessionally, each representing their different professional training;
- understand each other's curricula and professional body requirements;
- learn more about the methods of interprofessional education and how to manage group dynamics;
- establish intended learning outcomes relevant for all the participating professions;
- engage with frontline practitioners and individuals from the teams that will be attending the course;
- plan, where possible, for the involvement of patients and work with them in the early planning stages; and
- decide how the learning will influence practice.

Second, design teaching to align with the intended learning outcomes and assessment process:

- decide how the learning will take place;

- draw on theory to underpin the teaching; and
- agree an assessment strategy.

Third, evaluate the outcomes:

- use assessments to see whether the students have learnt from the event; and
- evaluate the impact of the learning event on all participants/stakeholders.

There are many questions to be addressed and these can be aligned to consideration of the 'presage', 'process' and 'product' of learning – the 3P model (Biggs 1993). Table 16.1 shows the 3P model as adapted for interprofessional education by Freeth and Reeves (2004).

Assessment of Interprofessional Competencies

The assessment of interprofessional competencies at both the undergraduate and postgraduate level is not an easy task. At the undergraduate level, students in mental health may be asked to reflect on learning opportunities. There has also been much work examining the use of reflective portfolios which can be used by a variety of different professionals, but which must align to both uniprofessional and interprofessional competencies (Domac et al. 2015). More recently, academics have been working to develop rigorous tools to formatively assess and give feedback to learners on their interprofessional competencies (Thistlewaite et al. 2016).

In postgraduate medical training in the UK there is some degree of assessment of team working skills in the various Royal College portfolios, including in 360 appraisals of competency and performance. Senior medical colleagues must also provide evidence of team working skills in order to revalidate.

The Future

There is still a need for interprofessional education to be firmly embedded for all trainee and consultant psychiatrists. We have offered one model, familiar to us at Leicester, which has been evaluated and adapted for use in mental health settings. Patient-centred models need to be further developed, especially where they offer the opportunity to improve practice. An alternative model that is popular in postgraduate education is the Quality Improvement Programme (Health Foundation 2012), although it is important to avoid delivering this in uniprofessional silos.

Psychiatrists Should Take the Lead

Psychiatrists involved in postgraduate training must work collaboratively with educators in other health and social care professions to forward interprofessional education. This would address concerns that medical faculties have been slow to support interprofessional education, in part because of the recognized imbalance of status and power (Hean et al. 2006; Curran et al. 2007).

Caution is needed not only to create a balance of those leading interprofessional education from across the professions, but also to ensure the right balance of students who attend. In their feedback on interprofessional education events, social work students continue to express concerns about the 'lack of respect' shown to them by medical students and the dominance of the medical model in assessing patient need (Smith and Anderson 2008). However, although individual research papers have highlighted a perceived lack of medical participation in

Table 16.1 Using the 3P model[a] to shape a learning event in interprofessional education

Presage	Process	Product
Factors such as: the context of learning, teacher characteristics, learner characteristics	*The impact of the learning on all stakeholders*	*Considers approaches to teaching and learning*
Decide which professions will take part.	Where will the learning take place: classroom or workplace?	Consider how the course will be assessed and evaluated.
Is this the first time these students have learnt interprofessionally? Preparation for the learning should reflect this.		
	If the course relates to the working of a CMHT[b] it should take place at a CMHT base.	Evaluation will offer insights into how to improve the learning, whereas assessments help show where learning has taken place.
Design teaching to take into account mental health services legislation.	Environment is important to help the learning.	
	Train facilitators to help them manage group dynamics, as the various professional groups will bring different values to their practice and different perceptions of power in clinical areas.	
Will the course meet the needs of the clinical directors?		
Involve management: they will be more likely to release staff if they can see that the learning might improve the way staff work together.		
	Structure the learning to enable participants to feel comfortable working and learning together.	
Design appropriate preparation materials.	How will the course materials (e.g., workbooks, e-tivities) help learning?	
Consider the ethical issues if patients are involved (e.g., consent).		

[a]The 3P model was proposed by Biggs (1993) and adapted for interprofessional learning by Freeth and Reeves (2004). [b]CMHT: community mental health team.

interprofessional education, the interprofessional education agenda both nationally and internationally has been supported by many prominent clinicians, including the late Dr John Horder, who founded the Centre for the Advancement of Interprofessional Education (CAIPE) and was a past president of the Royal College of General Practitioners.

Trusting the Evidence Base

There are several examples in the literature of the benefits of interprofessional education at both undergraduate and postgraduate level. These include learning events on breaking bad news (Wakefield et al. 2006), community healthcare (Anderson et al. 2003) and team working and communication (Parsell et al. 1998). The advantages of interprofessional education have included clarification of uniprofessional roles and responsibilities, and identifying where roles are similar and overlap. Interprofessional education allows students to experience clinically realistic team working situations, and allows potential conflicts to be identified and discussed. Few health and social care practitioners practise in isolation, and interprofessional education is a vehicle that allows students to experience collaborative working at an undergraduate or postgraduate level. There is longitudinal evidence that interprofessional education programmes at the undergraduate level produce attitudinal and behavioural changes that remain after graduation (Pollard and Miers 2008). Students trained in programmes that included interprofessional education were more confident in their interprofessional relationships and communication skills. If mental health services are to become more efficient and effective, interprofessional working and communication will be key to individual professional groups working together.

Interprofessional education is becoming increasingly common in health and social care undergraduate curricula (Hammick et al. 2007). The evidence for interprofessional education for undergraduates continues to grow and it is important that we develop relevant and interesting educational tools to teach different groups of postgraduates the skills necessary for teamwork and collaboration.

Controversies

While the authors are clearly strong supporters of interprofessional education as a means to improve collaborative care, there are controversies surrounding it, and new models of care. Not all healthcare professionals support changes to our individual uniprofessional roles, (e.g., non-medical prescribing), and it is important that these changes are carefully thought through before implanting wholesale changes to local or national service delivery.

Conclusion

There is a continuing drive to implement and embed interprofessional education in undergraduate curricula to help reinforce students' preparation for interprofessional team working after graduation (Barr et al. 2006). This focus has also shown that students can become agents of change, not only for individual patients but also, potentially, for future practice within the NHS and social care systems. Postgraduate education is in danger of being left behind, but interprofessional education at this level may be an opportunity to train and develop staff to implement the huge changes occurring in most NHS-based mental health teams and services. It may also give staff groups the space to reflect on changes to services and their own and their colleagues' roles in these changes.

Acknowledgements

For information, the original paper on which this chapter is based was: Kinnair, D., Anderson, E., Van Diepen, H., & Poyser, C. (2014). Interprofessional education in mental health services: Learning together for better team working. *Advances in Psychiatric Treatment*, *20*(1), 61–68. doi:10.1192/apt.bp.113.011429 We wish to acknowledge with thanks the contributions of Henderikus van Diepen and Cath Poyser to the original paper. Unfortunately, it was not possible to contact them during the preparation of the chapter, for which we apologise.

References

Anderson ES, Lennox A (2009) The Leicester Model of Interprofessional Education: developing, delivering and learning from student voices for 10 years. *Journal of Interprofessional Care*, 23: 557–73.

Anderson ES, Thorpe LN (2010) Learning together in practice: an interprofessional education programme to appreciate teamwork. *Clinical Teacher*, 7: 19–25.

Anderson ES, Lennox A, Petersen S (2003) Learning from lives: a model for health and social care education in the community context. *Medical Education*, 37: 59–68.

Anderson ES, Ford J, Thorpe LN (2011) Learning to listen: improving students' communication with disabled people. *Medical Teacher*, 32: 1–9.

Barnes D, Carpenter J, Bailey D (2000) Partnerships with service users in interprofessional education for community mental health: a case study. *Journal of Interprofessional Care*, 14: 189–200.

Barr H (2002) *Interprofessional Education Today, Yesterday and Tomorrow (Occasional Paper 1)*. Higher Education Academy, King's College London.

Barr H, Low H (2012) *Interprofessional Education in Pre-registration Courses: A CAIPE guide for Commissioners and Regulators of education*. CAIPE.

Barr H, Freeth D, Hammick M, et al. (2006) The evidence base and recommendations for interprofessional education in health and social care. *Journal of Interprofessional Care*, 20: 75–8.

Biggs J (1993) From theory to practice: a cognitive systems approach. *Higher Education Research and Development*, 12: 73–85.

Bleakley A (2006) Broadening conceptions of learning in medical education: the message from teamworking. *Medical Education*, 40: 150–7.

Cooper H, Spencer-Dawe E (2006) Involving service users in interprofessional education: narrowing the gap between theory and practice. *Journal of Interprofessional Care*, 20: 603–17.

Curran VR, Sharpe D, Forristall J (2007) Attitudes of health sciences faculty members towards interprofessional teamwork and education. *Medical Education*, 41: 892–6.

Curran VR, Sharpe D, Forristall J, et al. (2008) Student satisfaction and perceptions of small group process in case-based interprofessional learning. *Medical Teacher*, 30: 431–3.

Department of Health (1990) *The Care Programme Approach for People with a Mental Illness, Referred to Specialist Psychiatric Services* (HC(90)23/LASSL(90)). The Stationery Office.

Department of Health (2001) *Working Together–Learning Together: A Framework for Lifelong Learning for the NHS*. Department of Health.

Department of Health (2003) *Changing Workforce Programme: Pilot site Report*. The Stationery Office.

Department of Health (2005) *New Ways of Working for Psychiatrists: Enhancing Effective Person Centred Services through New Ways of Working in Multidisciplinary and Multiagency Contexts. Final Report but Not the End of the Story*. The Stationery Office.

Department of Health (2008) *Refocusing the Care Programme Approach: Policy and Positive Practice Guidance*. The Stationery Office.

Department of Health and Social Care (2021) Reforming the Mental Health Act. Available at:

www.gov.uk/government/consultations/reforming-the-mental-health-act/reforming-the-mental-health-act.

Domac S, Anderson ES, O'Reilly M, Smith R (2015). Assessing interprofessional competence using a prospective reflective portfolio. *Journal of Interprofessional Care*, **29**: 179–87.

Duggan M, Cooper A, Foster J (2002) *Modernising the Social Model in Mental Health: A Discussion Paper*. Social Perspectives Network.

Freeth D, Reeves S (2004) Learning to work together: using the presage, process and product (3P) model to highlight decisions and possibilities. *Journal of Interprofessional Care*, **18**: 43–56.

General Medical Council (2018) *Outcomes for Graduates*. General Medical Council.

General Medical Council (2019) *Ready for Revalidation: The Good Medical Practice Framework for Appraisal and Revalidation*. General Medical Council.

Glasby J, Lester H (2004b) Cases for change in mental health: partnership working in mental health services. *Journal of Interprofessional Care*, **18**: 7–16.

Hammick M, Freeth D, Koppel I, et al. (2007) A best evidence systematic review of interprofessional education (BEME Guide no 9). *Medical Education*, **29**: 735–51.

Health Foundation (2012) *Quality Improvement Training for Healthcare Professionals*. Health Foundation.

Hean S, MacLeod Clark J, Adams K, et al. (2006) Will opposites attract? Similarities and differences in students' perceptions of the stereotype profiles of other health and social care professional groups. *Journal of Interprofessional Care*, **20**: 162–81.

Hean S, O'Halloran C, Craddock D, et al. (2013) Testing theory in interprofessional education: social capital as a case study. *Journal of Interprofessional Care*, **27**: 10–7.

Kinnair DJ, Anderson ES, Thorpe LN (2012) Development of interprofessional education in mental health practice: adapting the Leicester model. *Journal of Interprofessional Care*, **26**: 189–97.

Knowles M (1978) *The Adult Learner: A Neglected Species*. Gulf Publishing.

Kolb DA (1984) *Experiential Learning: Experience as a Source of Learning and Development*. Prentice Hall.

Lennox A, Anderson ES (2007) The Leicester Model of Interprofessional Education: a practical guide for implementation in health and social care (Higher Education Academy Medicine, Dentistry and Veterinary Medicine Special Report 9). *Journal of Interprofessional Care*, **23**: 557–73.

Lennox A, Anderson ES (2012) Delivering improvements in patient care: the application of the Leicester Model of Interprofessional Education. *Quality in Primary Care*, **20**: 219–26.

Maranzan K. (2016). Interprofessional education in mental health: an opportunity to reduce mental illness stigma. *Journal of Interprofessional Care*, **30**: 370–7.

McCann E, Higgins A, Maguire G, et al. (2012) A survey of pedagogical approaches and quality mechanisms used in education programs for mental health professionals. *Journal of Interprofessional Care*, **26**: 383–9.

Parsell G, Spalding R, Bligh J (1998) Shared goals, shared learning: evaluation of a multiprofessional course for undergraduate students. *Medical Education*, **32**: 304–11.

Peck E, Dickinson H (2008) *Managing and Leading in Inter-Agency Settings*. Policy Press.

Pollard K, Miers M (2008) From students to professionals: results of a longitudinal study of attitudes to pre-qualifying collaborative learning and working in health and social care in the United Kingdom. *Journal of Interprofessional Care*, **22**: 399–416.

Prins H (2004) Mental health enquiries – 'Cui Bono'? In Stanley N, Manthorpe J (eds.), *The Age of the Inquiry: Learning and Blaming in Health and Social Care*. Routledge, pp. 19–38.

Reeves S, Freeth D (2006) Re-examining the evaluation of interprofessional education for community mental health teams with a different lens: understanding presage, process and product factors. *Journal of Psychiatric and Mental Health Nursing*, **13**: 765–70.

Reeves S (2008) Planning and implementing a collaborative clinical placement for medical, nursing and allied health students: a qualitative study. *Medical Teacher*, **30**: 699–704.

Royal College of Psychiatrists (updated 2017) A competency based curriculum for specialist core training in psychiatry: core training in psychiatry CT1–CT3. Available at: www .rcpsych.ac.uk/docs/default-source/ training/curricula-and-guidance/curricula-core-psychiatry-curriculum-april-2018.pdf? sfvrsn=881b63ca_2.

Smith R, Anderson L (2008) Interprofessional learning: aspiration or achievement? *Social Work Education*, **27**: 759–76.

Thistlethwaite J, Dallest K, Moran M, et al. (2016) Introducing the individual Teamwork Observation and Feedback Tool (iTOFT): development and description of a new interprofessional teamwork measure. *Journal of Interprofessional Care*, **30**: 526–8.

Towle A, Bainbridge L, Godolphin W, et al. (2009) Active patient involvement in the education of health professionals. *Medical Education*, **44**: 64–74.

UK Foundation Programme (2016) *The UK Foundation Programme Curriculum*. UK Foundation Programme.

Wakefield A, Cocksedge S, Boggis C (2006) Breaking bad news: qualitative evaluation of an interprofessional learning opportunity. *Medical Teacher*, **28**: 53–8.

Wenger E (1998) *Communities of Practice: Learning, Meaning and Identity*. Cambridge University Press.

Whittington C (2003) A model of collaboration. In Weinstein J, Whittington C, Leiba T (eds.), *Collaboration in Social Work Practice*. Jessica Kingsley Publishers, pp. 39–62.

World Health Organization (2010) *Framework for Action on Interprofessional Education and Collaborative Practice*. World Health Organization.

Zwarenstein M, Reeves S, Perrier L (2005) Effectiveness of pre-licensure interprofessional education and post-licensure collaborative interventions. *Journal of Interprofessional Care*, **19** (suppl 1): 148–65.

Portfolio-Based Learning in Medical Education

Antonina Ingrassia and Oliver Batham

Introduction

Portfolio-based learning is relatively new to medical education and, in many ways, quite far removed from the more traditional instructional pedagogy that has been associated with the education of doctors for centuries. Despite that, the use of portfolios has rapidly expanded in recent years. This increased popularity is clearly set against a background of important changes and new trends in medical education. Before considering further the use of portfolios, it is useful to understand some of these changes as the contextual factors on which the search for new and creative learning and assessment strategies (which include portfolio-based learning) is predicated. We will particularly focus on:

(1) increasing levels of accountability; and

(2) the professionalization of trainers.

Increasing Levels of Accountability

Standards are nothing new in the practice and teaching of medicine. The traditional Hippocratic Oath sets out practical and ethical standards to be upheld by the new physician, as well as a responsibility to teach and pass on the knowledge acquired. However, in recent years, the regulation of doctors and the quality assurance of undergraduate and postgraduate medical training and continuing professional development (CPD) have assumed an increasingly high profile in the UK (Fig. 17.1). It is therefore no surprise that medical education has become 'a place of increasing accountability and regulation' (Swanwick 2018). This process arguably started in 1993, when the Calman report, *Hospital Doctors: Training for the Future* (Calman 1993), recommended significant alterations to medical postgraduate training. Further changes and a clear move towards the establishment of a competency-based curriculum were introduced by *Modernising Medical Careers* in 2004 (Department of Health 2004).

Various organizations provide oversight of medication education. The Postgraduate Medical Education and Training Board (PMETB) was also established in 2005, drawing attention to learning and assessment in the workplace and external accountability. This focus has been maintained following the merger of PMETB and the General Medical Council (GMC) in April 2010. In another development, Health Education England (HEE) was established in 2012 to provide oversight of education and training of the health workforce in England, including medical education (HEE 2012), by continuing to review and develop training for junior doctors (HEE 2019). Within local areas, local educational and training boards (LETBs) assume responsibility for the training of clinical and non-clinical staff, and are committees of HEE (HEE 2017).

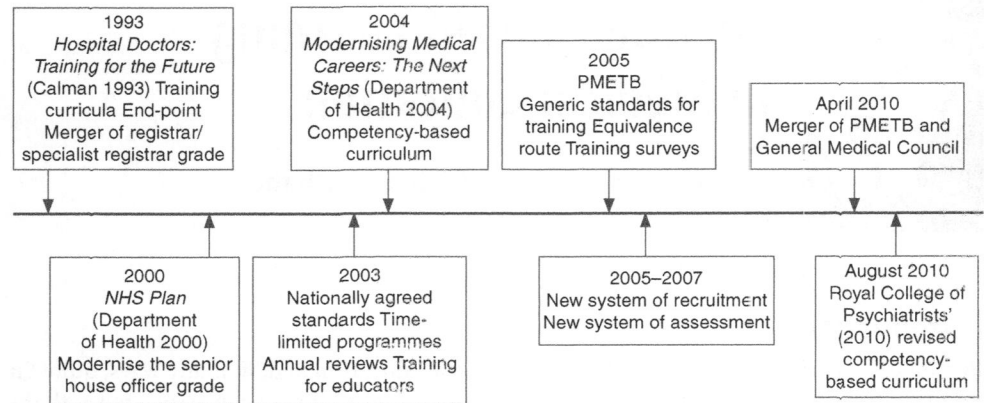

Fig. 17.1 Timeline of changes in medical education. PMETB, Postgraduate Medical Education Training Board.

Interestingly, Williamson (2011) argues that a well-maintained portfolio, by providing corroboration of the competencies achieved, also ensures public accountability, as patients can be confident that a doctor's ability to practise against agreed standards has been clearly evidenced. Given that increasing numbers of junior doctors are taking longer breaks before entering speciality training (GMC 2020), and portfolio careers are becoming more popular (Kemp 2020), portfolios also allow tracking and evidence of achievements and competencies, thereby contributing to increasing flexibility in medical training. General practitioners have long embraced the idea of a portfolio career.

Professionalization of Trainers

Education has always been an integral part of the working day of a consultant because medical education has rightly been centred on patient care. Nonetheless, as the demands and pressures on senior clinicians rapidly increase, is it feasible to expect that medical educators will simply 'find' the time to exercise their role? In addition, as we move away from traditional models of medical education to focus on the process, as well as the content, of learning, can trainers develop a better understanding of 'how best' to educate, an area where they have often had little or no training?

The process of formal recognition of trainers, which will effectively 'professionalize' the role of large numbers of medical educators, presents both challenges and opportunities to address some of these dilemmas. Under the powers of the Medical Act 1983, the GMC, through HEE and the LETBs, in England, but deaneries elsewhere in the UK, has been responsible for the selection and accreditation of general practitioner (GP) trainers for a number of years. This approach had a very positive impact on the quality of training for GPs and provided a useful template for postgraduate medical training in other specialties.

The Patel review (GMC 2010) suggested that 'the GMC should develop a framework for the accreditation of trainers'; after extensive consultation, a proposal to enhance the process of recognition for non-GP trainers was finalized and those initial arrangements came into place in 2013/2014 (GMC 2012a). The GMC do not directly approve trainers in undergraduate, foundation, or speciality training; this is instead the role of the LETBs who follow GMC standards (GMC 2015).

The new arrangements have been in place since 2013/2014 and require postgraduate deans and medical schools to formally recognize medical trainers undertaking these specific roles:

- undergraduate education;
- those responsible for overseeing students' progress at each medical school;
- lead coordinators at each local education provider;
- postgraduate training;
- named educational supervisors; and
- named clinical supervisors.

What a Portfolio Is and What It Is Not

A portfolio can be generally defined as (Paulson 1991: p. 60):

> a purposeful collection of student work that exhibits the student's efforts, progress, and achievements in one or more areas. The collection must include student participation in selecting contents, the criteria for selection, the criteria for judging merit, and evidence of student self-reflection.

In its widest use, the term portfolio has come to encompass a number of commonly used tools in the education and career development of doctors, despite the significant differences in structure and purposes. Therefore, a portfolio is not the same as:

- a logbook, which simply records specific activities undertaken;
- a curriculum vitae, which just provides a summary of an individual's employment history and qualifications;
- a course log, which records training and targeted activities for a specific course; or
- a training folder, which collects evidence of participation in training (e.g., certificates, programmes).

Snadden and Thomas (1998) provide a useful description for portfolios in postgraduate medical education as 'a documentation of learning and an articulation of what has been learned'. These authors suggest that a portfolio can include some of the things listed above as long as the learner also provides written reflective accounts of the events documented, reflections on problem areas, what has been learnt and plans for how new learning needs will be tackled. Driessen and van Tartwijk (2018) write that portfolios in medical education broadly serve three goals:

- to monitor and plan development (with a focus on achievement);
- assessment (with a focus on evidence that competencies are attained); and
- for reflection.

They further note that an individual portfolio may focus on one or a combination of the above goals.

Although a number of other different descriptions are available, it is clear that portfolios provide the best educational value for any learner when the following are achieved:

- the learner takes full responsibility for the creation and the development of the portfolio;

- the portfolio contains an account of the learning that has taken place as well as an articulation of what has been learnt;
- the learner's portfolio is reviewed with another individual (a supervisor, a peer, etc.) who can provide feedback; and
- the portfolio is closely linked to the learner's professional development plan.

Other professional groups have successfully used portfolios as part of their systems for accreditation and continuing education. For example, nurses and midwives consistently rely on the use of professional portfolios to evidence their skills and to support their career development. This process is helpful both in the preregistration stage, to demonstrate the achievement of competencies set out by the Nursing and Midwifery Council, and in the post-registration stage, to show a commitment to ongoing learning and CPD.

Portfolios are also useful springboards for the sort of experiential learning which is often associated with Kolb's learning cycle (Kolb 1984): a model of continuous spiral learning is presented, constantly moving between the realm of concrete experience, through observations and reflections on that experience, to abstract concepts (the theory), which are then tested, evaluated and redefined on the basis of further experience.

Clarke's (2010) suggestion of the use of practice notes (Box 17.1), although mainly directed at nurses, is a useful example of how the above outcomes can be achieved in everyday practice. Similarly, the Royal College of Psychiatrists' (2012) reflective templates for critical (significant) events (Box 17.2) provide a clear direction for any psychiatrist on how to begin to develop a portfolio, which can be used as a reflective tool, linking theory to practice, as well as for revalidation purposes.

What Is the Educational Value of a Portfolio?

Pitts (2010), referring to the growing literature on the use of portfolios, identifies six main purposes:

(1) CPD;
(2) enhanced learning;
(3) assessment;
(4) evaluation;
(5) certification and re-certification; and
(6) career advancement.

Box 17.1 Using practice notes in a portfolio (adapted from Clarke 2010)

A practice note is a way of describing experiences in everyday practice and what has been learnt from them, using the following three questions:

1. What have I done today in terms of patient care activities or team activities?
2. What have I learnt today about: my approach to . . .?

   how much I know about . . .?

   how skilled I am becoming in . . .?

3. What do I need to do now to enhance my knowledge, skills or approach?

> **Box 17.2** Significant event audit: structured reflective template (after Royal College of Psychiatrists 2012)
>
> **What happened?**
> (*Describe the significant event and the context for it*)
> I work with a team providing specialist mental health services to adolescents in the care of the local authority. These young people have had very unsettled lives, disappointing or abusive experiences with their families, and find change very unsettling. Our team is commissioned to see young people up to their 18th birthday and the transition to adult mental health services is often difficult.
>
> A number of our patients experience crises just before or after their 18th birthday. One of our patients was admitted under Section 2 of the Mental Health Act 1983 a week after their 18th birthday.
>
> **What could have been done better?**
> (*Identify triggers and opportunities for better practice*)
> Despite the fact that our team had made efforts to link up with adult mental health teams, our patients often voice concerns at the prospect of working with a set of different professionals. In response to our request for transfer, the adult team had been hesitant and unclear about their potential role. What changes have been agreed? (Identify opportunities for learning and actions to be taken forward)
>
> **Personally**
> Although I was aware of the difficulties of the transition process, this case highlighted the need to focus on the ending process much earlier in the work.
>
> **For the team**
> We have now put in place an even tighter process for transition to adult mental health, which includes a series of meetings with the prospective key worker in the months leading up to the 18th birthday, so that the young person can become familiar with the new treating team. We have also undertaken an audit of cases transferred and presented the results to colleagues in adult mental health to highlight potential difficulties and practice issues.

These items clearly have overlapping scopes and we summarize them in two broad areas of assessment and reflection.

A Portfolio as an Assessment Tool (Formative and Summative)

'The whole discussion about scoring, marking and standard setting is in fact all about finding the best possible way to throw away a substantial amount of measurement information.' (Schuwirth and van der Vleuten 2006: p. 297). This quotation highlights some of the difficulties of using traditional psychometric methods in the assessment of doctors' competence and performance. As it is increasingly recognized that valid assessment methods cannot rely just on the testing acquisition of knowledge and the reproduction of facts, portfolios have been put forward as a useful alternative.

Sturmberg Farmer (2009: p. e86) suggest that an 'assessment should aim to test or closely approximate the learner's capabilities, i.e. the attributes that the learner should demonstrate in actual clinical practice'. Consequently, they advocate the use of portfolios as a flexible and reliable way to demonstrate:

- clinical capability – as this is a reflection of a very complex interaction between knowledge, skills and attitudes, it is arguably best demonstrated through a gathering of 'real practice' examples such as patient letters, records of case-based discussions and peer-review meetings;
- reflective abilities – the building of the portfolio is predicated on the process of reflection, both at the beginning (in the purposeful and attentive collection of the actual material) and throughout the process when further learning needs can be identified on the basis of gaps, challenges and difficult encounters in clinical experience;
- organizational capability – these are the domains of practice often referred to as non-technical or non-clinical skills (e.g., leadership, the ability to work effectively as part of a team, awareness of one's role in a complex organization). These skills, which underpin and enhance any practitioner's technical skills and underline successful performance, are undoubtedly essential to mental health practitioners but notoriously hard to measure with traditional assessment tools. A portfolio has the significant advantage of incorporating elements of feedback which most closely reflect achievement in these areas of professional practice.

Portfolios have high face validity when used for formative and developmental assessments and this is probably the more widespread and uncontested use of portfolio-based learning.

Despite the advantages highlighted above, the use of portfolios for summative assessments in medical education is still relatively untested and a number of potential difficulties are reported in the literature. Snadden and Thomas (1998), on the basis of the findings of their study on portfolio learning in general practice vocational training, urge caution against portfolio-based summative assessment. This is because the presence of high-stakes external monitoring might fundamentally alter the nature and content of the material that the learners might include in a portfolio, at the expense of any problem areas or examples of 'less than excellent' practice, the very areas one would wish to usefully focus on in a formative, reflective portfolio.

In addition, as Challis (1999: p. 375) points out, 'the highly individual nature of each portfolio means that their assessment can present as many challenges as the building of the portfolio itself'. Therefore, issues concerning interrater reliability (how the scores of different examiners correlate), variability of content (how much freedom the learner should be allowed in the choice of content) and criterion-related validity (how portfolio-based assessments compare with other forms of assessment) are often quoted as barriers to a more widespread introduction of portfolio-based summative assessments.

A Portfolio as a Tool to Enhance Learning and Reflection

The process of reflection is a cornerstone of adult learning and, for medical practitioners, the necessary link between the academic knowledge acquired during years of rigorous training and the day-to-day experience of dealing with patients' illness and suffering. An often quoted analogy by Donald Schon (1984: p. 42) clearly illustrates the challenges of translating theoretical, evidence-based, technical solutions (what Shon describes as 'the high ground') to complex encounters with patients, the 'swampy lowlands of practice'.

Portfolio-based learning has clear value in helping practitioners develop that link, creating a bridge between theory and practice and encouraging further learning that arises directly from dilemmas in clinical practice. As Challis (1999: p. 371) points out:

> the building of the portfolio itself requires engagement in a process of reflection and critical self-awareness. Its creation therefore constitutes an educational process, and this aspect needs to be recognised over and above the outcomes of learning that are identified and evidenced in the physical material contained in the portfolio.

The examples in Boxes 17.1 and 17.2 use different approaches to illustrate the value of a reflective portfolio in promoting improvements in clinical practice and learning from challenging situations. By stimulating reflection and self-analysis, a portfolio provides the additional benefit of highlighting gaps in skills and knowledge, prompting practitioners at every level of experience and training to find creative solutions to address them.

How Are Portfolios Currently Used in the Professional Development of Doctors?

Foundation Training

All doctors in foundation must use an electronic portfolio, which serves as evidence of satisfactory learning. The UK Foundation Programme (2021) states that the foundation portfolio generally should contain:

- [a] personal development plan (PDP);
- meetings with your educational and clinical supervisors;
- assessments;
- supervised learning events (SLEs);
- reflective reports and other evidence; and
- [an] ARCP (annual review of competencies progression)

More detail on the foundation programme can be found in Chapter 16 of this volume. Some of the tensions, as well as the benefits, of using a portfolio are highlighted in this quote by a foundation year 1 doctor (Moore 2010: p. 20):

Finally, the temptation is to fill in the portfolio because it's a requirement, and you're running out of time by the end of the year. But this is something to be proud of, and ultimately should be a personal log of what you've become since passing medical school – a competent doctor.

Specialist Training

Portfolios, usually e-portfolios, are used to support and monitor the educational progress of doctors in a range of specialist training programmes.

The Royal College of Psychiatrists also has an e-portfolio, and all doctors in training are registered with it, as it supports the annual review of competence progression (ARCP). This is a mandatory process that reviews the ongoing progress of doctors in training through a portfolio of evidence, which is gathered in a structured way by the trainee and evaluated by a panel. The evidence collected in the portfolio compromises a number of workplace-based assessments (WPBA), multi-source feedback, reports from educational and clinical supervisors and evidence of mandatory training, among other items; these are subsequently mapped to the Royal College of Psychiatrists' training curriculum. An enhanced ARCP process, with clear responsibilities for the doctor in training, the responsible officer (the Postgraduate Dean in England, or equivalent role in the other UK countries) and the employing organization is the vehicle for the revalidation of doctors in training (GMC 2012b).

The 'Seasoned' Practitioner

In its revised CPD policy, the Royal College of Psychiatrists encourages a portfolio-based approach with self-accreditation as well as peer reviewing, with the College regularly auditing a sample of returns (Royal College of Psychiatrists 2015). Along similar lines, the GMC's guidance for CPD (GMC 2012c) also provides a good framework to think about the ongoing needs of doctors in a way that is both practical and reflective.

A model of portfolio-based accreditation, with a rolling three-year cycle of review, is promoted by Health Education England with their Professional Development Framework for Educators. It applies to all named supervisors (clinical and educational) within a trust or local education provider, in line with the GMC standards for named supervisors set out in *Promoting Excellence* (GMC 2015). The quality control for this accreditation process is generally within the role of the Director of Medical Education, though arrangements may vary.

Most importantly, the process of revalidation is also a key driver for the use of portfolios by medical professionals. This is because revalidation is dependent on a system of annual appraisals based on the Good Medical Practice Framework (GMC 2013, updated 2014) and therefore strongly relies on the doctor's ability to provide relevant supporting information in a structured and well-thought-out portfolio. This is not intended as a mere collection of evidence of the doctor's achievements – GMC guidance (GMC 2013: p. 1) clearly highlights the importance of the reflective process which underpins the development of any worthwhile portfolios:

> When you are preparing for your appraisal and collecting supporting information, you should review your practice and consider how the supporting information can demonstrate that you are continuing to meet the principles and values set out in Good Medical Practice [. . .] In most cases, your appraiser will be interested in what you did with the information and your reflections on that information, not simply that you collected it and maintained it in a portfolio. Your appraiser will want to know what you think the supporting information says about your practice and how you intend to develop or modify your practice as a result of that reflection.

In its own guidance on revalidation, the Royal College of Psychiatrists (2014) provides a detailed list of the sort of supporting information psychiatrists ought to include in their portfolio.

It is useful to consider the potential difficulties of introducing portfolios to experienced practitioners, as on one hand they may be less likely than trainees to be familiar with their use, and on the other they may be required, at any time, to maintain three different ones concurrently:

(1) a CPD portfolio;
(2) a supervisor's portfolio (for those in educational roles); and
(3) a revalidation portfolio.

In terms of the specific challenges for psychiatrists, the Royal College of Psychiatrists' and GMC's recommendations about the intents and purposes of such portfolios share a clear emphasis on the value of reflection, learning from experience and multi-source feedback. However, confusion about overlapping information and roles remain.

In terms of overlapping information, is the CPD portfolio just a subsection of the revalidation portfolio? How much of the information in the supervisor's portfolio is repeated in the CPD portfolio? Do the purposes of the individual portfolios overlap? Heeneman and Driessen (2017) acknowledge the problems of keeping one large portfolio, and that the purposes of portfolios will overlap, but argue that these problems can be overcome with proper portfolio design and clear objectives for all those involved with the portfolio, including supervisors and educators.

In terms of overlapping roles, is the Director of Medical Education performing the same role of the responsible officer in appraising supervisors? How does the three-yearly educational appraisal for supervisors relate to the general appraisal, given that most consultants also have supervisory roles?

These issues are still left to be addressed at local levels.

Practical Considerations

Although it is clear that a number of developments in educational theory underpin the value of portfolio-based learning, the introduction of portfolios in the medical profession has been met by mixed responses. A study assessing the knowledge, attitudes and pattern of use of portfolios by psychiatric trainees (Seed et al. 2007) showed that although doctors' attitudes to the use of portfolios were broadly neutral, their understanding of their actual purpose and benefits was very limited. Relatively few trainees had included in their portfolios examples of reflective practice, despite the available evidence that portfolios are probably most effective as reflective tools. Similarly, a more recent study of psychiatric trainees' views on portfolios (Halder et al. 2012) shows large variations in the use and appreciation of the usefulness of this learning tool. A systematic review of portfolio use in medical, nursing and allied health professional undergraduate education (Buckley et al. 2009) found several benefits of portfolio use, including in promoting acquisition of knowledge and the use of reflection, but also noted that the additional time needed to keep portfolios could have a negative impact on engagement with it.

A systematic review of the use of portfolios (Driessen et al. 2007) highlight several potential issues which may account for the 'mixed success':

- poor introduction;
- time constraints;
- lack of clarity about structure;
- lack of adequate support; and
- the issue of assessment.

Although now widely used, the response to e-portfolios remain mixed, with one study of core medical trainees showing broad suspicion of the value of the e-portfolio as an educational tool (Tailor et al. 2014). Driessen emphasizes that users' views of portfolio-based learning are mixed, and that incorrectly used portfolios and e-portfolios can appear more like bureaucratic exercises than educational tools when not implemented appropriately.

These issues are echoed by Davis et al. (2013), who note that:

- keeping portfolios and e-portfolios can be time-consuming;
- the purpose of the portfolio must be clearly defined;
- assessors must be trained;
- there may be ownership issues around evidence, the possibility of plagiarism needs to be considered, and if they are to be used as summative assessments 'the triangulation of contents with other sources is desirable' (Davis et al. 2013: p. 74); and
- the relevance of reflective work may not be clear to portfolio creators or assessors.

Moreover, concern about the possibility of having to release reflective writing from portfolios following legal requests has led to the Academy of Medical Royal Colleges providing additional guidance on writing reflective notes, which can be found at www.aomrc.org.uk/wp-content/uploads/2016/11/Academy_Guidance_on_e-Portfolios_201916-5.pdf.

Some of the cautions about the use of portfolios as summative assessment tools will undoubtedly apply to revalidation portfolios, particularly with regard to the nature and content of the material included. This will only partially be chosen by the doctor, who will have to engage with a variety of service-related information that does not always reflect individual performance (e.g., DNA data and cancellation reports, data on outcome measures, bed usage and serious untoward incidents) and a range of organizational priorities affecting individual performance (staffing levels and funding, support for developmental activities in job plans, etc.).

It has been proposed that some of the practical challenges can be overcome by the use of e-portfolios; for example, having access to electronic devices for timely recording is known to increase the frequency of reflection (Macaulay and Winyard 2012). This is indeed promising but the expectations about accessibility and functionality cannot be underestimated, as highlighted by Pathiraja (2012):

> the ePortfolio is far from perfect. The end user is typically generation Y and expects technology to have the beautiful aesthetics and seamless functionality of their i-products.

Conclusion

A portfolio-based approach fits very well with ideas about adult learning; a well-maintained portfolio, by allowing the learner to retain a high degree of flexibility and control over their own learning, is clearly one of the educational strategies that promote the development of self-directed learning. Although the reliance on the learner's ability to identify and effectively address learning needs has been questioned (Davis et al. 2006), other sources for their identification are recognized in the literature, including peer review, external observation, gap or discrepancy analysis. All of those methods, alongside self-assessment and self-direction, strengthen and complement a portfolio- based approach to learning and would enhance any professional portfolio.

Barriers to the use of portfolios, both practical and ideological, are often quoted. This is despite the trend towards their increasing usage, which is based on sound educational principles and, most importantly, mirrors changing values and expectations about training (including increased flexibility), assessment and CPD within the profession and among the general public.

Although there are clearly no straightforward answers for these dilemmas, it is important for all psychiatrists to actively seek to engage in this dialogue about changing values and expectations, as suggested by Bhugra (2008: p. 282):

In the 21st century, it is only appropriate that psychiatry as a profession revisits what society expects from the profession and in turn what we expect from society. Complacency, paternalism, arrogance, inability to self-regulate and poor leadership have no place in our profession.

The use of portfolios as an example of 'authentic', real-life assessments gives us yet another opportunity to do just that. In addition, the use of portfolios calls for medical educators to rethink some of the paradigms on which traditional examinations and appraisals have been based, to make room for a different set of educational values and prioritize learning from reflective practice which 'accepts the subjectivity of data and interpretations, and focuses on individual insights and developments [...] values creativity and, importantly, allows and understands the possibility of being wrong' (Pitts 2010: p. 104).

References

Bhugra D (2008) Renewing psychiatry's contract with society. *Psychiatrist*, **32**: 281–3.

Buckley S, Coleman J, Davison I., et al. (2009) The educational effects of portfolios on undergraduate student learning: a Best Evidence Medical Education (BEME) systematic review. BEME Guide No. 11. *Medical Teacher*, **31**: 282–298. https://doi.org/10.1080 /01421590902889897

Calman K (1993). *Hospital Doctors: Training for the Future. The Report of the Working Group on Specialist Medical Training.* HMSO.

Challis M (1999) AMEE Medical Education Guide No. 11 (revised): portfolio-based learning and assessment in medical education. *Medical Teacher*, **21**: 370–86.

Clarke AC (2010) How to compile a professional portfolio 1: aims and intended learning outcomes. *Nursing Times*, **106**: 41.

Davis DA, Mazmanian PE, Fordis M, et al. (2006) Accuracy of physician self-assessment compared with observed measures of competence. *JAMA*, **29**: 1094–102.

Davis M, Forrest K, McKimm J (2013) Portfolios. In Davis M, Forest K and McKimm J (eds.), *How to Assess Doctors and Health Professionals.* John Wiley & Sons, 68–80.

Department of Health, Scottish Executive, Welsh Assembly Government, et al. (2004) *Modernising Medical Careers: The Next Steps. The Future Shape of Foundation, Specialist and General Practice Training Programmes.* Department of Health. Available at: https://webarchive.nationalarc hives.gov.uk/ukgwa/20130107105354/http:// www.dh.gov.uk/assetRoot/04/07/95/32/ 04079532.pdf.

Driessen E (2017) Do portfolios have a future? *Advances in Health Sciences Education*, **22**: 221–8.

Driessen E, van Tartwijk J (2018) Portfolios in personal and professional development. In Swanwick T, Forrest K, O'Brien BC (eds.), *Understanding Medical Education.* John Wiley & Sons, Inc., pp. 255–262.

Driessen E, van Tartwijk J, van der Vleuten C, et al. (2007) Portfolios in medical education: why do they meet with mixed success? A systematic review. *Medical Education*, **41**: 1224–33.

GMC (2010) *Final Report of the Education and Training Regulation Policy Review: Recommendations and Options for the Future Regulation of Education and Training.* General Medical Council.

GMC (2012a) *Recognising and Approving Trainers: The Implementation Plan.* General Medical Council.

GMC (2012b) *Information for Doctors in Training.* General Medical Council.

GMC (2012c) *Continuing Professional Development: Guidance for All Doctors*. General Medical Council.

GMC (2013) *The Good Medical Practice Framework for Appraisal and Revalidation.* General Medical Council.

GMC (2015) *Promoting Excellence: Standards for Medical Education and Training*. General Medical Council.

GMC (2020) *The State of Medical Education and Practice in the UK 2020*. General Medical Council.

Halder N, Subramanian G, Longson D (2012) Trainees' views of portfolios in psychiatry. *Psychiatrist*, **36**: 427–33.

HEE (2012) *Introducing Health Education England*. Health Education England.

HEE (2017) Our leaders and structure. Available at: www.hee.nhs.uk/about/ how-we-work/our-leaders-structure (accessed 21 July 2021).

HEE (2019) Reforming medical education for the good of all. Available at: www.hee.nhs .uk/news-blogs-events/blogs/reforming-medical -education-good-all.

HEE (2020) *Professional Development Framework for Educators 2020–2021*. Health Education England.

Heeneman S, Driessen EW (2017) The use of a portfolio in postgraduate medical education: reflect, assess and account, one for each or all in one? *GMS Journal for Medical* Education, **34**: 57.

Kemp N (2020) Portfolio careers: the 'new normal'? Available at: www.bma.org.uk/ news-and-opinion/portfolio-careers-the-new-normal.

Kolb DA (1984) *Experiential Learning: Experience as a Source of Learning and Development*. Prentice Hall.

Macaulay CP, Winyard PJW (2012) Reflection: tick box exercise or learning for all? *BMJ*, **345**: e7468.

Moore CG (2010) *The Rough Guide to the Foundation Programme*, 3rd ed. The UK Foundation Programme Office.

Pathiraja F (2012). The ePortfolio and generation Y. *BMJ Group Blogs*, 25 July. Available at: http://blogs.bmj.com/bmj/2012/ 07/25/fiona-pathiraja-the- eportfolio-and-generation-y.

Pitts (2010) Portfolios, personal development and reflective practice. In Swanwick T (ed.), *Understanding Medical Education: Evidence, Theory and Practice*. Wiley-Blackwell, pp. 99–110.

Paulson FL, Paulson PR, Meyer CA (1991) What makes a portfolio a portfolio? *Educational Leadership*, **48**: 60–3.

Royal College of Psychiatrists (2012). *Revalidation Guidance for Psychiatrists (College Report CR172).* Royal College of Psychiatrists.

Royal College of Psychiatrists (2014). *Supporting Information for Appraisal and Revalidation: Guidance for Psychiatrists (College Report CR 194)*. Royal College of Psychiatrists.

Royal College of Psychiatrists (2015) Continuing professional development: guidance for psychiatrists (College Occasional Paper OP98). Available at: www.rcpsych.ac.uk/docs/ default-source/members/cpd/members-cpd-op98.pdf?sfvrsn=1de40c5f_4.

Schon D (1984) *The Reflective Practitioner: How Practitioners Think in Action*. Basic Books.

Schuwirth LWT, van der Vleuten CPM (2006) A plea for new psychometric models in educational assessment. *Medical Education*, **40**: 296–300.

Seed K, Davies L, McIvor RJ (2007) Learning portfolios in psychiatric training. *Psychiatrist*, **31**: 310–12.

Snadden D, Thomas ML (1998) Portfolio learning in general practice vocational training: does it work? *Medical Education*, **32**: 401–6.

Sturmberg JP, Farmer L (2009) Educating capable doctors: a portfolio approach. Linking learning and assessment. *Medical Teacher*, **31**: e85–9.

Swanwick T (2018) Understanding medical education. In Stanwick T Forrest K, O'Brien BC (eds.), *Understanding Medical Education*. John Wiley & Sons, Inc., pp. 1–6.

Tailor A, Dubrey S, Das S (2014) Opinions of the ePortfolio and workplace-based assessments: a survey of core medical trainees and their supervisors. *Clinical Medicine*, 14: 510–16; doi: https://doi.org/10.7861/clinmedicine.14-5-510.

UK Foundation Programme Office (2021) E-Portfolio. Available at: https://foundationprogramme.nhs.uk/curriculum/e-portfolio/ (accessed 21 July 2021).

Williamson A (2011) Building a portfolio. *BMJ Careers*, 15 September.

Bringing Smartphone Technology into Undergraduate and Postgraduate Psychiatry

Chapter 18

Melvyn W. B. Zhang, Cyrus S. H. Ho, Christopher C. S. Cheok and Roger C. M. Ho

Introduction

Over the past decade, there have been massive developments in web-based and internet technologies, along with the introduction of smartphones. Smartphones represent a new generation of mobile technology that has fundamentally changed telecommunications (Abboudi and Amin 2011). They are equipped with immense computing capabilities that allow constant access to the internet and they enable more than just voice- and text-based communication. Smartphones are generally regarded as handheld computers rather than merely mobile telephones (Abboudi and Amin 2011). The release of Apple's iPhone in 2007 most likely sparked a revolution in the telecommunications and information technology arena. The launch of the Apple App Store in July 2008 is also regarded as a pivotal moment in the advancement of smartphone technologies (Payne et al. 2012). The store enables users to download smartphone-based applications (apps) – computer programs that give smartphones capabilities and functions beyond accessing the internet.

A literature review that we conducted in July 2014 revealed no rigorous studies of the use of web-based e-learning technologies and smartphone-based technologies in the education of medical students and junior doctors (residents). Hence, there is a paucity of research looking into the application of the latest web-based and, in particular, smartphone technologies in psychiatry education. The purpose of this chapter is to highlight what other medical specialties have done in terms of research into educational smartphone apps and what psychiatry could potentially do for its trainees to make the most of smartphone and web-based technologies for education.

Medical Students' and Trainees' Perspectives on Smartphones

Recent studies have examined medical students' and trainees' ownership, usage and perspectives on smartphones. In 2012, a questionnaire-based survey was distributed among interns in the Republic of Ireland (O'Connor et al. 2014). This study demonstrated that smartphones were widely adopted and that they were being used daily by interns to help them perform their regular duties. The British National Formulary was the most commonly used app. Another study in the same year (Payne et al. 2012) found a high level of smartphone ownership among the 257 UK medical students and 131 junior doctors surveyed. The majority of the participants owned between one and five medically related apps. Compared with other platforms, iPhone users were more likely to own apps. App use was similar for both the students and the trainee doctors, the majority using them for

212

20–30 minutes a day. The most frequently used apps were those for disease diagnosis and management and drug reference.

In 2013, Robinson et al. carried out a questionnaire-based study looking into smartphone usage and acceptability among clinical medical students at the University of Birmingham, UK (Robinson et al. 2013). In all, 361 students took part; 59 per cent of them owned a smartphone and 37 per cent of these reported using the device to help them in their learning. Importantly, the students had generally positive attitudes towards the concept of using smartphones as future educational aids, with at least 84 per cent of them believing the devices to be useful. However, it is also important to note that about 64 per cent of these students felt that smartphones might be too costly to introduce in clinical education.

The studies described above were largely limited to an examination of smartphone and app ownership and usage rates, and the general views of medical students and trainees on smartphones and apps. There has been a paucity of research looking at apps themselves, for example, students' evaluation and views of a particular educational app that their tutors have asked them to use. This gap in terms of research evidence has recently been addressed by Payne et al. (2014). This research group conducted a pilot study to investigate the effect of a hospital-specific smartphone app on the work of a cohort of British junior doctors. The investigators created an iPhone app that contained mainly disease management and antibiotic dosing guidelines specific to the hospital and tested it with 39 foundation year doctors for four months. Their results showed that participants felt generally positive towards the availability of such an app, with 68 per cent reporting that it helped them save time when performing clinical activities.

In a study among orthopaedic trainees, Al-Hadithy et al. (2012) noted that smartphones allowed them to complete their work-based assessments without the need for computer access, which might increase completion rates and reliability. More journals now provide podcasts and video tutorials that can be accessed on smartphones, which is particularly useful for higher examinations.

Smartphone Use for Education in Medical Specialties

Franko and Tirrell (2012) conducted an email survey of smartphone and smartphone app use by medical providers in the US Accreditation Council for Graduate Medical Education (ACGME) training programmes. Of the 3,306 respondents, 1,397 were residents, 524 fellows and 1,385 attending physicians. More than 85 per cent of the respondents used a smartphone. Importantly, the study highlighted that the app types most frequently requested by the respondents were associated with textbook/reference materials, classifications, treatment algorithms and general medical knowledge. Out of the 134 psychiatry respondents, 84 per cent used a smartphone and 63 per cent of them used apps. The study found no association between the level of training and the use of apps.

Given the generally positive attitudes and perspectives that trainees and medical students have towards smartphones and smartphone apps, more specialties are actively embracing the smartphone as an educational tool (Box 18.1).

Current Use of Technology in Psychiatric Training and Education

For over a decade, journals such as *Academic Psychiatry* have noted that knowledge and skills in medical informatics are essential for lifelong learning and modern psychiatric

Box 18.1 How other medical specialties are using smartphone apps

Nephrology

In their review paper, Bhasin et al. (2013) identified several online learning resources that improve medical students' and residents' knowledge about the complications of chronic kidney disease.

Despite the existence of several nephrology apps, such as calculators for nephrology-based equations and drug information for kidney dosing, there is still a lack of nephrology education tools for clinicians and medical trainees.

Ophthalmology

Hassani et al. (2013) searched through the Apple App Store and the Android Play Store and identified 342 apps relevant to ophthalmology, some intended for patients, some for ophthalmologists. It might be inferred that some of these apps might be helpful in education and in enhancing ophthalmologists' clinical skills.

Orthopaedics

Al-Hadithy et al. (2012) noted the potential of the smartphone not only in education but also as an invaluable tool in clinical care. Commonly used educational apps include AO Surgery Reference and Zollinger's Atlas of Surgical Operations, which provide immediate access to information pertaining to surgical procedures, and iSpineOperations, which provides three-dimensional animations of cervical and lumbar spine procedures.

Paediatrics

Hawkes et al. (2013) identified a lack of current studies demonstrating the usefulness of smartphones and smartphone apps in teaching of core clinical skills. Twenty paediatric trainees evaluated NeoTube, a smartphone neonatal intubation instructional app. Use of the app resulted in an increase in the trainees' overall skills score and a reduction in the duration of each intubation attempt.

Pharmacology

Haffey et al. (2014) noted that many pharmacology-themed apps offer the potential to improve the ease and accuracy of oral dose calculations and intravenous dose calculation and delivery, and that the current wealth of apps also allows users greater ease of access to popular pharmacological textbooks, guides and journals. However, textbook-based educational apps tend to be very expensive and are not affordable for all users.

Plastic Surgery

Al-Hadithy and Ghosh (2013) give a comprehensive guide to mobile-based educational websites, podcasts, videos and electronic books for plastic surgeons. There are at least 16 apps of educational value for plastic surgeons, including Mersey Burns, a free app for calculating burn area percentages and the amount of fluids that should be prescribed.

Urology

Abboudi and Amin (2011) highlight apps that can help urologists in their daily clinical practice and several apps (such as Urology Flashcards) have been developed specifically for educational purposes. They describe how an app based on the widely used Oxford Handbook series has potential educational benefits, offering quick access to relevant information for residents and trainees.

> **Box 18.2** Current use of technology in psychiatry education
>
> - Personal digital assistants (PDAs) to check for evidence-based information
> - Online e-learning modules and learning resources such as the Royal College of Psychiatrists' CPD Online (https://psychiatry-training.com/) and Trainees Online (tron .rcpsych.ac.uk)
> - Videos to enable students to gain insight into psychiatric disorders
> - Tele-technologies in the supervision of junior doctors during psychodynamic psychotherapy training

practice (Hilty et al. 2006) (Box 18.2). A needs-based assessment was conducted, and it was previously proposed that the existing psychiatry curriculum needs to integrate with the advancement in technologies. A 2006 pilot study of users' perceptions of technology in medicine demonstrated that residents and medical students believed technology skills to be integral to their medical training (Briscoe et al. 2006). Participants indicated a preference for the use of PDAs as these provide immediate access to critical information pertinent to the clinical care of patients. More recent research has looked into the use of e-learning in the teaching of psychiatry to medical students (Weninger et al. 2009). This particular feasibility trial, at the University of Ulm, Germany, showed that child and adolescent psychiatry case studies could successfully be added to an e-learning system primarily oriented towards somatic disease. In another German study, psychiatric educators at the Hamburg Medical School used 'cinemeducation' to help students gain a deeper understanding of psychiatric illnesses (Kuhnigk et al. 2012).

The latest advancement in technology is the application of unique teletechnologies to help augment resident training in psychodynamic psychotherapy (Katzman 2015).

A Framework for Psychiatry to Adopt

Although our literature search for this article revealed no recent reviews of apps specific to psychiatric training, there are many apps for academic purposes in the commercial app stores. A quick search using the keywords 'psychiatry education' reveals 266 apps in the Apple App Store and 240 in the Android Play Store.

A scoping review was recently conducted by Boydell et al. (2014) to assess the use of technology (such as videoconferencing, mobile phone apps and websites) in delivering mental health services to children in Canada. They carried out a descriptive numerical summary and thematic analysis of the reviewed literature. They concluded that technology did indeed play a major role in the service and support provided to children; it also played a role in the prevention, assessment, diagnosis and treatment of psychiatric disorders.

It might be worth carrying out more scoping reviews in psychiatry. One might analyse peer-reviewed studies on education in psychiatry, to summarize the key findings of current research and to identify knowledge gaps. Another might assess the application of technology in the specialty, which would be essential for understanding the breadth and impact of current research. A scoping review could also consider commercial psychiatry-related educational apps that are currently available in app stores and highlight their common themes.

Haffey et al. (2014) have suggested two ways of overcoming the lack of evidence-based educational apps in pharmacology that would serve well in psychiatry (Box 18.3). The first

---

Box 18.3 A framework that psychiatry could adopt for educational needs

- Conduct a scoping review to identify the current gaps in psychiatry education and commercially available educational apps in psychiatry
- Enable clinicians and educators to develop their own 'in-house' educational apps
- Enable clinicians and educators to identify suitable educational apps through a systematic peer-review process

---

involves encouraging universities and healthcare organizations to create their own 'in-house' apps. They suggest that in-house apps have inherent advantages, including the fact that they could focus on current shortfalls in clinical education or deficiencies in the competencies of medical students or junior doctors. The second is for universities and healthcare organizations to compile lists of apps that have been peer-reviewed and deemed suitable for use by medical students or junior doctors.

Developing In-house Educational Apps

As regards Haffey et al.'s first suggestion, clinicians in universities could play a greater role by using existing easy-to-follow software to develop simple web-based apps. This strategy has been described by Subhi et al. (2014), who show how to create a simple web-based mobile app using just an internet browser and a text editor. The jQuery Mobile builder (jquerymobile.com) leads the clinician through a step-by-step process of creating a custom app. The builder automatically generates codes based on the content that the clinician has included and the clinician pastes these into a text-editor file, thereby creating a simple smartphone-based web app. They can thus create their own apps for the dissemination of information they feel is pertinent for the educational needs of medical students and junior doctors. Elsewhere (Zhang 2014a,b), we describe in greater detail how psychiatrists could be app developers and introduce two other cost-effective methods for app development. Here, we outline two educational portals and apps for undergraduate and postgraduate education with which we have been involved.

The Mastering Psychiatry Portal

In collaboration with colleagues around the world, we used the method described above to develop the Mastering Psychiatry online portal and smartphone app (masteringpsychiatry .wordpress.com). The portal, which went online in 2013, was originally conceived to help Singapore's medical undergraduates, giving them access to a free online textbook and simulated patient videos (Fig. 18.1). By August 2014, there had been 15,803 views and 2,109 downloads of the online textbook (Zhang 2014c).

The app, which was developed between August and December 2013, was supported by an educational grant and subjected to a user survey to evaluate students' perceptions of it. A total of 185 students participated in the survey. Results showed that a high proportion of the students would like an educational psychiatry smartphone app to have the following features: textbook-based content, clinical videos of objective structured clinical examinations (OSCEs) and an event notification service. A high proportion of the students concurred with the perception that a smartphone app would be helpful in psychiatry education and that smartphones can be a viable and good alternative to a book.

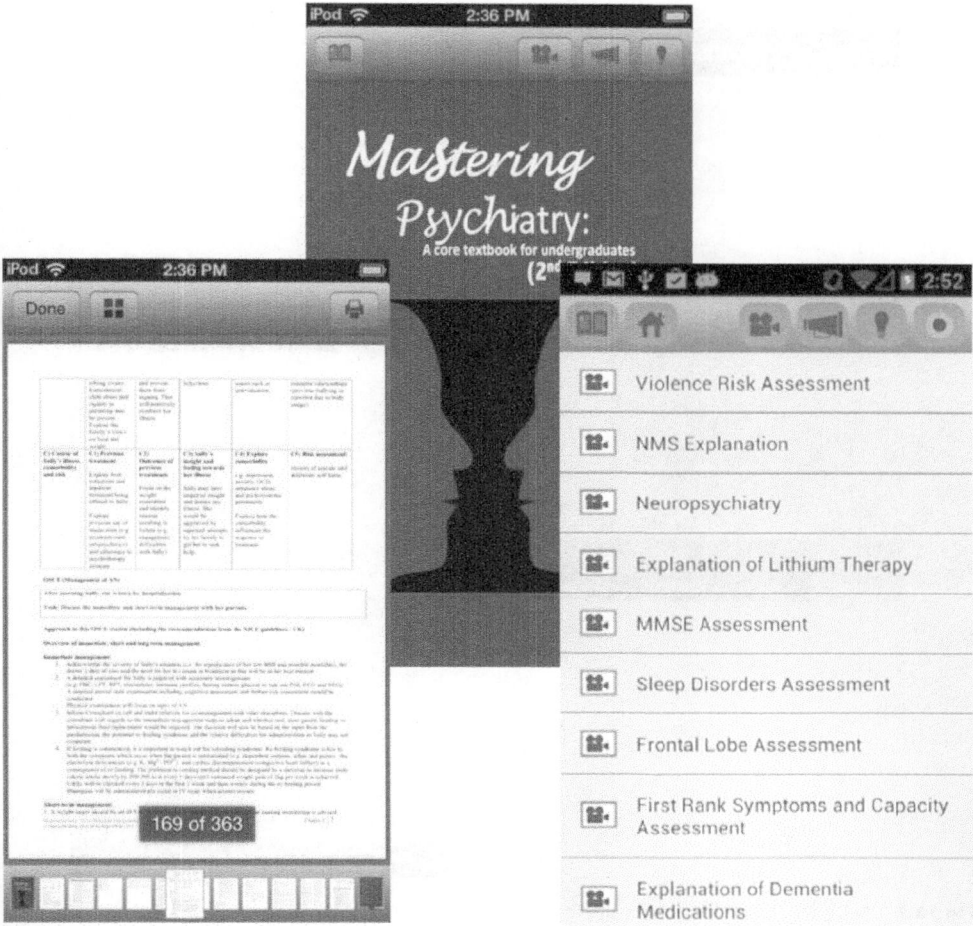

Fig. 18.1 The Mastering Psychiatry textbook and online portal (www.masteringpsychiatry.com).

The CASC Feedback Portal and the Deja Vu CASC App

Another international collaboration, this between the Singapore MRCPsych CASC Consortium and the Cornwall Partnership NHS Foundation Trust in the UK, resulted in the CASC Feedback portal (cascfeedback.org) and the Deja Vu CASC smartphone app (https://dejavucascsg.wordpress.com/) (Fig. 18.2). The latter is now available from the Google Play app store. These were developed between January and April 2014 using methods similar to that outlined above for the creation of web-based apps. Their purpose is to help trainees master the Member of the Royal College of Psychiatrists (MRCPsych) Clinical Assessment of Skills and Competencies (CASC), which is the final examination towards obtaining membership of the Royal College of Psychiatrists.

By August 2014, there had been 57 downloads of the app from the web link made available to trainees via the PsychClub website (www.psychclub.com). In addition, there have been 225 views of the videos deployed within the app. Since the launch of the CASC

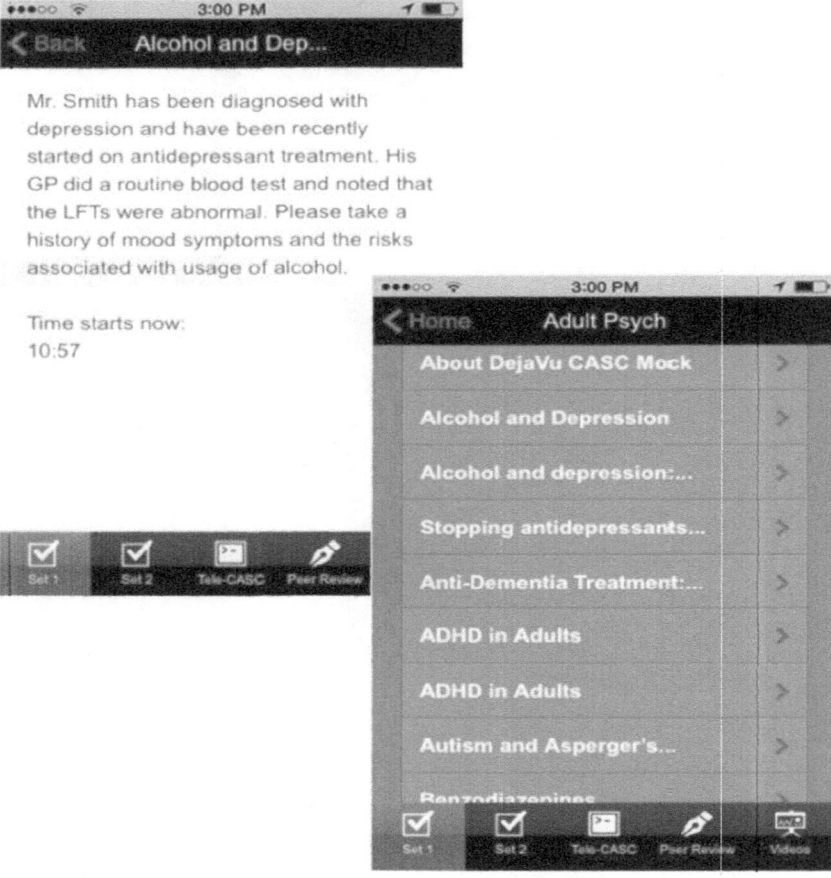

Fig 18.2 The Deja Vu CASC smartphone app (https://dejavucascsg.wordpress.com/).

feedback portal, there have been 65 visitors to the site, the majority of whom are from the UK (n = 36) and Singapore (n =18). These early data, in particular the number of downloads of the app, show that trainees are willing to consider using such a system.

Identifying Suitable Educational Apps through Systematic Peer Review

The second suggestion made by Haffey et al. is for universities and healthcare organizations to compile lists of peer-reviewed apps that educators and clinicians deemed to be suitable for use. Lewis (2013) has suggested criteria for conducting such peer review of smartphone medical apps using a self-certification model. The model (Table 18.1) builds on what has been developed by the Health on the Net Foundation (www.healthonnet.org/HONcode/) to assess the reliability and credibility of the information presented on medical and health websites. Note that the self-certification model provides criteria for evaluating the reliability of the information contained in an app – more work is needed to further a set of criteria to determine the educational value of the app.

Table 18.1 A self-certification model for the review of smartphone apps

Criteria	Description of criteria
Nature of the information in the app	All medical information in the app must be attributed to an author The level of training of the author in his or her specialty must be clearly presented in the app
Purpose of the app	There should be a statement documenting the main purpose of the app and the intended target audience
Confidentiality	The app must include a privacy policy indicating how confidential, private or semi-private information such as email addresses and the contents of emails received are treated The app must inform users whether their data will be recorded in any databases
Information	All medical information within the app must show a specific date of creation, a last modification date and appropriate references
Justification of claims	If there is information about the benefits or performance of any treatment (whether medical or surgical), it has to be supported by scientific evidence
Contact details	There must be a specific way to contact the developer and this information must be included within the app
Disclosures	Apps should disclose their sources of funding, for example, government agencies, private companies or donations Developers should state any conflicts of interest
Advertising policy	Apps that display paying banners need to have an advertising policy: this policy should explain how the app distinguishes between editorial and advertising content and which advertisements are accepted

Before developing new apps, psychiatrists need to assess the increasing numbers of psychiatry-related apps in the app stores to identify those (whether educational or clinical) that are safe and might be of value in their specialty and to reveal current needs and knowledge gaps. The self-certification model can help in such assessments. The literature review on apps that we conducted for this article showed that most papers are limited merely to the identification of apps and have not begun to use models for their peer review and evaluation. If more psychiatrists become involved in the review of psychiatry-related apps and more related publications appear in informatics journals psychiatry as a specialty, this area will advance further.

Advantages and Disadvantages of the Proposed Framework

Advantages

The adoption of the proposed framework for app development and review in psychiatry education has a number of potential advantages:

- there would be more clinician involvement in app building, which would help ensure the quality of content within the apps;

- clinicians and educators could take charge and develop apps that fulfil specific educational needs in their organizations;
- clinicians and educators would be able to systematically review apps and would also have a collection of apps deemed suitable for their universities or organizations;
- clinicians and educators could help to ensure that their collection of apps is evidence-based and safe for use in education;
- use of smartphone technology would enhance students' perceptions of psychiatry as a modern specialty;
- these technologies could facilitate students' mastery of core concepts in psychiatry;
- these technologies would augment current teaching methods; and
- use of smartphone technology would facilitate student's mastery of knowledge 'on the go'.

Disadvantages

The most obvious disadvantages are:

- additional commitments (in terms of time) required to create new educational apps; and
- potential duplication of content.

Conclusion

There have been massive developments and advancements in the use of smartphones and their related apps for education in other medical specialties. Psychiatry should also consider their utilization, given their inherent benefits in education. Two core approaches have been reviewed in this article: equipping psychiatrists with the necessary skills to develop apps themselves; and equipping them with a framework for reviewing existing apps to enable them to create lists of apps that are evidence-based and can be used in their educational setting. Implementation of these two approaches would do much to advance psychiatry as a specialty.

References

Abboudi H, Amin K (2011) Smartphone applications for the urology trainee. *BJU International*, **108**: 1371–5.

Al-Hadithy N, Ghosh S (2013) Smartphones and the plastic surgeon. *Journal of Plastic, Reconstructive and Aesthetic Surgery*, **66**: e155–66.

Al-Hadithy N, Gikas PD, Al-Nammari SS (2012) Smartphones in orthopaedics. *International Orthopaedics*, **36**: 1543–7.

Bhasin B, Estrella MM, Choi MJ (2013) Online CKD education for medical students, residents, and fellows: training in a new era. *Advances in Chronic Kidney Disease*, **20**: 347–56.

Boydell MK, Hodgins M, Pignatiello A, et al. (2014) Using technology to deliver mental health services to children and youth: a scoping review. *Journal of the Canadian Academy of Child and Adolescent Psychiatry*, **23**: 87–99.

Briscoe GW, Fore Arcand LG, Lin T, et al. (2006) Students' and residents' perceptions regarding technology in medical training. *Academic Psychiatry*, **30**: 470–9.

Franko OI, Tirrell TF (2012) Smartphone app use among medical providers in ACGME training programs. *Journal of Medical Systems*, **36**: 3135–9.

Haffey F, Brady RRW, Maxwell S (2014) Smartphone apps to support hospital prescribing and pharmacology education: a review of current provision. *British Journal of Clinical Pharmacology*, **77**: 31–8.

Hassani TJR, Sanharawi EM, Dupont-Monod S, et al. (2013) Smartphones in ophthalmology [article in French]. *Journal Français d'Ophtalmologie*, 36: 499–525.

Hawkes CP, Walsh BH, Ryan CA, et al. (2013) Smartphone technology enhances newborn intubation knowledge and performance amongst paediatric trainees. *Resuscitation*, 84: 223–6.

Hilty DM, Hales DJ, Briscoe G, et al. (2006) APA Summit on Medical Student Education Task Force on Informatics and Technology: learning about computers and applying computer technology to education and practice. *Academic Psychiatry*, 30: 29–35.

Katzman J, Abbass A, Coughlin P, et al. (2015) Building connections through teletechnologies to augment resident training in psychodynamic psychotherapy. *Academic Psychiatry*, 39: 110–13.

Kuhnigk O, Schreiner J, Reimer J, et al. (2012) Cinemeducation in psychiatry: a seminar in undergraduate medical education combining a movie, lecture, and patient interview. *Academic Psychiatry*, 36: 205–10.

Lewis TL (2013) A systematic self-certification model for mobile medical apps. *Journal of Medical Internet Research*, 15: e89.

O'Connor P, Byrne D, Butt M, et al. (2014) Interns and their smartphones: use for clinical practice. *Postgraduate Medical Journal*, 90: 75–9.

Payne KFB, Wharrad H, Watts K (2012) Smartphone and medical related App use among medical students and junior doctors in the United Kingdom (UK): a regional survey. *BMC Medical Informatics and Decision Making*, 12: 121.

Payne KFB, Weeks L, Dunning P (2014) A mixed methods pilot study to investigate the impact of a hospital-specific iPhone application (iTreat) within a British junior doctor cohort. *Health Informatics Journal*, 20: 59–73.

Robinson T, Cronin T, Ibrahim H, et al. (2013) Smartphone use and acceptability among clinical medical students: a questionnaire-based study. *Journal of Medical Systems*, 37: 9936.

Subhi Y, Todsen T, Ringsted C, et al. (2014) Designing web-apps for smartphones can be as easy as making slideshow presentations. *BMC Research Notes*, 7: 94.

Weninger L, Keller F, Fegert JM, et al. (2009) Docs'n Drugs – an E-learning program for medical students; feasibility and evaluation of the acceptance in student training in child and adolescent psychiatry at the University Hospital in Ulm [article in German]. *Zeitschrift für Kinder und Jugendpsychiatrie und Psychotherapie*, 37: 123–8.

Zhang M, Cheow E, Ho CS, et al. (2014a) Application of low-cost methodologies for mobile phone app development. *JMIR Mhealth and Uhealth*, 2: e55.

Zhang MW, Tsang T, Cheow E, et al. (2014b) Enabling psychiatrists to be mobile phone app developers: insights into app development methodologies. *JMIR Mhealth and Uhealth*, 2: e53.

Zhang MWB, Ho CSH, Shankar R, et al. (2014c) *Mastering Psychiatry: A Core Textbook for Undergraduates*, 3rd ed. Lulu.

Evidence-Based Mental Health and E-Learning

Katharine A. Smith, Katherine E. Stevens, Andrea Cipriani and John R. Geddes

Introduction

'E-learning' can be defined broadly as the use of internet technologies to deliver teaching and to enhance knowledge and performance. It is also referred to as web-based, online, distributed or internet-based learning (Ruiz et al. 2006). Many sites use 'blended learning', where e-learning is combined with in-person or virtual face-to-face instructor-led training.

The increase in portability, power and connectivity of devices means that most smartphones can easily access information in real time (Marzano et al. 2017) and, of internet users worldwide, 93% access the internet via mobile devices (Johnson 2021). This means that access to the internet to gather information about mental health is immediate, but the vast number of information sites can easily become overwhelming for both patients and clinicians. A simple search for a single mental health topic generates a huge number and range of results. These vary from reviews of the evidence and primary research articles, to news articles and advertisements for treatment centres. The internet user is swamped with an array of sites of variable (and often unknown) quality, which are neither necessarily relevant to the original question nor ranked in order of reliability.

The large number of sites and amount of information mean that although clinicians have many questions regarding patient care, they only pursue answers to these questions via the internet in half of cases. The commonest reason for clinicians not researching an answer is the perception that they will not be able to find it among the multitude of possible information sites (Ely et al. 2005). This is confirmed, as in a quarter of cases when clinicians do look for an answer, they cannot find it (Ely et al. 2007). Time pressure together with a lack of searching skills and awareness of accessible sources are reported as frequent barriers (Daei et al. 2020).

By contrast, the immediate access provided via the internet can mean that people assume the retrieved information is the most up to date. For example, a study of emergency doctors showed that when they used internet search engines to answer clinical questions, their accuracy in gaining the correct information was only 59%, but their confidence much higher, with 92% of answers rated as reliable enough to use in patient care (Krause et al. 2011). A key challenge, therefore, is not whether information is available via the internet, but how to manage it in a way that allows access to data which are of high quality and evidence-based.

Web-based resources can be divided either by the format in which they deliver knowledge, or by the primary group for which the information has been prepared.

Types of Evidence-Based Mental Health Knowledge Accessed via the Internet

Summary Sites

Giving clinicians access to user-friendly summaries improves clinical knowledge and reduces error (Hoogendam et al. 2009). However, clinicians are often not aware of reliable sources of evidence or feel that time pressures prevent them from exploring new sites which are less familiar. Brief targeted interventions may be helpful to increase the use and application of knowledge from evidence-based sites (Atkinson et al. 2017).

The summary websites listed in Table 19.1 are suggested as a starting point for exploration of sites of this type. There is overlap between sites primarily for clinicians and those for the public, with many sites providing information to both. These lists are not exhaustive, as websites are rapidly superseded and sites change in content, methodological rigour and frequency of updates (Banzi et al. 2011; Kwag et al. 2016). Given the changing nature and quality of sites we would encourage all clinicians to practice 'evidence-based-ly' (Cipriani and Furukawa 2014), by applying the tools of evidence-based medicine (EBM) to assess the quality of sites before using them or recommending to patients and carers.

Institutional websites, web pages and e-journals providing summaries of knowledge are the most easily and frequently accessed first port of call for clinicians and patients to update themselves quickly. Systematic reviews in the Cochrane Library, NICE guidance and evidence-based search engines such as the TRIP database (see Table 19.1) provide a quick and easy reference guide. The advantage of these sites is that the evidence presented has been carefully appraised, synthesized and summarized by qualified experts who follow rigorous methodological guidance and make stringent efforts to avoid bias as far as possible (Higgins et al. 2022). In addition, many also provide plain language summaries for the public.

Although a quick and generally reliable source of information, these summaries do not usually create an actively dynamic environment for engaging an audience in mental health learning. The evidence is presented in a concise and technical way, which can make for dense reading. Even if regularly updated (at varying time periods depending on the site) there is little real-time interaction or opportunity for dynamic feedback.

Static summary sites also take time to develop resources and may be slow to reflect changes in evidence and to respond to feedback. However, it is possible to combine evidence-based methods with a more timely and dynamic interaction with users. For example, in response to the COVID-19 global pandemic, researchers from the Oxford Precision Psychiatry Lab (part of the National Institute for Health Research Oxford Health Biomedical Research Centre: https://oxfordhealthbrc.nihr.ac.uk/our-work/oxppl/) responded to urgent questions from clinicians and senior managers in areas of management specific to mental health. Within two weeks, using evidence-based techniques, guidance had been extracted and summarized on an open access web page in an easy-to-use question-and-answer format. In the following months this expanded to include international collaborations, with translations and adaptations in foreign languages (Smith et al.2020a).

Interactive Summary Sites

In general, learning is greatly enhanced by interaction. For example, a systematic review of continuing education meetings showed that interactive workshops result in moderately large changes, while didactic sessions alone are unlikely to change professional practice (Forsetlund et al. 2009). Some information resources offer interactive features (see Table 19.1). Examples include 'Students 4 Best Evidence', an online community of students posting reviews of evidence-based resources, online discussions and blogs, and 'The Mental Elf' via online meetings, webinars, live streaming on YouTube and conversations across social media platforms. The advantages are that the interaction makes learning engaging and can be individualized to the learner's needs. However, as with all interactive modes of learning, particularly in real time, there is less option for editing: the experience relies heavily on the expertise and skills of those who engage in the process.

New Ways to Access Mental Health Information

As internet access has dramatically increased, so has the role of internet users in developing content. In 2022, 94% of UK adults reported having internet access at home, with 21% accessing the internet exclusively via a smartphone (Ofcom 2022). Some are primarily or solely consumers (finding information, using email, online shopping) but many are also contributors. In the last 10 years or so there has been a dramatic increase in the use of blogs and social media by clinicians, researchers and the general public. This is also true worldwide: in 2019, 6 in 10 phone users in emerging economies had used their phones to look up healthcare information in the previous 12 months (Silver and Huang 2019). This democratization of research has expanded the discussion about new evidence well beyond the traditional intellectual and literal paywalls of publishers and academic journals. Access to full-text research remains a barrier in some cases, although open-access publication of research is increasing. Some funders, such as Wellcome, have made open access mandatory, to ensure that knowledge and discoveries resulting from the projects they fund are shared and used in a way that maximizes their benefit. Good science bloggers also provide an alternative free-access way of keeping up to date with the latest relevant and reliable evidence.

Social media is an immediate route for debating current areas of interest, including new mental health research. There are a multitude of platforms, such as Facebook, Twitter, LinkedIn, YouTube, Google Plus and others (Hootsuite 2022), each with a slightly different focus but all used to share information, opinions and comments. For example, Twitter subscribers can create personalized feeds of information to follow organizations and individuals and include real-time Tweet chats (e.g., #WeNurses) and live tweeting from conferences (e.g., #RCPsychIC).

Webinars

Webinars allow users to meet experts and be updated about recent advances, using livestreaming or videoconferencing platforms such as GoToMeetings, Microsoft Teams, Google Meet and Zoom. These meetings are hosted by a range of organizations, some of which are open access (such as the public campfires organized by the National Elf Service) whereas others require membership or subscription (such as the BMJ masterclasses, https://master classes.bmj.com).

Gamification

Game-based learning is accessible and engaging. An example is the Mental Elf (see Table 19.1) where members' website activity is automatically compiled using gamification

Table 19.1 A selection of websites, including information on evidence-based mental health, which are aimed at clinicians' and the public

Name	Website
Clinician focused:	
BMJ Best Practice	https://bestpractice.bmj.com/info/
Centre for Evidence Based Mental Health	https://www.cebm.net
Cochrane Library	www.cochranelibrary.com
CPD Online (Royal College of Psychiatrists)	https://elearning.rcpsych.ac.uk
DynaMed	www.dynamed.com
Evidence-Based Mental Health	www.ebmh.bmj.com
Health Evidence	www.healthevidence.org/default.aspx
King's Fund	www.kingsfund.org.uk
The National Elf Service (The Mental Elf)	www.nationalelfservice.net
NHS Confederation	www.nhsconfed.org
NICE (National Institute for Health and Care Excellence)	www.nice.org.uk
Students 4 Best Evidence	https://s4be.cochrane.org
Trainees Online (TrOn) (Royal College of Psychiatrists)	https://tron.rcpsych.ac.uk
TRIP database	www.tripdatabase.com
Information via professional organizations:	
General Medical Council (GMC)	www.gmc-uk.org
British Association for Psychopharmacology (BAP)	www.bap.org.uk
Royal College of Psychiatrists (RCPsych)	www.rcpsych.ac.uk
Royal College of General Practitioners (RCGP)	www.rcgp.org.uk
Royal College of Nursing (RCN)	www.rcn.org.uk
The British Psychological Society (BPS)	www.bps.org.uk
British Association for Behavioural and Cognitive Psychotherapies (BABCP)	www.babcp.com
British Association for Counselling and Psychotherapy (BACP)	www.bacp.co.uk
Public and patient focused:	
Alzheimer's Society	www.alzheimers.org.uk
Anxiety UK	www.anxietyuk.org.uk
Bipolar UK	www.bipolaruk.org
Carers UK	www.carersuk.org
Centre for Mental Health	www.centreformentalhealth.org.uk

Table 19.1 (cont.)

Name	Website
Depression Alliance	www.depressionalliance.org
Driving and medical conditions	www.gov.uk/browse/driving/disability-health-condition
healthtalk.org	www.healthtalk.crg
Mental Health Foundation	www.mentalhealth.org.uk
Mind	www.mind.org.uk
MindEd	www.minded.orc.uk
The National Elf Service (The Mental Elf)	www.nationalelfservice.net
NHS Health A–Z	www.nhs.uk/conditions
NICE (National Institute for Health and Care Excellence)	www.nice.org.uk
Rethink Mental Illness	www.rethink.org
Royal College of Psychiatrists, Mental Health Resources	www.rcpsych.ac.uk/mental-health
SANE	www.sane.org.uk
Time to Change	www.time-to-change.org.uk
Togetherall (formerly Big White Wall)	https://togetherall.com/en-gb
Young Minds	https://youngminds.org.uk

Sites are listed alphabetically and are suggestions as a starting point for exploration of sites which may be of interest. We would therefore encourage all readers to appraise sites for themselves for quality before using or recommending them. NHS England has provided guidance on standards and best practice guidance for creating high quality health content at www.england.nhs.uk/tis.

techniques, so users can learn about new research while progressing through an engaging 'game'. Educational apps are a popular way of providing learning to the public (see the apps section) and can also be useful for professionals. For example, the Resuscitation Council (UK) has developed Lifesaver (www.life-saver.org.uk), a live action movie accessible via the website or an app, for professionals and the public to learn cardiopulmonary resuscitation by choosing what to do next in a real-life scenario. The user learns by doing, as the video shows the positive and negative consequences of each decision.

Information Directed Primarily at Practitioners/Clinicians

Websites

The accessibility of the internet means that information is no longer categorized purely as suitable for one group or another (unless the website has a restricted access), and many sites are used by both professionals and the public, incorporating lay information and summaries.

Many websites also deliver training and learning packages, including those developed to help clinicians meet their continuing professional development (CPD) requirements. These packages vary in how they deliver learning. Some use methods similar to a traditional lecture, whilst the other end of the spectrum is represented by multimedia online CPD. This may incorporate video and/or audio tools and can be enhanced by reflective learning, and the facility for the user to personalize and adapt outputs. For example, the GMC's learning disabilities website (www.gmc-uk.org/ethical-guidance/ethical-hub/learning-disabilities) helps health professionals to learn about good and bad practice through interactive video tutorials and reflective learning. CPD web-based teaching is also often combined with face-to-face teaching as blended learning, for example completing online resuscitation learning before a hands-on practical assessment. The route of access to learning also varies. Some CPD can be accessed free via the internet, whilst some is restricted to particular groups, or may require an extra subscription.

Online Courses Specifically Aimed at Learning Evidence-Based Medicine

The advantages of e-learning, including its flexibility and accessibility, have also been applied to the teaching of EBM. Traditionally, EBM has been taught through 'stand-alone' courses, conferences, workshops, journal clubs or educational meetings, but a potential criticism has been that these are insufficiently integrated into daily clinical practice and clinical postgraduate training. Systematic reviews show that 'stand-alone' education improves basic knowledge of EBM, but not necessarily an improvement in practice (Coomarasamy and Khan 2004; Hecht et al. 2016). Clinically integrated e-learning courses for teaching EBM (Kulier et al. 2009; Hadley et al. 2010; Weberschock et al. 2013) show similar effectiveness to traditional teaching with reduced cost, increased ease of updating and good acceptance rates. EBM teaching in mental health can also be combined online with problem-based learning. For example, medical students from London and Somaliland met online to work through mental health clinical cases together using a problem-based learning approach to access and evaluate relevant evidence. Feedback was positive, with effective delivery of online learning to a setting within low- and middle-income countries (Murphy et al. 2017).

Resources for Patients, Carers and the General Public

Information Websites

The public are increasingly making use of online resources to support their own health and supplement their knowledge. Studies of mental health information sites for the public have often highlighted poor usability and quality (Reavely and Jorm 2011). The readability of information (the complexity of its vocabulary and syntax) is often set at a high level of difficulty, preventing a significant proportion of users from accessing it (Gralton et al. 2010) and its quality can be variable (Ferreira-Lay and Miller 2008). However, an increasing number of evidence-based sites, some with specific lay versions, have been developed in recent years (see Table 19.1). Users can also assess quality themselves using checklists such as DISCERN (www.discern.org.uk). Organizational codes of conduct or self-applied quality labels may also be present. Quality assessment in general is discussed in more detail later in the chapter.

Websites directed at the public can also help to inform professionals and policy makers about the views of patients and carers. For example, healthtalk.org provides information about health issues by sharing people's real-life experiences. It is aimed at the public, but the patient experiences have also been useful in training health professionals. Online communities such as the Side by Side forum run by Mind, and Togetherall (see Table 19.1), allow users to talk online and gain support and advice from within the group.

Web-Based Treatment Programmes

Web-based programmes can also be used to deliver treatments such as cognitive behavioural therapy. A full discussion is beyond the scope of this chapter; however, as an example it is worth mentioning the new digitally enabled therapy assessment programme for NHS England, where many digital therapy products are assessed for use in NHS Improving Access to Psychological Therapies (IAPT) services (www.england.nhs.uk/mental-health/adults/iapt/digital-therapy-selection). In general, despite the existence of numerous effective interventions, the transition of computerized interventions into care had been slower than expected, perhaps because of a perception that users prefer face-to-face treatment (Musiat et al. 2014). The move to digital technology, virtual consultations and remote treatment was massively accelerated by the COVID-19 pandemic and associated restrictions on in-person contact. Clinicians and patients rapidly moved to consultations using virtual media, such as telephone or videoconferencing. Evidence-based guidance summaries on telepsychiatry have been published and are available to help with the new skills required (Smith et al. 2020b).

Monitoring Systems

The combination of smartphone technology, email and the Internet has allowed the development of remote monitoring systems of symptoms, where day-to-day feedback from patients can supplement the clinical consultation and provide active evidence for clinicians and patients to decide together on treatment plans. For example, digital mood tracking is available via systems which collect mood ratings in real time (Goodday et al. 2020). These data can also be combined with behavioural and physiological monitoring. This allows detection of minute-to-minute changes as well as capturing a longitudinal perspective of an individual's illness, which enables more collaborative and personalized care (Malhi et al. 2017). Wearable devices and smartphone sensors can collect high-dimensional objective information (e.g., blood pressure, heart rate, activity). Using machine-learning techniques, these complex data can be translated into clinically meaningful patient-generated symptoms and signs, which can then be used to improve individual early detection and surveillance of illness and aid more efficient clinical decision making (Goodday et al. 2021).

Apps

Mobile health apps have many advantages. They are easily accessible with the increasing prevalence of smartphones, have increasing precision and therapeutic potential and can provide unique insights into physical and cognitive behaviour (Rodriguez-Villa and Torous 2019). However, as they are developed and shared at a fast rate, it is hard to assess clinical efficacy, safety, security and relative quality beyond star ratings on retailers' websites and the subjective feedback of other users (Mercurio et al. 2020). Many mental health apps make claims that appear medical, but it is difficult to identify a core set of features to accurately assess app quality (Wisniewski et al. 2019). For example, a recent systematic evaluation of 278 current mental health apps (Lagan et al. 2021) showed that ratings such as app stars and downloads do not correlate with more clinically relevant metrics related to privacy/security, effectiveness and engagement. Many of these mental health apps offered similar functionality to each other and only a minority were regularly updated. This evidence supports the difficulties that clinicians and patients may find as they struggle to distinguish helpful tools from unreliable or even harmful ones.

Regulatory bodies such as the US Food and Drug Administration regulate mobile medical apps (www.fda.gov/media/106331/download). However, they focus on apps that directly control medical devices or function as these, which excludes most mental-health-related resources. In the UK, the NHS Apps Library (www.nhs.uk/apps-library/?page=4) was originally set up to contain recommended digital health tools. The initial version in 2013 was withdrawn in 2015, after concerns that only a minority provided evidence of patient-reported outcomes or applied validated metrics (Leigh and Flatt 2015). The library was relaunched in 2017, evaluating resources with advice rather than recommendation, but then decommissioned in December 2021.

The NHS also collaborates with the National Institute for Health and Care Excellence (NICE) to establish credentials for digital health tools or digital health technologies (www.nice.org.uk/about/what-we-do/our-programmes/evidence-standards-framework-for-digital-health-technologies). NICE assesses the evidence base as well as its financial footprint. In response to the challenges of the COVID-19 pandemic, Public Health England also produced specific guidance for developers on evaluating digital health products (www.gov.uk/guidance/rapid-evaluation-of-digital-health-products-during-the-covid-19-pandemic).

Users can also refer to evaluation websites such as Psyberguide, MindTools.io or ORCHA (Rodriguez-Villa and Torous 2019). However, these generally show a lack of concordance between ratings of the same apps, are quickly out of date and assessment measures are often qualitative. The American Psychiatric Association app evaluation framework (www.psychiatry.org/psychiatrists/practice/mental-health-apps) suggests that users (patients and clinicians) ask questions across four areas, in order of descending importance: safety and privacy, evidence, ease of use and interoperability (www.psychiatry.org/psychiatrists/practice/mental-health-apps/the-app-evaluation-model). This could also be supplemented with a self-certification checklist completed by developers or volunteers on a frequent basis. Ideally, this would be a public, interactive approach, so that a patient could filter categories for app choices that meet their standards in terms of privacy, level of evidence, usability based on peer reviews and clinical integration (e.g., https://apps.digitalpsych.org/).

It remains challenging to implement digital mental health tools in care settings. Clinicians and patients find practical implementation difficult and, whilst smartphone ownership has increased, users often struggle to access their full functionality. One potential solution might be the introduction of a 'digital navigator', a new care team member who could bridge the gap, developing expertise in relevant apps and helping patients to use and summarize the data they collect to guide their clinical care effectively (Wisniewski and Torous 2020).

What Are the Advantages of E-Learning?

Accessibility, Transparency and Democracy

A key advantage of e-learning is that it can be accessed at any time and is immediately available to anyone with a connection to the Internet. Geography is no barrier and in theory there is no physical limit to the numbers attending a course or accessing information. This immediate access is crucial, as learning is often an unplanned experience, prompted by clinical dilemmas in diagnosis or treatment (Ward et al. 2001).

E-learning can be accessed anonymously, allowing the learning to be more transparent and democratic than traditional communications. It can inform the wider community and policy makers. For example, during the 2014–2016 Ebola outbreak, media coverage in the USA and UK was criticized for being factually misleading and overly focused on the small number of cases outside West Africa. A Twitter chat hosted by the *Lancet* showed that social media can help to balance the trend for biased reporting, as 'all voices are equal' (Lancet 2014). In only an hour, more than 300,000 views of tweets and many new ideas emerged from experts and the public. The separation between scientists, health professionals and policy makers was reduced, creating a new diverse community where everyone has a voice, can contribute and rate the experience on different parameters.

Immediacy

Online learning is instantly accessible and can be updated or revised frequently. Feedback is a key element of learning (Forsetlund et al. 2009). This can be synchronous, where instructors and learners communicate in real time (e.g., internet chat forums and instant messaging) or asynchronous, where learners pace themselves and feedback is delivered via email, online bulletin boards, newsgroups or other technologies (Ruiz et al. 2006).

Individualizing Learning

At a basic level, users might select only the modules of a course that are relevant to them. With more advanced sites, users interact with tutors to create their own learning programme. This individualized approach is usually not possible in group face-to-face teaching, where the needs of the group take precedence. However, it is important, because more active engagement and personalization of the learning experience motivates learners to become more engaged with the content (Clark 2002).

Standards and Accountability

E-learning standardizes course content and delivery. Automated tracking and reporting of learners' activities reduces the administrative burden. Outcome assessments can be incorporated, to determine whether learning has occurred. Sites often incorporate automated log-keeping and assessments, providing proof of learning for professional development logs. These can be personalized, with individual learning aims created by the user and reflections on the learning achieved.

Use of Innovative Methods

Innovative methods include the use of virtual patients, or multimedia and interactivity. For example, the GMC good medical practice in action (www.gmc-uk.org/gmpinaction/get-started) website helps doctors improve the care they offer by using case studies, and their resources around people with learning disabilities (www.gmc-uk.org/learningdisabilities) also contain best practice examples from the GMC guidance, alongside video interviews with experts in the field (patients and professionals).

Potential Disadvantages of E-Learning

Variable Quality

The quality and regulation across different sites vary significantly. Accessibility can also be a disadvantage when inaccurate or misleading information is rapidly disseminated before it can be corrected (Cook 2007). Users are often left to assess the quality of websites themselves. DISCERN is a 16-item checklist (Charnock 1999), designed to be used by consumers without content expertise to assess the quality of healthcare information. It primarily assesses the reliability of information and is less focused on other important elements such as accessibility and usability. Although applicable to the Internet, it was not specifically designed for internet-based information. Specific online tools are also available, such as the Lida instrument, which uses a series of questions to assess the accessibility, usability and reliability of information presented on healthcare websites via a set of free tools to help website developers (www.minervation.com/welcome-to-the-lida-blog).

NHS England provides guidance on standards and best practice for creating high quality health content (www.england.nhs.uk/tis), which indicates whether the methodology used to produce the information may be considered reliable. Some sites display a quality label such as Health On the Net Foundation (www.hon.ch) (Wilson 2002) but these provide guidance only, rather than certification or regulation. It is therefore still key that clinicians assess the quality of sites themselves, before recommending to patients and carers. It is also important to remember that the use of evidence-based terminology (such as 'systematic review', 'randomized controlled trial') is not a guarantee of quality. Critical appraisal tools such as the Critical Appraisal Skills Programme checklists (www.casp-uk.net) can help readers decide how much weight to give to a particular study or summary.

Usability

Although there is potential for innovative and exciting learning, some websites have a poor design, with a static interface and little interaction. Setting up high-quality web-based learning can be costly (e.g., funding multimedia additions, actors simulating patients) and time-consuming (e.g., maintaining online discussion forums). Quality can vary, as live discussions depend on the quality of the participants and the nominated 'expert'. Technological problems can mean the teaching is not available, either unintentionally or because many NHS trusts do not allow access to certain sites or technology.

For those with severe mental illness in particular, digital literacy can be a barrier to access. Whilst many patients may own smartphones, just like clinicians, they do not always feel confident in using their full functionality. For example, in a US study of inpatients, 83 per cent owned a smartphone. Only 25 per cent reported using a mental health app, but more than 50 per cent expressed interest in using such apps in the future (Iliescu et al. 2021). Teaching smartphone skills as part of mental health rehabilitation strategies in severe mental illness can improve not only digital literacy but also functional outcomes (Rodriguez-Villa et al. 2021).

Conclusion

The Internet has great potential as an immediately accessible source of high-quality evidence-based information on mental health, but there are potential pitfalls. To avoid an overwhelming array of sites, most users turn to summary sites for information or inter-action. These sites are only as reliable as the methods used to synthesize the information, and so it is the responsibility of the clinician or user to assess each site ⟨and to continue to do so as more information is added) to evaluate the quality and 'evidence-based' credentials it claims. However, there is no way back, and the advantages of embracing the new digital age in mental health are worth actively pursuing: creative and interactive use of the internet and digital technology allows the dissemination, sharing and discussion of clinical information in an easily accessible and democratic format.

Acknowledgements

For information, the original paper on which this chapter is based was: Smith K, Tomlin A, Cipriani A, Geddes J (2016). Evidence-based mental health and e-learning: a guide for clinicians. *BJPsych Advances*, 22, 55–63. The authors wish to acknowledge with thanks the contribution of André Tomlin to the original paper.

KAS and AC are supported by the National Institute for Health Research (NIHR) Oxford cognitive health Clinical Research Facility and by the NIHR Oxford Health Biomedical Research Centre (grant BRC-1215-20005). AC is supported by the National Institute for Health Research (NIHR) Research Professorship (grant RP-2017-08-ST2-006), and by the National Institute for Health Research (NIHR) Applied Research Collaboration (ARC) Oxford and Thames Valley. The views expressed are those of the authors and not necessarily those of the United Kingdom National Health Service, the NIHR, or the United Kingdom Department of Health.

References

Atkinson LZ, Forrest A, Marriner L, Geddes J, and Cipriani A (2017) Implementing tools to support evidence-based practice: a survey and brief intervention study of the National Elf Service across Oxford Health NHS Foundation Trust. *Evidence-Based Mental Health*, **20**: 41–5; doi: https://doi.org/10.1136/eb-2017-102665.

Banzi R, Cinquini M, Liberati A, et al. (2011) Speed of updating online evidence based point of care summaries: prospective cohort analysis. *BMJ*, **343**: d5856; doi: https://www.bmj.com/content/343/bmj.d5856.

Charnock D, Shepperd S, Needham G, et al. (1999) DISCERN: an instrument for judging the quality of written consumer health information on treatment choices. *Journal of Epidemiology and Community Health*, **53**: 105–11; doi: https://www.ncbi.nlm.nih.gov/pmc/articles/PMC1756830/.

Cipriani A, Furukawa TA (2014) Advancing evidence-based practice to improve patient care. *Evidence Based Mental Health*, **17**: 1–2; doi: https://doi.org/10.1136/eb-2014-101722.

Clark D (2002) Psychological myths in e-learning. *Medical Teacher*, **24**: 598–604; doi: https://doi.org/10.1080/0142159021000063916.

Cook DA (2007) Web-based learning: pros, cons and controversies. *Clinical Medicine*, 7: 37–42; doi: https://doi.org/10.7861/clinmedicine.7-1-37.

Coomarasamy A, Khan KS (2004) What is the evidence that postgraduate teaching in evidence-based medicine changes anything? A systematic review. *BMJ*, **329**: 1017; doi: https://www.bmj.com/content/329/7473/1017.

Daei A, Soleymani MR, Ashrafi-Rizi H, Zargham-Boroujeni A, Kelishadi R (2020) Clinical information seeking behavior of physicians: a systematic review. *International Journal of Medical Informatics*, **139**: 104144; doi: https://www.sciencedirect.com/science/article/pii/S138650561930187X.

Ely JW, Osheroff JA, Chambliss MA, et al. (2005) Answering physicians' clinical questions: obstacles and potential solutions. *JAMIA*,

12: 217–24; doi: https://www.ncbi.nlm.nih.gov/pmc/articles/PMC551553/.

Ely JW, Osheroff JA, Maviglia SM, et al. (2007) Patient-care questions that physicians are unable to answer. *JAMIA*, **14**: 407–14: doi: https://www.ncbi.nlm.nih.gov/pmc/articles/PMC2244897/.

Ferreira-Lay P, Miller S (2008) The quality of internet information on depression for lay people. *Psychiatric Bulletin*, **32**: 170–3; doi: https://doi.org/10.1192/pb.bp.107.016188.

Forsetlund L, Bjørndal A, Rashidian A, et al. (2009) Continuing education meetings and workshops: effects on professional practice and health care outcomes. *The Cochrane Database of Systematic Reviews*, **2**: CD003030; doi: https://doi.org/10.1002/14651858.CD003030.pub2.

Goodday SM, Atkinson L, Goodwin G, et al. (2020) The true colours remote symptom monitoring system: a decade of evolution. *Journal of Medical Internet Research*, **22**: e15188; doi: https://doi.org/10.2196/15188.

Goodday SM, Geddes JR, Friend SH (2021) Disrupting the power balance between doctors and patients in the digital era. *The Lancet Digital Health*, **3**: e142–3; doi: https://doi.org/10.1016/S2589-7500(21)00004-2.

Gralton E, Sher M, Lopez CD (2010) Information and readability issues for psychiatric patients: e-learning for users. *The Psychiatrist*, **34**: 376–80; doi: https://doi.org/10.1192/pb.bp.109.027102.

Hadley J, Kulier R, Zamora J, et al. (2010) Effectiveness of an e-learning course in evidence-based medicine for foundation (internship) training. *Journal of the Royal Society of Medicine*, **103**: 288–94; doi: https://doi.org/10.1258/jrsm.2010.100036.

Hecht L, Buhse S, Meyer G (2016) Effectiveness of training in evidence-based medicine skills for healthcare professionals: a systematic review. *BMC Med Education*, **16**: 103; doi: https://doi.org/10.1186/s12909-016-0616-2.

Higgins JPT, Thomas J, Chandler J, et al. (2022) Cochrane Handbook for Systematic Reviews of Interventions. Available at: www.training.cochrane.org/handbook.

Hoogendam A, de Vries Robbé PF, Stalenhoef AF, Overbeke AJ (2009) Evaluation

of PubMed filters used for evidence-based searching: validation using relative recall. *Journal of the Medical Library Association*, **97**: 186–93; doi: https://doi.org/10.3163/1536-5050.97.3.007

Hootsuite (2022) Global Social Media Statistics. Available at: https://datareportal.com/social-media-users.

Iliescu R, Kumaravel A, Smurawska L, Torous J, Keshavan M (2021) Smartphone ownership and use of mental health applications by psychiatric inpatients. *Psychiatry research*, **299**: 113806; doi: https://doi.org/10.1016/j.psychres.2021.113806.

Johnson J (2021) Worldwide digital population as of January 2021. Available at: www.statista.com/statistics/617136/digital-population-worldwide/ (accessed 16 April 2021).

Krause R, Moscati R, Halpern S, Schwartz, DG, Abbas J (2011) Can emergency medicine residents reliably use the internet to answer clinical questions? *The Western Journal of Emergency Medicine*, **12**: 442–7; doi: https://doi.org/10.5811/westjem.2010.9.1895.

Kulier R, Coppus SF, Zamora J. et al. (2009) The effectiveness of a clinically integrated e-learning course in evidence-based medicine: a cluster randomised controlled trial. *BMC Med Educ*, **9**: 21; doi: https://doi.org/10.1186/1472-6920-9-21.

Kwag KH, González-Lorenzo M, Banzi R, Bonovas S, Moja L (2016) Providing doctors with high-quality information: an updated evaluation of web-based point-of-care information summaries. *Journal of Medical Internet Research*, **18**: e15; doi: https://doi.org/10.2196/jmir.5234.

Lagan S, D'Mello R, Vaidyam A, Bilden R, Torous J (2021). Assessing mental health apps marketplaces with objective metrics from 29,190 data points from 278 apps. *Acta Psychiatrica Scandinavica*, **144**: 201–10; doi: https://doi.org/10.1111/acps.13306.

Lancet (Editorial) (2014) The medium and the message of Ebola. *Lancet*, **384**: 1641; doi: https://doi.org/10.1016/S0140-6736(14)62016-X.

Leigh S, Flatt S (2015) App-based psychological interventions: friend or foe? *Evidence-Based Mental Health*, **18**: 97–99; doi: https://doi.org/10.1136/eb-2015-102203.

Malhi GS, Hamilton A, Morris G, et al. (2017) The promise of digital mood tracking technologies: are we heading on the right track? *Evidence-Based Mental Health*, 20: 102–107; doi: https://doi.org/10.1136/eb-2017-102757.

Marzano L, Hollis C, Cipriani A, et al. (2017) Digital technology: coming of age? *Evidence-Based Mental Health*, 20: 97; doi: http://dx.doi.org/10.1136/eb-2017-102821.

Mercurio M, Larsen M, Wisniewski H, et al. (2020). Longitudinal trends in the quality, effectiveness and attributes of highly rated smartphone health apps. *Evidence-Based Mental Health*, 23: 107–11.

Murphy R, Clissold E, Keynejad RC (2017) Problem-based, peer-to-peer global mental health e-learning between the UK and Somaliland: a pilot study. *Evidence-Based Mental Health*, 20: 142–6; doi: https://doi.org/10.1136/eb-2017-102766.

Musiat P, Goldstone P, Tarrier N (2014) Understanding the acceptability of e-mental health: attitudes and expectations towards computerised self-help treatments for mental health problems. *BMC Psychiatry*, 14: 109; doi: https://doi.org/10.1186/1471-244X-14-109.

Ofcom (2022) Adults' media use & attitudes, report 2022. Available at: www.ofcom.org.uk/__data/assets/pdf_file/0020/234362/adults-media-use-and-attitudes-report-2022.pdf .

Reavley NJ, Jorm AF (2011) The quality of mental disorder information websites: a review. *Patient Education and Counseling*, 85: e16–e25; doi: https://doi.org/10.1016/j.pec.2010.10.015.

Rodriguez-Villa E, Torous J (2019) Regulating digital health technologies with transparency: the case for dynamic and multi-stakeholder evaluation. *BMC Med*, 17, 226; doi: https://doi.org/10.1186/s12916-019-1447-x.

Rodriguez-Villa E, Camacho E, Torous J (2021) Psychiatric rehabilitation through teaching smartphone skills to improve functional outcomes in serious mental illness. *Internet Interventions*, 23: 100366; doi: https://doi.org/10.1016/j.invent.2021.100366.

Ruiz JG, Mintzer MJ, Leipzig RM (2006). The impact of e-learning in medical education. *Academic Medicine: Journal of the Association of American Medical Colleges*, 81: 207–12; doi: https://doi.org/10.1097/00001888-200603000-00002.

Silver L, Huang C (2019) Social activities, information seeking on subjects like health and education top the list of mobile activities. Pew Research Centre. Available at: www.pewresearch.org/internet/2019/08/22/social-activities-information-seeking-on-subjects-like-health-and-education-top-the-list-of-mobile-activities.

Smith K, Ostinelli E, Cipriani A (2020a) Covid-19 and mental health: a transformational opportunity to apply an evidence-based approach to clinical practice and research. *Evidence-Based Mental Health*, 23: 45–6; doi: https://doi.org/10.1136/ebmental-2020-300155.

Smith K, Ostinelli E, Macdonald O, Cipriani A (2020b) COVID-19 and telepsychiatry: development of evidence-based guidance for clinicians. *JMIR Mental Health*, 7: e21108; doi: https://doi.org/10.2196/21108.

Ward JP, Gordon J, Field MJ, Lehmann HP (2001) Communication and information technology in medical education. *Lancet*, 357: 792–6; doi: https://doi.org/10.1016/S0140-6736(00)04173-8.

Weberschock T, Sorinola O, Thangaratinam S, et al. (2013) How to confidently teach EBM on foot: development and evaluation of a web-based e-learning course. *Evidence-Based Medicine*, 18: 170–2; doi: https://doi.org/10.1136/eb-2012-100801.

Wilson P (2002) How to find the good and avoid the bad or ugly: a short guide to tools for rating quality of health information on the internet. *BMJ*, 324: 598–602; doi: https://doi.org/10.1136/bmj.324.7337.598.

Wisniewski H, Torous J (2020) Digital navigators to implement smartphone and digital tools in care. *Acta Psychiatr Scandinavia*, 141: 350–5; doi: https://doi.org/10.1111/acps.13149.

Wisniewski H, Liu G, Henson P, et al. (2019) Understanding the quality, effectiveness and attributes of top-rated smartphone health apps. *Evidence-Based Mental Health*, 22: 4–9; doi: https://doi.org/10.1136/ebmental-2018-300069.

PowerPoint: Avoiding the Slide to Damnation

Guy Undrill and Fiona McMaster

Introduction

Psychiatrists are often called on to do presentations, of which PowerPoint slides are usually an expected component. Even more frequent is the experience of 'death by PowerPoint': sitting in someone else's presentation and simultaneously experiencing both intense boredom and cognitive overload. This phenomenon has been cited for more than 20 years: 'poor documents are so common that deciphering bad writing and bad visual design have become part of the coping skills needed to navigate in the so-called information age' (Schriver 1997, p. xxiii). Mayer's (2009) text is seminal in describing how this arises: there are dual channels for processing (the visual and the auditory), which both have limited capacity. The death by PowerPoint experience happens when one channel is overloaded and one channel is ignored: typically, a presenter reading text from a screen (cognitive overload – the audience cannot read and listen simultaneously) and boredom (there is no visual stimulation).

Coupled with this, there is great pressure to distribute slides to students. This can have the effect of minimizing cognitive effort by listeners in the presentation – cognitive effort (e.g., by taking notes) that is key to understanding and retention (see also Brown et al. 2014 on the centrality of cognitive effort in successful learning). Hill et al. (2012) make the interesting point that there sometimes a dilemma between pedagogical commitment and career pragmatism: presentations that involve effort from students may get poorer feedback than those that don't.Mayer (2014) suggests that the key to good presentation is to divide cognitive effort into 'extraneous processing, which drains limited cognitive processing capacity without contributing to learning; essential processing, which involves selecting relevant information and organizing it as presented in working memory; and generative processing, which involves making sense of the material by reorganizing it into a coherent structure and integrating it with relevant prior knowledge', with the aim being to minimize the first (e.g., by clear, visual slide design) and to foster the other two. Badly designed PowerPoint can make for extraneous cognitive effort that distracts a potential learner (Craig and Amernic 2006; Harden 2008) and reduces learning (Kjeldsen 2006). Good PowerPoint functions as a tool for engagement, a way of directing learner attention (Wecker 2012) and a way of controlling the flow of information, such that the presentation supports essential and generative cognitive effort.

Kosslyn (2012) suggests that most people can recognize bad PowerPoint but that they may not necessarily be able to say why it is bad: that is to say, the presentation design is neither obvious nor intuitive, and most people need to spend some time learning it. In some respects this is harder than it may seem: bad practices in PowerPoint use are partially driven by the anxiety of beginner presenters but can easily develop into habits – an anxious beginner may have their anxiety assuaged by reading from the slide in a dimmed room or turning their back to the audience to look at their slide (and avoid audience gaze) but none of these practices make for good audience experience (Hertz et al. 2015). Nevertheless, we believe that the basic principles of slide design and presentation are simple and can be learned relatively easily. We have illustrated this chapter with some slides relating to the material of the chapter, which are accompanied with a sample text of what a presenter might say in presenting the slide in a hypothetical presentation on slide design.

There are many current uses for PowerPoint slides. For this discussion, we are assuming the reader is either:

- training psychiatrists in a formal setting;
- presenting to peers in a journal club/case presentation setting; or
- presenting at a conference.

Before You Switch On

Tufte (2006) points out that PowerPoint is intrinsically presenter centred. Making it content centred (better) or audience-centred (best) requires effort, and the first part of that effort is to plan your presentation away from the computer. If you start too early with PowerPoint, you will probably end up both wasting your time and having a message that is less clear.

Tufte (2006) recommends answering two questions: (1) what's my point? and (2) why does it matter? Think about these questions from the perspective of your prospective audience and then start to jot down some answers.

As you brainstorm ideas, allow patterns to emerge. Some people prefer to do this on paper by drawing mind maps; others use index cards or post-it notes, which can be rearranged into groups. A third group may use these approaches to develop a storyboard looking at where the presentation may go, and thinking deeply about its key messages. Whatever the approach, throw away all but the best ideas as you begin to winnow down each group to a few key points. These patterns and groups will be the basis of the structure for the presentation. Structure (Box 20.1) is important for providing a memorable presentation because it leverages the principle of chunking to increase the chances of people remembering your presentation (Atkinson 2007). A good and transparent structure also allows people to lose concentration briefly and then pick up your train of thought. Well-designed slides should be understandable 'as a single thought, while at the same time, we grasp their relationship to the narrative or argument in which they are embedded' (Gross and Harmon 2009: p. 121).

The goal is to have a series of main points, each consisting of two to four sub-points or ideas, which you can now transform into visuals and lastly put onto your slides.[1]

Key Principles of Slide Design

Slide design is largely a matter of aesthetics. It is possible to have ugly but memorable slides, or beautiful but ineffective slides. However, where aesthetic questions and practical research overlap, the research often pulls in the same direction as the aesthetic principles. The basic principles of design are easy to learn and apply.

---

[1] Variants of this process are described in more detail in Duarte (2010) and Atkinson (2007).

Box 20.1 Structure

(1)Â Hierarchical

This is the most important organizing principle. Some degree of hierarchical relationship is usually necessary in a presentation, if only in the arrangement of headings and subheadings. More than three levels of headings rarely work.

An inverted pyramid is a way of organizing information that puts crucial information first, with less important elaborative information lower down. It can work against narrative methods of organizing information as it precludes suspense and surprise, though a well-made summary can draw people to the main body of the presentation.

(2)Â Sequential

Sequential organizations include chronologies and narratives.

Simple sequential structures work on binaries such as problem–solution, compare–contrast, cause–effect or advantage–disadvantage.

Most more complex sequences of organization are explicitly or implicitly narrative.

(3)Â Arbitrary

There are various other principles by which you can organize information, with varying degrees of arbitrariness. Arbitrary structures include alphabetical or by location

Box 20.2 Mayer's principles

1. **Dual channels:** people have separate 'channels' for processing pictorial and auditory/verbal material
2. **Limited capacity:** people can only process a few pieces of information in each channel at any one time
3. **Active processing:** learning occurs when people engage in active cognitive processing during learning.
4. **Transfer:** new knowledge and skills must be retrieved from long-term memory during performance

1. Less Is More

Use fewer slides and put less on each slide. Give less of your presentation from slides and more from yourself. Meyer's principles of multimedia learning (Box 20.2) (Clark and Mayer 2007) are good guidelines to apply. Clark and Mayer also suggest that people can't read and listen simultaneously and that retention is better for what is spoken rather than what is read, so prioritize what you are saying over than what is on the screen.

Use fewer 'features' (animations, transitions, etc.). Animations can be useful to control the flow of information (Cyphert 2004) and to direct attention, for example building up a complex diagram piece by piece. Use fewer colours (two to four) and typefaces (three maximum). If you are able to access newer iterations of PowerPoint, there are some good design guidelines that appear as options (these usually present as a pop-up to the right of the window) while you are creating the slides.

Within each slide, pare away everything that is extraneous to the core message. Bradshaw (2003) found that extraneous elements (fancy fonts, garish colours or sounds at slide transition) generally (but not consistently) reduced retention of information. *Everything in your presentation should be there for a purpose.*

A specific instance of less being more is to use what designers call negative space. Empty space on a slide doesn't need to be crammed with information. Slides will often look better if empty areas are consolidated into a single region.

As with all rules, 'less is more' should be broken where appropriate: a complicated graph can sometimes work better using animation to bring in one element at a time. Different transitions can be used between sections and within sections of your presentation to give a subtle additional cue to your audience as to where you have got to in your argument. Some dynamic presenters use very many slides per minute, though this is difficult to pull off convincingly and requires a large amount of preparation (e.g., look at the work of Larry Lessig and his TED talks).

2. Type Elements

Serif typefaces, such as Minion Pro, the face used in this book, have small lines or spurs added to the ends of strokes. Sans serif typefaces (such as Myriad Pro Condensed) don't have these markings (for more on the anatomy of type see Williams (2014), or for more detail a short typography primer such as Lupton (2010) or Squire (2006)). Often, designers recommend sans serif typefaces, such as Gill Sans or Calibri, for use in slides, sometimes justifying this by saying that the serifs are poorly rendered at typical screen resolutions. Although this opinion is often heard, the evidence from readability studies is equivocal. Mackiewicz (2006) asked audience members to rate various typefaces on four variables: comfortable-to-read; professional; interesting; and attractive. Gill Sans came out well on all four variables. Hoffman et al. (personal communication, 2005) showed that the differences between typefaces in terms of subjective preference are greater than the differences between typefaces in respect of the objective measure of time taken to read a passage, which is actually minimally different between the typefaces he examined. Verdana came out well in his study: this typeface was designed for screen use and one of its main distinguishing characteristics is a relatively loose letter spacing. Hoffman (2010, personal communication) recommends bearing this in mind when using other typefaces and opening up the letter spacing ('positive tracking') slightly for readability when using them on screen.

There is some evidence that people's subjective preferences for readability are actually a poor guide to choice of typeface. Reber et al. (2004) use the term 'hedonic fluency hypothesis' to refer to the general principle that people prefer easily processed stimuli. However, stimuli that are more difficult to process *may* in some circumstances be preferable if the disfluency leads people to process information more deeply, perhaps because disfluency acts as a cue that one does not have mastery over the material, which in turn (see Mayer's third principle, above) leads to more effortful and effective processing. Diemand-Yauman et al. (2011) have shown that this is the case and that, in some circumstances, a less readable typeface can increase retention of information at testing. We do not recommend choosing hard-to-read typefaces as a standard strategy and prefer to think of typeface choice as being better governed by Mayer's suggestion of reducing extraneous effort: clarity is a good principle.

In summary, there is no strong reason for restricting your choice of typeface purely on the basis of audience preference, readability or retention and (within limits) it is reasonable to choose typefaces according to the mood you wish to portray (for guidance on typeface and mood see Reynolds 2020). However, Gill Sans is a good default and is supported by the little research there is. The PowerPoint default of Calibri is probably also a good choice.

The single most important aspect of typography for presentations is size. The 'font size' drop-down menu in PowerPoint refers to the 'caps height', the height of capital letters measured in points (there are 72 points to an inch). It is difficult to give hard and fast rules about what size to set the text, as both readability and subjective size vary not just with the size at which the text is set but also with the relative height of the lower-case letters in the particular typeface (the 'x-height'). A good principle is to 'design for the back of the room' – if you find yourself apologizing that something is too small to be read by anyone in your audience, it has no place on your slide. A tip for checking this at the design stage is to switch to slide-sorter view in PowerPoint. If you can't read the text, people at the back of the room may not be able to either.

For readability, 'sentence case' (where the first word is capitalized and the latter words start with lower case) is generally thought to be preferable to capitals or 'title case' (where all words in the sentence have initial capitals). This is repeated as a truism in many primers on typography and is usually justified that the shape of words is easier to recognize in lower case.

Use complete sentences rather than sentence fragments as headlines on your slides where possible as this improves retention of the information in the audience (Alley et al. 2006).

Create a typographic hierarchy coordinated with the structure and conceptual hierarchy you have adopted for your presentation. It is rare to need more than two typefaces, and often more effective to keep to one and vary the weight or colour of the type (e.g., see how this book uses Minion Pro for the body text, and Myriad Pro Condensed for titles, section headings and so on). When combining typefaces, use faces that are sufficiently different: for example a sans serif such as Gill Sans for titling with an old style serif face like Caslon. Mixing similar faces (such as Times New Roman with Caslon) will clash and look like a mistake. Avoid using underlining: use a heavier weight of the same face. In general, drop shadows reduce readability.

As a general rule, aim for high levels of contrast between text and background (Bradshaw 2003). Not all PowerPoint templates promote a high level of contrast between background and text, and some of the templates are conspicuously 'noisy', with the worst also reducing the amount of screen space available for meaningful information with large colourful margins. For this reason and to achieve some of the other recommendations around typography, we follow the advice of Duarte (2008) and suggest you start with a blank white slide with no layout or background and to put the text you want where you want it at the size you want it.

How much text should you put on each slide? This has been a heavily contested question in recent years. Tufte (2006) has been particularly caustic about the '6 × 6' rule (six lines of text, six words per line), comparing the results to a 'first grade reading primer'. Clark and Mayer (2007) suggest that visuals should be explained through text on screen or through narration but not both ('the redundancy principle') and that words presented as narration have a higher rate of retention ('the modality principle'), which would tend to suggest less text (and more visuals) on screen. Not all research has supported this: Blokzijl and Andeweg (2007) found that although text-intensive slides support a lecture as well as visualizations, visualization is strongly preferred by learners. We suggest that the choice of how much text to be put on a slide should be made mindfully: there may be times when a visually engaging slide is needed where the amount of text could be usefully reduced. However, slides with relatively large amounts of text on them are sometimes needed and probably do not have a major impact on understanding or retention.

3. Image and Colour

The basic principle in using graphics is to respect Mayer's first principle. More information can be transferred from presenter to audience and subsequently retained if both of the limited capacity channels are used. The 'death by PowerPoint' experience of simultaneous boredom and cognitive overload comes from ignoring one channel (the visual) and over-loading the other (text on screen replicated by the spoken presentation). A relevant picture, diagram or graphic should ideally be displayed on the screen as the presenter talks about it. In this way, the visual channel and auditory/verbal channel are both used. Ideally, to integrate the information from the two channels with pre-existing knowledge, a certain amount of effort and cognitive processing is required.

The background of the slide should be a single colour or a gentle gradient. Avoid bright, busy or complicated backgrounds and avoid slide templates that take up large amounts of screen space with graphic elements unrelated to your presentation. Text should have a high contrast with the background – again, not all of the templates provided with PowerPoint provide this high contrast. The one exception to the high-contrast rule is to avoid relying on a red/green contrast because of the high prevalence of red/green colour blindness. Use colour deliberately and with care: for example, use colour as part of your organizational hierarchy, or as emphasis for particular points. Few (2004: p. 109) describes this as including only 'visual differences that correspond to actual differences in meaning'. Different colours carry different emotional associations. A presentation in shades of candy pink will not look as professional as a presentation that uses a palette of desaturated blues. Detailed discussion of colour palettes is beyond the scope of this article: the interested reader is referred to Reynolds (2020).

Two background colours deserve specific mention as having particular strengths. A plain white background is useful when adding stock photographs as many of these will be objects photographed on a plain white background. Placing these image elements on a white background avoids problems with ugly borders round images (Fig. 20.1). Black text on white provides maximum contrast. Think about whether you will be standing in front of a set of slides, or if you will be sharing a screen and consider the contrast implications of your slides. A slide with a white background can throw your face into shadow; a black background may allow the audience to see you better.

It is important that any picture or graphic is relevant. It is now well established that irrelevant pictures can actually have a negative effect on learning (Bartsch and Cobern 2003), something Mayer (Clark and Mayer 2007: p. 133) calls the 'coherence principle' (Fig. 20.2). Clark and Mayer regard this as perhaps the single most important recommen-dation in their book: 'spicing up' a presentation by adding pictures, videos, animations or sounds that don't relate to the material at hand reduces learning. This is a good example of

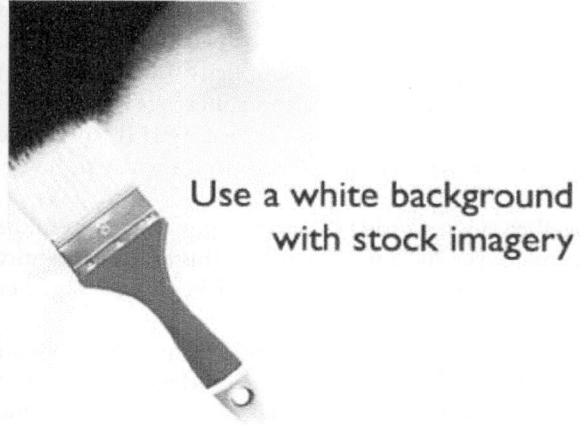

Fig. 20.1 Using stock imagery.

A plain white background allows for high-contrast text and makes it easier to drop commercial stock imagery (which is frequently provided with a white background) onto the slide. In this example, the slide is white and a stock image of a paintbrush is used to illustrate the point. Note how there is no image border around the paintbrush, which sits directly on the background. The image is of a high enough resolution that it is not jagged or pixellated and has no jpeg artefact, neither is it stretched in one dimension.

Mayer regards the coherence principle as one of his most important recommendations. Keep your slides uncluttered and remove any elements that are not central to the content of the presentation. Extraneous graphics that are not relevant can harm the retention of information, so try to resist the temptation to 'spice up' your presentation with pictures. In this slide, a single complete sentence is coupled with a simple graphic, which the presenter explains verbally in more detail. Note also the contrasting white text on a black background and the use of a heavier text weight to emphasise the key point. The slide is divided into thirds for a coherent look. The text font (on the full-size slide) is 72 point Gill Sans and the graphic is made from the font Infobits.

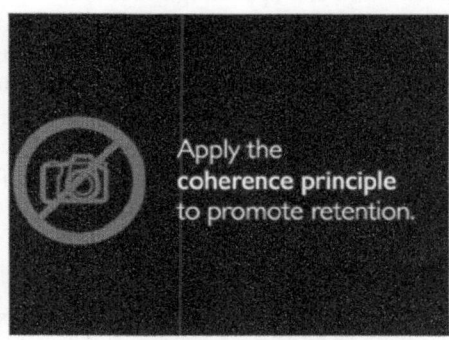

Fig. 20.2 A notional talk on slide design showing spoken text with an example slide, in this case covering the coherence principle.

how design principles often parallel empirical evidence about PowerPoint: Clark and Mayer encourage us to 'weed' our slides for empirically derived, pedagogical reasons; Reynolds encourages us to design visuals 'with an eye towards simplicity' (Reynolds 2020) for aesthetic reasons. It is perhaps also worth noting that the coherence principle is commonly violated by designers of UK National Health Service (NHS) corporate PowerPoint templates, who usually place the organization's logo prominently on every slide.

When using graphics and text together, align words to the corresponding diagram or element in the graphic. Mayer (Clark and Mayer 2007: p. 77) refers to this as the contiguity principle – information that belongs together conceptually should be placed together spatially.

The design of graphs and tables is a topic in itself. The classic text is Tufte (2001) though Few (2004) is often more practical (if business rather than science orientated). One of Tufte's contributions is the now well-known concept of 'data ink'. He rates graphs by the proportion 'non-erasable data ink' displaying data information to the total ink used to print the graphic. The principle transfers well to PowerPoint (the 'data–pixel ratio'). PowerPoint sadly offers the temptation of many three-dimensional decorations for graphs which reduce the data–pixel ratio and can have a substantial negative impact on the clarity of the data presented. Mackiewicz (2007) lends support for Tufte's recommendations in research that suggests two-dimensional rather than three-dimensional graphs are better understood and suggests good contrast between graph and background is also important. Few (2004: p. 60) also suggests avoiding three-dimensional graphs of any description (whether the third dimension is decorative or ostensibly informative) and also eschews pie charts as they communicate data poorly.

In using graphics, different approaches may need to be used depending on whether the prime function of the slide is engagement or information transfer. Reynolds (2020) suggests using a 'full bleed', that is, taking the photograph right to the edge of the slide, using empty space in the photograph for text for maximum impact (Fig 20.3). Alley (2003) recommends using photographs and diagrams at smaller size and combining them with text on the slide. Both are feasible approaches, and represent different poles along the spectrum of appealing to emotion and appealing to reason.

In recent years, PowerPoint's own internal graphics have much improved. If you haven't looked at the options for generating diagrams and graphics recently, we suggest this is worth doing. It is now possible to search for images and icons with a Creative Commons license from within PowerPoint. In addition, there are now a plethora of sites on the Internet offering free or very low cost photos and graphics. (Unsplash, Pixabay, Burst by Shopify and Pexels are four of our favourites. For something a bit different, icons8 is also worth a look.)

4. Layout

The commonest cause of untidy looking slides is poor alignment of elements on the slide (Williams 2014). Every element of the slide should be visually connected to something else. The best way to achieve this is to use a grid for your slides (Reynolds 2020), and the simplest grid is made by dividing the slide into three, both vertically and horizontally (Fig. 20.2). Aim to either place key elements at the intersections of the lines (familiar to photographers as the

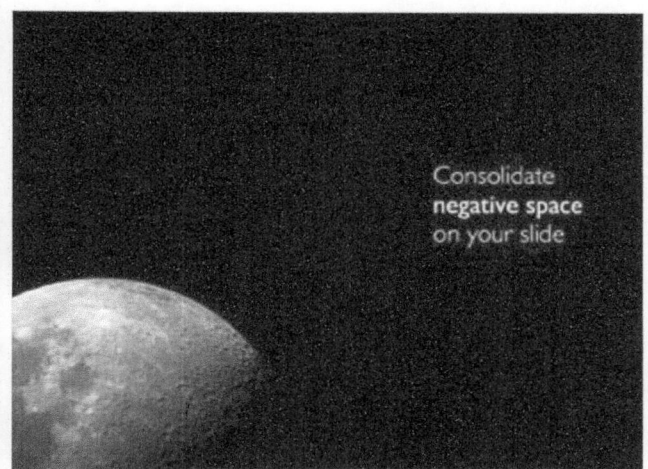

Fig. 20.3 Using negative space .

This slide uses the metaphor of outer space to represent space on the slide. All slides comprise a frame, positive space (the content) and negative space (empty space), and it is worth thinking about both the positive and negative components when considering design. Only two of the nine cells formed by the '3 × 3' layout grid are used here, one for the graphic and one for the text. The slide has an uncluttered and calm feel. Note also how the image 'bleeds' off the slide, suggesting how it continues beyond the frame of the slide. If you're looking for images with negative space for text, iStockphoto allows you to search their collections.

'rule of thirds') or to divide the slide into consistently used zones (e.g., for picture and text). Other grids may also work well applied consistently across slides.

Slides that are crowded with information may be unclear or feel like a visual assault. If you have got empty space (negative or 'white' space) on slides, aim to consolidate this – visually, it is better to have one large area of empty space rather than multiple smaller areas of empty space (Fig. 20.4).

Diversity, Inclusion and International Audiences

Be mindful of your audience in choosing images: for example, images with predominantly white Caucasian faces can send a meta message that the content of the presentation is not relevant to a predominantly non-Caucasian audience, or that the content in a medical context is focused around a particular ethnic group. Colour associations can be culture specific: for example, green features widely in Islamic cultures across the Indian subcontinent and parts of Africa (McCandless 2010); red is associated with good luck in the Chinese

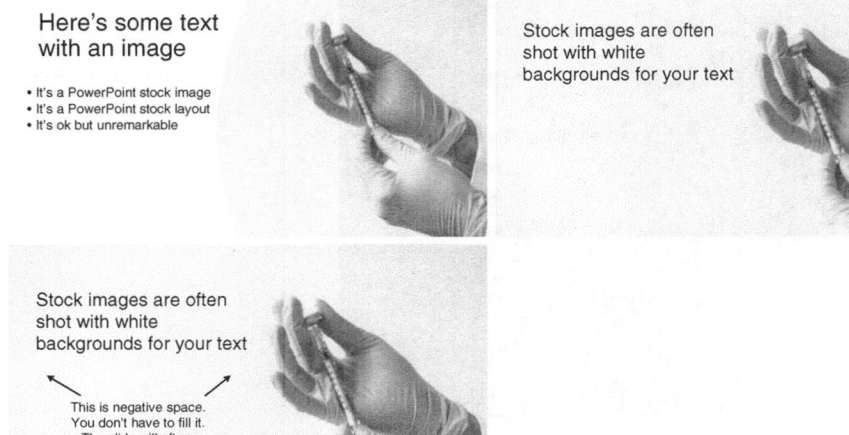

Fig. 20.4 Try to make sure that each slide has some negative space. It helps visually if the negative space is consolidated into once place.

diaspora. In presenting for audiences and those for whom English is a second or other language, we suggest modifying some of the principles above. We also recommend increasing the amount of text on slides when presenting to an international audience who then have 'two chances' at understanding your message, particularly if you have an accent that may be unfamiliar to your audience.

Presentation Factors

Perhaps the most common mistake to make is to assume that the slides are the presentation: they aren't. The slides are a presentation *aid*. Making your presentation audience centred means trying to build a relationship with an audience and to have conversational and interactional elements in what you are saying, with slides supporting this process. Our example slides in this article are accompanied by what might be the presenter's spoken text: there is more detail in the 'spoken' text than is on the slide. Clark and Mayer (2007: pp. 157–180) present evidence that a conversational style improves learning and theories that this may be because social cues lead people to 'work harder to understand material when they feel they are in a conversation with a partner rather than simply receiving information'. Come out from behind the podium and talk to the audience (Fig. 20.5).

In building a relationship with your audience, think about the location of the screen, whether behind you in an auditorium, or sharing through a videoconference: if you need to look at notes, learn how to use the presenter view in PowerPoint (called presenter display in Apple's Keynote), which allows you to look at detailed notes on the screen while your audience sees only the slide. Especially with videoconferencing, try to practice in the target environment to avoid unexpected issues that could detract from your overall message.

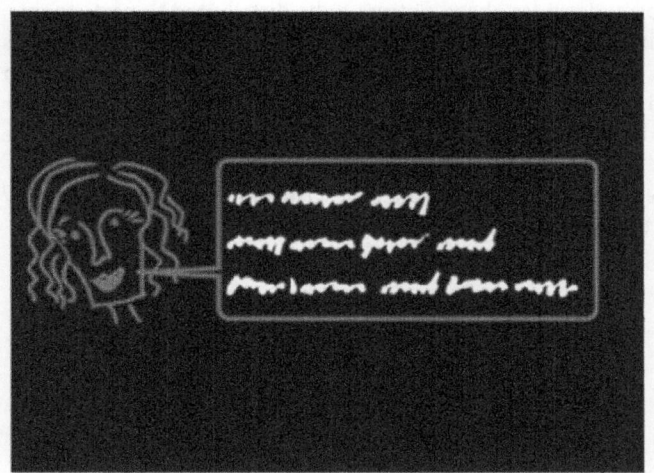

Fig. 20.5 Mayer's modality principle.

According to Mayer, retention is better from spoken words than written words, something he calls the modality principle. The bulk of your message should come from your mouth, not your slide. If you are using graphics, the narration of your presentation should explain the graphic on the slide. Absolutely the worst option is simply to read extensive text from a slide. Mayer explains the modality effect by his 'dual channel, limited capacity' model: a good presentation should engage both the verbal and the visual channels. This slide uses the free font The Written Word for the obscured text. The graphic of a head is from 'Ann's characters', an inexpensive font available from MyFonts.com. The slide is laid out in a grid based on thirds. The spoken narration explains the slide. The slide also illustrates why well-designed slides make poor handouts: it is meaningless without the presentation it is designed to accompany.

The corollary of the rule that PowerPoint is a presentation aid is that your slides (if well designed) make very little sense outside the context of a presentation. Avoid the temptation to use PowerPoint to make handouts, pseudo-documents that Reynolds (2020) disparages as 'slideuments'. Similarly, even when put under pressure to do so, don't distribute your slides on their own for people who didn't make it to your presentation – these days, you will probably be recorded so both audio and visual will be accessible to the participant, giving the opportunity to watch the presentation asynchronously. Despite urging from administrators and conference organizers to provide slides ahead of time to be distributed to participants, try to supply an alternative handout. While time consuming to make, a handout that has been prepared with the specific needs of the audience can further support learning (Kinchin 2006) and address cultural and special educational needs of audience members. Write your handouts separately and include the level of detail (such as reading lists) that doesn't make sense on well-designed slides (Fig. 20.6): so for example, a handout covering the information in Fig. 20.3 might include not only a more detailed description of grids, but also key references and web links. The top reasons to avoid slide handouts (Race 2010) are:

(1) Learners are more likely to switch off when they have the slides.

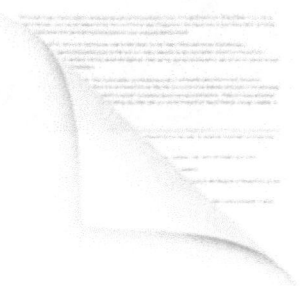

Fig. 20.6 Making handouts from slides.

The presentation is not the handout

PowerPoint and other slideware programs are there to make visual aids. They are very poor document creation tools. We have all had handouts of slides with paragraphs of text that are so small you need a magnifying glass to read them. It does not have to be this way! Write a handout that provides background to your slides with more detail and with elements that do not belong in the presentation itself such as a reading list. You might even explain things in a slightly different way to push learners to 'cognitive effort' in consolidating the presentation and the notes, remembering that this promotes deeper and more effective learning. This slide uses stock imagery of a page turn to suggest a handout 'behind' the slide, picking up the metaphor of the handout as background to the slide. It is deliberately too small to read as it is not meant to be read as part of the presentation.

(2) Many learners never look at the slides again.

(3) Slides are often information – learning only happens when information is processed.

(4) With slide handouts, the audience may get distressed at 'missed' or 'missing' slides.

If we consider any presentation as a potential forum for adult learning, all presenters should avoid a 'just the facts' approach (Knowles et al. 2005). Scientists could seek to incorporate some of the 'artistic stream' of learning as being 'led in discussion' (Lindeman 1925). In the past five years, increasing numbers of universities have encouraged recording and posting of lectures to allow students and participants to return to more challenging content in the format in which it was delivered. Since the COVID-19 lockdowns, this has been widespread, with a clear indication that asynchronous learning (sometimes referred to as the 'flipped classroom') may be adopted more widely in UK contexts, leaving face-to-face learning more reserved for practical skill development.

Today, it is suggested that learning is 'fundamentally social' (Connolly 2008), with active learners (Fink 2003) who are engaging in a 'dialogue' with their peers, the material and even with themselves (Leonard and Swap 2004). We recommend every effort to promote social learning: many of our presentations are to large groups where there is a temptation to assume that interaction is impossible, even more so with videoconference-based sessions. Race (2010) proposes that, even within a large group, it is possible to challenge and develop learners' thinking by encouraging feedback and participation, but without lecturing, and with interactive add-ons that integrate with PowerPoint (such as PollEverywhere and Padlet), there are possibilities for safer and even more honest interactions. Within medical learning environments, there is evidence that active learning assists recall whether the 'activity' is in providing material beforehand (Moravec et al. 2010) or in getting immediate feedback from the audience (Collins 2004; Stahl and Davis 2009; Hoyt et al. 2010). In these discussions of active learning, PowerPoint features prominently, but is largely limited to papers suggesting technical ways of accommodating different learner styles through inserting audio and video clips (Mixer et al. 2008; Myers et al. 2008; Gunderman and McCammack 2010; Henkel 2010).

Continuous Improvement

Making good visual aids is not difficult, but nor is it something that comes naturally. Very few people who use PowerPoint are trained in it. More than ever, there are resources to enable you to develop your PowerPoint skills, often using design features embedded within the software, such as the 'design ideas' feature, or the enhanced ability to use a variety of fonts or icons to create simple infographics. We hope that this chapter will encourage the reader to look at their own use of PowerPoint critically, read more about what works visually, and ultimately help their audience engage with the content. There is an online supplement to this article at https://static.cambridge.org/content/id/urn:cambridge.org:id:article:S1355514600017065/resource/name/S1355514600017065sup001.pdf with links to other resources including good examples of PowerPoint and providers of images.

References

Alley M (2003) *The Craft of Scientific Presentations: Critical Steps to Succeed and Critical Errors to Avoid.* Springer.

Alley M, Schreiber M, Ramsdell K, Muffo J (2006) How the design of headlines in presentation slides affects audience retention.

Technical Communication,
53: 225–34.

Atkinson C (2007) *Beyond Bullet Points: Using Microsoft® Office PowerPoint® 2007 to Create Presentations That Inform, Motivate, and Inspire.* Microsoft Press.

Bartsch R, Cobern KM (2003) Effectiveness of PowerPoint presentations in lectures. *Computers & Education,* **41**: 77–86.

Blokzijl W, Andeweg B (2007) The effect of text slides compared to visualizations on learning and appreciation in lectures. In Proceedings of the 2007 IEEE International Professional Communication Conference, Seattle, WA, 1–3 October, pp. 1–9.

Bradshaw A (2003) Effects of presentation interference in learning with visuals. *Journal of Visual Literacy,* **23**: 41–60.

Brown P, Roediger H, McDaniel M (2014) *Make It Stick: The Science of Successful Learning.* Harvard University Press.

Clark RC, Mayer RE (2007) *E-Learning and the Science of Instruction: Proven Guidelines for Consumers and Designers of Multimedia Learning,* 2nd ed. Jossey Bass.

Collins J (2004) Education techniques for lifelong learning: giving a PowerPoint presentation: the art of communicating effectively. *RadioGraphics,* **24**: 1185–92.

Connolly B (2008) *Adult Learning in Groups.* McGraw Hill Open University Press.

Craig RJ, Amernic JH (2006) PowerPoint presentation technology and the dynamics of teaching. *Innovative Higher Education,* **31**: 147–60.

Cyphert D (2004) The problem of PowerPoint: visual aid or visual rhetoric? *Business Communication Quarterly,* **67**: 80–4.

Diemand-Yauman C, Oppenheimer DM, Vaughan EB (2011) Fortune favors the bold (and the italicized): effects of disfluency on educational outcomes. *Cognition,* **118**: 111–15.

Duarte N (2008) *Slideology: The Art and Science of Creating Great Presentations: The Art and Science of Presentation Design.* Pragma.

Duarte N (2010) *Resonate: Present Visual Stories That Transform Audiences.* John Wiley & Sons, Inc.

Few S (2004) *Show Me the Numbers: Designing Tables and Graphs to Enlighten.* Analytics Press.

Fink LD (2003) *Creating Significant Learning Experiences: An Integrated Approach to Designing College Courses.* Jossey Bass.

Gross A, Harmon J (2009) The structure of PowerPoint presentations: the art of grasping things whole. *IEEE Transactions on Professional Communication,* **52**: 121–37.

Gunderman RB, McCammack KC (2010) PowerPoint: know your medium. *Journal of the American College of Radiology,* **7**: 711–4.

Harden RM (2008) Death by PowerPoint-the need for a 'fidget index'. *Medical Teacher,* **30**: 833–5.

Henkel CK (2010) Creating interactive learning objects with PowerPoint: primer for lecture on the autonomic nervous system. *Medical Teacher,* **32**: e355–9.

Hertz B, van Wooerkum C, Kerkhof P (2015) Why do scholars use PowerPoint the way they do? *Business and Professional Communications Quarterly,* **78**: 273–91.

Hill A, Arford T, Lubitow A, Smollin L (2012) 'I'm ambivalent about it': the dilemmas of PowerPoint. *Teaching Sociology,* **40**: 242–56.

Hoffman B, White A, Aquino N (2005) Screen text readability: ease, accuracy, and speed of some common computer typefaces. In Proceedings of The International Visual Literacy Association (IVLA) Annual Conference.

Hoyt A, McNulty JA, Gruener G, et al. (2010) An audience response system may influence student performance on anatomy examination questions. *Anatomical Sciences Education,* **3**(6), pp. 295–299.

Kinchin IM (2006) Developing PowerPoint handouts to support meaningful learning. *British Journal of Education Technology,* **37**: 647–50.

Kjeldsen JE (2006) The rhetoric of PowerPoint. *International Journal of Media Technology and Lifelong Learning,* **2**; doi https://doi.org/10.7577/seminar.2523.

Knowles MS, Holton EF, Swanson RA (2005) *The Adult Learner,* 6th ed. Elsevier.

Kosslyn S, Kievit R, Russel A, Shepher J (2012) PowerPoint presentation flaws and failures: a psychological analysis. *Frontiers in Psychology*, **3**: 1–22.

Leonard D, Swap W (2004) Deep smarts. *Harvard Business Review*. Available at: https://hbr.org/2004/09/deep-smarts.

Lindeman EC (1925) Adult education, a creative opportunity. *Library Journal*, **50**: 445–57.

Lupton E (2010) *Thinking with Type, Second Revised and Expanded Edition: A Critical Guide for Designers, Writers, Editors, and Students* 2nd ed. Princeton Architectural Press.

Mackiewicz J (2006) Audience perceptions of fonts in projected PowerPoint text slides. In Proceedings of the 2007 IEEE International Professional Communication Conference, Seattle, WA, 1–3 October, pp. 68–76.

Mackiewicz J (2007) Perceptions of clarity and attractiveness in PowerPoint graph slides. *Technical Communication*, **54**: 145–56.

Mayer R (2009) *Multimedia Learning*, 2nd ed. Cambridge University Press.

Mayer R (2014) Research-based principles for designing multimedia instruction. In Benassi VA, Overson CE, Hakala CM (eds.), *Applying Science of Learning in Education: Infusing Psychological Science into the Curriculum. Society for the Teaching of Psychology.* Available at: http://teachpsych .org/ebooks/asle2014/index.php.

McCandless D (2010) *Information is Beautiful.* Collins.

Mixer SJ, McFarland MR. McInnis LA (2008) Visual literacy in the online environment. *The Nursing Clinics of North America*, **43**: 575–82.

Moravec M, Williams A, Aguilar-Roca N, O'Dowd DK, 2010. Learn before lecture: a strategy that improves learning outcomes in a large introductory biology class. *CBE: Life Sciences Education*, **9**: 473–81.

Myers DR, Sykes C, Myers S (2008) Effective learner-centered strategies for teaching adults: using visual media to engage the adult learner. *Gerontology & Geriatrics Education*, **29**: 234–8.

Race P (2010) *Making Learning Happen: A Guide for Post-Compulsory Education*, 2nd ed. Sage Publications Ltd.

Reber R, Schwarz N, Winkielman P (2004) Processing fluency and aesthetic pleasure: is beauty in the perceiver's processing experience? *Personality and Social Psychology Review*, **8**: 364–82.

Reynolds G (2020) *Presentation Zen Design: Simple Design Principles and Techniques to Enhance Your Presentations*, 3rd ed. New Riders.

Schriver KA (1997) *Dynamics in Document Design: Creating Texts for Readers*. John Wiley & Sons, Inc.

Squire V (2006) *Getting It Right with Type: The Do's and Don'ts of Typography*. Laurence King.

Stahl S, Davis R (2009) Applying the principles of adult learning to the to teaching of psychopharmacology: overview and finding the focus. *CNS Spectrums*, **14**: 170–82.

Tufte E (2001) *The Visual Display of Quantitative Information*, 2nd ed. Graphics Press.

Tufte E (2006) *The Cognitive Style of PowerPoint: Pitching Out Corrupts Within*, 2nd ed. Graphics Press.

Wecker C (2012) Slide presentations as speech suppressors: when and why learners miss oral information. *Computers and Education*, **59**: 260–73.

Williams R (2014) *The Non-Designer's Design Book*, 4th ed. Peachpit Press.

Virtual Teaching and Learning in Psychiatric Medical Education

Thomas Hewson, Sridevi Sira Mahalingappa
and Subodh Dave

Introduction

Broadly speaking, virtual learning refers to the delivery of education via the use of digital technology. It encompasses a broad range of learning techniques, communication methods and electronic media to provide a learning experience that is flexible, engaging and learner centred (Ellaway and Masters 2008).

Virtual learning has been possible since the invention of the Internet in the late twentieth century. In 1969, the Open University pioneered the use of emerging digital technologies to increase the accessibility of higher education. Since its inception, the Open University has provided remote learning opportunities for over two million students (The Open University 2021). Over the past few decades, virtual teaching and learning have become increasingly popular within medical education, but their use has been particularly accelerated by the COVID-19 pandemic (He et al. 2020). Since the onset of coronavirus, medical educators have used virtual learning to safeguard the delivery of medical curricula, whilst also abiding by social distancing precautions and protecting staff and students from disease transmission. This has been akin to the global upsurgence in the use of telehealth and remote delivery of physical and mental healthcare (Monaghesh and Hajzadeh 2020).

Many of the same principles of face-to-face education apply to virtual teaching and learning, but the virtual setting brings new benefits, challenges and considerations. In virtual learning, the learner and educator are separated by time and/or space, and it is therefore rooted in 'distance education' (Moore et al. 2011). The term 'transactional distance' has been coined to describe the 'social, psychological, and relational distance between teachers and learners that is fluid and manageable based on a function of dialogue and structure' (Rhim and Han 2020: p. 176, referring to Moore 1993). Online educators must maintain effective interactions with learners in the virtual setting and deliver course content flexibly to account for individual needs and reduce their transactional distance (Rhim and Han 2020). When transactional distance is reduced, learning processes are likely to become more individualized.

Cognitive, Social and Teaching Presence

Although not physically present in the virtual setting, learners must be supported to achieve 'cognitive' and 'social' presence (Rhim and Han 2020). Cognitive presence refers to the degree to which learners can construct meaning through sustained communication with others in the virtual platform (Anderson 2008). For example, brainstorming ideas and debating concepts with colleagues are both means of achieving cognitive presence, whereby learners can express their thoughts and reflections to others. 'Social presence' involves connectedness between peers and educators (Anderson 2008; Rhim and Han 2020). Furthermore, it entails the creation of a sense of community and supportiveness among those in the learning environment. This can be achieved through encouraging collaboration between learners and the sharing of personal feelings, emotions and characteristics. The acquisition of social presence is essential for reducing feelings of isolation and loneliness that students may feel when physically separate from their peers (Song et al. 2004). Another important concept is 'teaching presence', which is defined as 'the design, facilitation, and direction of cognitive and social processes for the purpose of realising personally meaningful and educationally worthwhile learning outcomes' (Anderson et al. 2001: p. 5). It is important that educators immerse themselves in the online learning environment, and 'lead by example' by modelling the behaviours and contributions expected from learners. Regularly monitoring and commenting on student's online postings and work can maintain interest and engagement, while reducing the transactional distance between learner and educator.

Synchronous and Asynchronous Learning

An important distinction exists between synchronous and asynchronous learning. The former refers to when persons engage in learning at the same time, whereas asynchronous learning allows learners to complete education separately. For example, live-streamed lectures and live chatting between students and educators both constitute synchronous teaching and learning, whereas pre-recorded presentations, email exchanges and independent completion of e-learning modules represent asynchronous educational methods. The flexibility provided by asynchronous learning is a particular benefit to adult learners with competing commitments, allowing them to regularly adapt their learning schedules (Boulos et al. 2005). However, synchronous student–student and student–teacher interactions can build team working capabilities, enhance learning communities and facilitate social integration. Improved educational performance has also been associated with the integration of synchronous learning opportunities within distance education programmes (Boulos et al. 2005). For these reasons, many virtual learning courses integrate synchronous and asynchronous learning.

Tips for Organizations Implementing Virtual Learning

Organizations must ensure that learners and educators have access to suitable equipment for engagement in virtual learning. A laptop or computer with a good internet connection, reliable Wi-Fi network, microphone and webcam are typically minimally required (Sharp et al. 2021). Various online platforms and learning management systems may be used for the delivery of course content, the most popular of which include Microsoft Teams (www.microsoft.com/en-gb/microsoft-teams), Zoom (https://zoom.us), Blackboard (www.blackboard.com) and Moodle (https://moodle.org). Individual organizations will often require their own policies regarding the use of different platforms and online communication methods. For example, within healthcare, virtual teaching sessions involving the discussion of sensitive information or patient interaction warrant greater data security procedures and attention to information governance and GDPR regulations (Ramkisson et al. 2020).

Organizations must ensure that learners and educators feel comfortable using the required technologies and have adequate digital literacy to effectively educate and/or learn in the virtual setting. Digital literacy is defined by Health Education England as "those capabilities that fit someone for living, learning, working, participating and thriving in a digital society" (Health Education England 2021). To promote digital literacy among learners and educations, organizations can deliver tutorials and virtual tours explaining the use of online platforms, and/or hold digital skills sessions in addition to standard teaching topics. With the increasing use of telemedicine in modern healthcare, equipping healthcare professionals with adequate digital literacy is of increasing importance, and has the potential for improving patient care and outcomes (Health Education England 2021); furthermore, this could support the democratization of learning and help to address differential attainment in undergraduate and postgraduate medical education.

Preparing for Virtual Learning

Both learners and teachers should carefully consider the physical environment from which they engage in and/or deliver education. The room should ideally be free from distractions, with adequate lighting so that the person is easily viewed through their webcam. Some applications, such as Zoom, permit the use of 'neutral' backgrounds for these reasons. Indirect lighting is generally recommended during videoconferencing to avoid excess luminance, and reliance on natural light should be avoided as this may fluctuate throughout the educational encounter (Zoom Video Communications 2021). The learner and educator may additionally wish to consider how they present themselves in the virtual environment, in the same way that they would ensure appropriate attire for attendance at classroom learning (Sharp et al. 2020). It is beneficial to ensure that notepads, water bottles, pens and other items that may be needed during learning are within close proximity of the electronic device being utilized; although many people engage in virtual learning from home environments where such items are easily accessible, obtaining them during synchronous teaching can interrupt the flow of learning and communication. Logging into the online platform several minutes in advance of synchronous teaching can allow learners and educators time for troubleshooting any technical difficulties, such as ensuring adequate functioning of their webcam and microphone (Sharp et al. 2020). Early attendance at synchronous teaching sessions can additionally create opportunities for informal peer-to-peer and learner-to-educator conversations, which facilitate social cohesion and support the cognitive and social presence of learners in the virtual setting (Tu and McIsaac 2002; Sharp et al. 2020).

Delivering and Engaging in Virtual Learning

Knowing and understanding the expectations of educators may help learners to feel more comfortable and confident in immersing themselves in virtual platforms. As such, educators should set ground rules for engagement with virtual learning. These rules might include asking learners to mute themselves when not speaking to reduce background noise, and/or keeping their webcams switched on, where possible, to encourage engagement and build familiarity with colleagues. Importantly, learners should be made aware of the expected format in which to ask questions or make comments (Sharp et al. 2020). For example, learners could be instructed to use the virtual 'raise hand' function, type messages in the virtual chat box or unmute themselves and speak aloud. All of these methods have different advantages and disadvantages (Sharp et al. 2020). For example, the 'raise hand' function can facilitate turn-taking and distribution of learner participation but can reduce the spontaneity of communication. Alternatively, typing questions and comments in virtual chat boxes can instantly clarify confusion and provides all learners the option to answer, thus boosting engagement and accountability, but requires the careful attention of educators to monitor this whilst focusing on pedagogy (Khan et al. 2021). The use of a second teaching facilitator to monitor the chat and encourage engagement from learners can improve the interactivity and effectiveness of virtual teaching (Khan et al. 2021).

Educators should also consider the different features available within online learning platforms and how these can be utilized to improve the learning experience (Mukhopadhyay et al. 2020; Sharp et al. 2021). For example, 'breakout rooms' involve the allocation of learners to small peer groups for a set amount of time before re-joining the entire class (Khan et al. 2021) These can be used for promoting teamwork, socialization and discussion between learners, particularly during group learning exercises (McDaniels et al. 2016). The 'share screen' function also allows the presenter to display content on their computer screen to others, which may involve multimedia videos, PowerPoint slides and graphics (Mukhopadyay et al. 2020). Polling during virtual learning can assess knowledge acquisition and augment interactivity (Dong et al. 2020).

When considering both the 'ground rules' and features available for virtual learning, educators must remember that a range of learning styles and preferences are likely to exist among students. For this reason, educators should be prepared to adapt these in response to the needs of students and use a range of online teaching methods to capture the interests of all learners (Zapalska and Brozik 2006).

Advantages and Disadvantages of Virtual Learning

Virtual learning offers several advantages compared to traditional face-to-face education (Song et al. 2004; Dung 2020). Perhaps the greatest advantage of virtual learning is the transcendence of usual geographical boundaries, allowing virtual teaching programmes to include educators and learners from various locations. This has the potential to improve collaboration between educational institutions on an international scale and to increase the accessibility of medical education. Virtual learning also provides increased flexibility and convenience, particularly asynchronous learning methods, by eliminating requirements for travel and allowing adjustment of learning schedules according to people's preferred times and locations (Song et al. 2004). Reduced travel requirements may additionally result in improved environmental sustainability. A further benefit of virtual learning is improved cost-effectiveness, largely attributable to reduced travel costs and lesser use of physical infrastructure (Dung 2020). Virtual teaching can additionally expose learners to a broader range of learning styles and online resources, while equipping them with skills in digital literacy for their future careers (Dung 2020).

Despite the above benefits of virtual learning, there are additionally drawbacks and barriers to its implementation (Song et al. 2004; Dung 2020). First, concerns exist regarding the extensive time that learners and educators can spend staring at computer screens (Dung 2020). This can result in tiredness and loss of concentration, which has recently been termed 'Zoom fatigue' (Fosslein and Duffy 2020; Sharp et al. 2020). To overcome this issue, educators should consider using short, well-timed breaks throughout virtual sessions (Sharp et al. 2020; Khan et al. 2021). Virtual learning additionally reduces opportunities for non-verbal communication and social interaction, including informal conversations between colleagues that usually aid learning and support wellbeing (Dung, 2020). Consequently, it is important that educators embed socialization functions into teaching and encourage collegiality and peer support before, during and after educational interventions. As with all technology, there is always the possibility of technical glitches and difficulties, which can interrupt the flow of learning, cause stress and anxiety among learners and educators and detract from learning time (Song et al. 2004). The potential for technical problems highlights a further need for effective digital literacy and for availability of support from information technology teams. Some students may also have difficulties directing their own learning and suffer from decreased motivation outside of face-to-face learning environments, thus requiring additional, personalized support (Dung 2020).

Examples of Virtual Teaching Methods

Below are some specific examples of virtual teaching methods, to which many of the above tips for preparing and engaging in virtual learning can be applied.

Online Webinars

Webinars are live virtual events hosted on the Internet that learners can log into and attend remotely, including online presentations, workshops and seminars (Topor and Budson 2020). As well as being delivered synchronously, webinars can be recorded and stored for later asynchronous viewing. Various platforms can be utilized for hosting online webinars. Educators should confirm the choice of virtual platform with session organizers prior to the event, including the various features available for learner interaction (Topor and Budson 2020). When planning online webinars, it is also important to consider specific learning needs within the audience. For example, educators can support trainees with sensory and visual impairments by using closed captions, subtitles and provision of screen readers. Microsoft (2021) provide various guidance for making PowerPoint slides accessible to persons with disabilities. For example, a strong contrast should be achieved between text and background to accommodate persons with low vision. Various changes may need to be made to presentations that have previously been designed for face-to-face delivery. Clear and engaging slides are particularly important since there is typically greater focus on these in online platforms, where it is more difficult to simultaneously view both presentation content and the presenter (Topor and Budson 2020). Learners may use a range of electronic devices with different screen sizes to access webinars, including mobile phones. Educators must, therefore, use sufficiently large, clear fonts and avoid including too much content per presentation slide (Topor and Budson 2020). Images can incorporate variety into presentations and visually demonstrate concepts but should be of high quality for effective online viewing (Topor and Budson 2020). Furthermore, the use of animations, sound effects and videos should be sufficiently tested in the online setting prior to learner engagement to minimize the likelihood of technical difficulties (Topor and Budson 2020). In face-to-face teaching, paper handouts are often delivered to learners to highlight key concepts, increase engagement and improve concentration (Wongkietkachorn et al. 2014). This can be mirrored in online webinars by making handouts available for virtual download and/or emailing these to participants prior to the event (Lieser et al. 2018). Finally, any interactive activities during the webinar should be enacted to maximize the involvement of all learners. For example, educators should consider reading aloud any comments from the 'chat box' to involve persons who are participating by audio only and generate further discussion (Topor and Budson 2020). Box 21.1 provides a summary of tips for delivering online webinars.

The Flipped Classroom

The traditional learning format usually involves learners listening to course content and lecture materials in a group-based setting, and subsequently independently applying their learning during homework activities. The 'flipped classroom' describes a pedagogical model where this traditional learning format is inverted. In this model, students familiarize themselves with course content remotely at home and then engage in deeper meaningful learning and problem solving with educators and peers during class time. This enables students to learn at their own pace and increases interactivity between students and educators, allowing class time to be reserved for student-centred, active learning (Long et al. 2017). The 'flipped classroom' can be utilized to blend synchronous and asynchronous learning. For example, students could listen to pre-recorded lectures and videos to learn about the different components of the mental state examination in their own time, before then practicing and evaluating difficult mental state examinations synchronously with peers and educators. A recent meta-analysis (Hew and Lo 2018) demonstrated a significant improvement in student health professionals learning through use of the flipped classroom model over traditional instructional methods. Furthermore, this approach is popular among students (Ramanan and Pound 2017; Hew and Lo 2018). The effectiveness of the flipped classroom model may be enhanced using quizzes at the beginning of synchronous teaching to motivate student engagement and address any misunderstandings of pre-class materials (Hew and Lo 2018).

Ward Rounds

Ward rounds provide an excellent opportunity for trainees to learn about patient presentations and healthcare journeys, as well as how the multidisciplinary team formulate clinical management plans. Traditionally, ward-round teaching has always occurred face to face; however, during the COVID-19 pandemic, innovations have been made to provide this experience virtually. For example, the Imperial College of London has digitalized the ward-round experience for their medical students (Hagana et al. 2021). Clinicians wore Microsoft HoloLens headsets, involving mixed reality smartglasses, whilst conducting patient interactions. This technology allowed them to live stream ward-round consultations to multiple students who attended the session virtually. Learning may be enhanced during virtual ward rounds by providing virtual images of relevant clinical information, such as radiographs and electrocardiograms, which students can interpret and use to practice their clinical skills

(Hagana et al. 2021). Learner involvement may also be maximized by asking students to remotely conduct ward-round tasks, such as practicing prescribing relevant medications, and providing designated time for asking questions and following up patients (Hoernke et al. 2020; Hagana et al. 2021). A major benefit of virtual ward rounds is the potential to record and showcase a greater variety of clinical presentations than may otherwise be seen in face-to-face learning. However, this teaching method is limited by the lack of direct patient contact for students (Hagana et al. 2021). It is paramount that educators obtain explicit informed consent from any patients involved in virtual ward rounds, and all students must be mindful of where and how they access this learning opportunity to avoid breaches of patient confidentiality. There is minimal literature on the use of virtual ward rounds in psychiatry, where some patients may be too mentally unwell to provide informed consent for their involvement.

Reverse Ward-Round Model

In this model, junior doctors are encouraged to take the lead in conducting ward rounds by interviewing patients, liaising with team members and formulating diagnoses and management plans (Royal College of Physicians and Royal College of Nursing 2021). Consultants can take up other roles, such as documentation of the consultation and providing observation and feedback for the trainee(s). Although this experience can be daunting for learners, consultants must prepare trainees for independent clinical practice and support the development of leadership skills and senior decision-making capabilities. Debriefing is essential after reverse ward rounds to support trainees and consolidate learning from the session (Royal College of Physicians and Royal College of Nursing 2021). The principles of this model can be applied to online learning environments to maximize the learning opportunities for trainees, and to increase learner engagement in virtual ward rounds.

Virtual Expert Patient Clinics

The Royal College of Psychiatrists' Person-Centred Training and Curriculum Scoping Group (Royal College of Psychiatrists 2018) highlight the need to actively involve patients in the design and delivery of medical education.

An 'expert patient' is somebody who has gained significant knowledge of their illness and its management through their own experiences of that illness and accessing healthcare (Cordier 2014). Expert patients can share their knowledge, skills and experiences to support medical students and healthcare professionals in improving their understanding and management of chronic health conditions, empathy and appreciation of the psychosocial impacts of illness. The Expert Patient Programme at Derbyshire Healthcare NHS Foundation Trust is an award-winning initiative involving people with lived experience of mental illness in medical student teaching. During COVID-19, weekly virtual expert patient clinics were established to provide remote clinical experience to approximately 12 medical students per session. These teaching sessions were co-led by expert patients and clinical educators. Initially, expert patients and students were briefed about the format and delivery of the teaching, and students were reminded of requirements to maintain patient confidentiality. Students observed expert patients speaking about their illness and being interviewed by clinicians, who demonstrated all aspects of initial psychiatric assessment including history taking, mental state examination and risk assessment. Subsequently, students witnessed follow-up consultations with expert patients in outpatient settings to reflect the entire treatment pathway. To maximize participant engagement, all learners received active observation sheets and were instructed to observe and evaluate specific clinical skills and tasks during the session. Group discussion and debriefing was essential to consolidate learning and facilitate consideration of the patient perspective. The major advantage of this virtual teaching format is the ability to impart technical skills in an 'authentic' clinical setting, albeit one that has been specifically created for the purposes of medical education. These sessions additionally allow students to practice communication skills and ask questions with patients in a safe, supportive environment prior to direct patient contact. Similar models can be applied to postgraduate training and may be particularly useful for reinforcing attitudes and values of person-centred care among clinicians, which should be reflected in clinical practice (Boardman and Dave 2020).

Virtual Assessments

Assessment is an important aspect of undergraduate and postgraduate medical education. Formative assessments are 'low-stakes' assessments that provide timely feedback on learner's knowledge and skills, with the aim of aiding self-reflection and the identification of knowledge gaps for subsequent remediation. On the other hand, summative assessments refer to 'high-stakes' assessments that determine a learner's success or failure to progress to subsequent stages of training. Although digital technologies have increasingly been used to deliver undergraduate and postgraduate medical assessments in recent years, these have typically been administered in the context of large examination halls or test centres with multiple persons present. Since COVID-19, medical schools and Royal Colleges have innovatively delivered remote, online formative and summative examinations. For example, Imperial Medical School tested final year medical students using online, remote open-book assessments (Monaghan 2020). Meanwhile, the Royal College of Psychiatrists has conducted remote, online theory examinations and utilized videoconferencing technology to test trainees' clinical skills remotely in the Clinical Assessment of Skills and Competencies (CASC) examination (Royal College of Psychiatrists 2021).

Online assessments offer several advantages compared to face-to-face administration. First, they may be more convenient for both leaners and educators, reduce travel time and avoid the anxiety that is associated with attending large test centres. Second, the Internet permits a broader range of question formats and assessment methods to be utilized, with options for various media to be incorporated into assessment processes (Walsh 2015). For example, rather than answering paper-based questions about psychopathology, students can watch online videos of mental state examinations and demonstrate application of their learning by identifying relevant psychiatric phenomena. Online assessments also provide scope for continuous and real-time feedback for learners, thus potentially improving their pace of learning and development (Walsh 2015).

A potential limitation of online assessments is the reliability of technological systems being utilized. Difficulties with computer hardware, software, Wi-Fi connection and power supply all have the potential to sabotage a learner's examination, causing considerable stress and anxiety (Walsh 2015). To avoid and promptly troubleshoot such issues, information technology support should be readily available for learners completing online examinations remotely, which is frequently provided by online invigilators or via telephone. Security issues and greater potential for academic misconduct are also frequently voiced concerns associated with remote online assessments (Walsh 2015); these can be addressed through online proctoring systems whereby invigilators oversee candidates' movements and physical environments through their webcams and monitor people's computers via screen sharing software.

The Future of Virtual Learning

It is presently unclear what role virtual learning will have in medical education post-pandemic. Blended learning involves the combination of virtual and classroom-based face-to-face educational activities to complement each other and improve student learning outcomes (Graham 2006). This approach has been suggested to maximize the benefits of face-to-face and virtual education while minimizing their respective limitations, and it has been shown to be effective in medical education (Kaur 2013; Liu et al. 2016). To successfully implement blended learning, educators must consider which teaching methods, whether they be face-to-face or virtual, are best suited to the delivery of specific course content and attainment of specific learning objectives. This approach offers the potential for addressing multiple needs and different learning styles across a diverse group of learners, while instilling variety within teaching programmes (Kaur 2013).

With the rapid advancement of digital technology, methods for delivering and engaging in virtual education are likely to further expand over the coming years; as this happens, educational institutions will need to evolve and adapt. Innovations in areas such as artificial intelligence and virtual reality are already beginning to diversify online teaching, creating potential for more immersive and personalized learning. For example, artificial intelligence can be used to detect specific gaps in people's knowledge and provide teaching that addresses their individual needs. It is vital that medical learners and educators remain abreast of the latest digital technologies to maximize their potential applications and benefits to medical education.

References

Anderson T (2008) Teaching in an online learning context. In Anderson T (ed.), *The Theory and Practice of Online Learning*, 2nd ed. AU Press, pp. 343–66.

Anderson T, Rourke L, Garrison DR, Archer W (2001) Assessing teaching presence in a computer conferencing context. *Journal of Asynchronous Learning Networks*, 5; doi: http://dx.doi.org/10.24059/olj.v5i2.1875.

Boardman J, Dave S (2020) Person-centred care and psychiatry: some key perspectives. *BJPsych International*, 17: 65–8; doi: https://doi.org/10.1192/bji.2020.21.

Boulos MNK, Taylor AD, Breton A (2005) A synchronous communication experiment within an online distance learning program: a case study. *Telemedicine and e-Health*, 11: 583–93.

Cordier JF (2014). The expert patient: towards a novel definition. *European Respiratory Journal*, 44: 853–7; doi: https://doi.org/10.1183/0903193 6.00027414.

Dong C, Lee DW, Aw DC (2020) Tips for medical educators on how to conduct effective online teaching in times of social distancing. *Proceedings of Singapore Healthcare*, 30: 59–63; doi: https://doi .org/10.1177%2F2010105820943907.

Dung DTH (2020) The advantages and disadvantages of virtual learning. *IOSR Journal of Research and Method in Medical Education*, 10: 45–8; doi: https://doi.org/10.9790/7388-1003054548.

Ellaway R, Masters K (2008) Part 1: Learning, teaching and assessment. In Ellaway R, Masters K (eds.), *E-Learning in Medical*

Education. Association for Medical Education in Europe.

Fosslein L, Duffy MW (2020) How to combat Zoom fatigue. Harvard Business Review. Available at: https://hbr.org/2020/04/how-to-combat-zoom-fatigue.

Graham CR (2006 Blended learning systems: definition, current trends and future directions. In Bonk CJ, Graham CR (eds.), *Handbook of Blended Learning: Global Perspectives, Local Designs*. Pfeiffer.

Hagana A, Behranwala R, Aojula N, Houbby N (2021) Digitalising medical education: virtual ward rounds during COVID-19 and beyond. *BMJ Simulation and Technology Enhanced Learning*, 7: 271; doi: http://dx.doi.org/10.1136/bmjstel-2020-000742.

Health Education England (2021) Digital literacy of the wider workforce. Available at: www.hee.nhs.uk/our-work/digital-literacy.

He S, Lai D, Mott S, et al. (2020) Remote e-work and distance learning for academic medicine: best practices and opportunities for the future. *Journal of Graduate Medical Education*, 12: 256–63; doi: https://dx.doi.org/10.4300%2FJGME-D-20-00242.1.

Hew KF, Lo CK (2018) Flipped classroom improves student learning in health professions education: a meta-analysis. *BMC Medical Education*, 18: 38; doi: https://doi.org/10.1186/s12909-018-1144-z.

Hoernke K, McGrath H, Tey JQ, Salazar O (2020) Virtual learning innovations for continuing clinical education during COVID-19. *Medical Science Educator*, 30: 1345–6; doi: https://doi.org/10.1007/s40670-020-01090-0

Khan RA, Atta K, Sajjad M, Jawaid M (2021) Twelve tips to enhance student engagement in synchronous online teaching and learning. *Medical Teacher*, 1–6; doi: https://doi.org/10.1080/0142159X.2021.1912310.

Kaur M (2013) Blended learning: its challenges and future. *Procedia Social and Behavioral Sciences*, 9: 612–17; doi: https://doi.org/10.1016/j.sbspro.2013.09.2.

Lieser P, Taff S, Murphy-Hagan A (2018) The Webinar Integration Tool: a framework for promoting active learning in blended environments. *Journal of Interactive Media in Education*, 1: 7; doi: http://doi.org/10.5334/jime.453.

Liu Q, Peng W, Zhang F, et al. (2016) The effectiveness of blended learning in health professions: systematic review and meta-analysis. *Journal of Medical Internet Research*, 18: e2; doi: https://doi.org/10.2196/jmir.4807.

Long T, Cummins J, Waugh M (2017) Use of the flipped classroom instructional model in higher education: instructors' perspectives. *Journal of Computing in Higher Education*, 29: 179–200; doi: https://doi.org/10.1007/s12528-016-9119-8.

McDaniels M, Pfund C, Barnicle K (2016) Creating dynamic learning communities in synchronous online courses: one approach from the Center for the Integration of Research, Teaching and Learning. *Online Learning Journal*, 20: 110–29.

Microsoft (2021) Make your PowerPoint presentations accessible to people with disabilities. Available at: https://support.microsoft.com/en-us/office/make-your-powerpoint-presentations-accessible-to-people-with-disabilities-6f7772b2-2f33-4bd2-8ca7-dae3b2b3ef25?ui=en-us&rs=en-us&ad=us.

Monaghan AM (2020) Medical teaching and assessment in the era of COVID-19. *Journal of Medical Education and Curricula Development*, 7; doi: https://doi.org/10.1177/2382120520965255.

Mukhopadhyay S, Booth AL, Calkins SM, et al. (2020) Leveraging technology for remote learning in the era of COVID-19 and social distancing. *Archives of Pathology and Laboratory Medicine*, 144: 1027–36; doi: https://doi.org/10.5858/arpa.2020-0201-ED.

Monaghesh E, Hajzadeh A (2020) The role of telehealth during COVID-19: a systematic review based on current evidence, *BMC Public Health*, 20: 1193; doi: https://doi.org/10.1186/s12889-020-09301-4.

Moore JL, Dickson-Deane C, Galyen K (2011) E-Learning, online learning, and distance learning environments: are they the same?. *The Internet and Higher Education*, 14: 129–35; doi: https://doi.org/10.1016/j.iheduc.2010.10.001.

Moore MG (1993) Theory of transactional distance. In Keegan D (ed.), *Theoretical Principles of Distance Education*, pp. 23–8.

Ramnanan CJ, Pound LD (2017) Advances in medical education and practice: student perceptions of the flipped classroom. *Advances in Medical Education and Practice*, 8: 63–73; doi: https://doi.org/10.2147/AMEP.S109037.

Ramkisson R, Dave S, Abraham S, et al. (2020) Remote psychiatric consultations: top tips for clinical practitioners. *Progress in Neurology and Psychiatry*, 24: 20–5; doi: https://doi.org/10.1002/pnp.674.

Rhim HC, Han H (2020) Teaching online: foundational concepts of online learning and practical guidelines. *Korean Journal of Medical Education*, 32: 175–83; doi: https://doi.org/10.3946/kjme.2020.171.

Royal College of Psychiatrists (2018) Person-centred care: implications for training in psychiatry (College Report CR215). Available at: www.rcpsych.ac.uk/docs/default-source/improving-care/better-mh-policy/college-reports/college-report-cr215.pdf?sfvrsn=7863b905_2.

Royal College of Psychiatrists (2021) CASC online: webinar. Available at: www.rcpsych.ac.uk/training/exams/preparing-for-exams/casc-online-webinar.

Royal College of Physicians and Royal College of Nursing (2021) Modern ward rounds: good practice for multidisciplinary inpatient review. Available at: www.rcn.org.uk/professional-development/publications/rcn-modern-ward-rounds-good-practice-for-multidisciplinary-inpatient-review-uk-pub009566.

Sharp EA, Norman MK, Spagnoletti CL, Miller BG (2021) Optimising synchronous online teaching sessions: a guide to the 'new normal' in medical education, *Academic Pediatrics*, 21: 11–15; doi: https://doi.org/10.1016/j.acap.2020.11.009.

Song L, Singleton ES, Hill JR, Koh MH (2004) Improving online learning: student perceptions of useful and challenging characteristics. *The Internet and Higher Education*, 7: 59–70; doi: https://doi.org/10.1016/j.iheduc.2003.11.003.

The Open University (2021) About the OU. Available at: www.open.ac.uk/about/main.

Topor DR, Budson AE (2020) Twelve tips to present an effective webinar. *Medical Teacher*, 42: 1216–20; doi: https://doi.org/10.1080/0142159X.2020.1775185.

Tu C, McIsaac M (2002) The relationship of social presence and interaction in online classes. *The American Journal of Distance Education*, 16: 131–50; doi: https://doi.org/10.1207/S15389286AJDE1603_2.

Walsh K (2015) Online assessment in medical education: current trends and future directions. *Malawi Medical Journal*, 27: 71–2; doi: https://doi.org/10.4314/mmj.v27i2.8.

Wongkietkachorn A., Prakoonsuksapan J, Wangsaturaka D (2014) What happens when teachers do not give students handouts? *Medical Teacher*, 36: 789–93; doi: https://doi.org/10.3109/0142159X.2014.909921.

Zapalska A, Brozik D (2006) Learning styles and online education. *Campus-Wide Information Systems*, 23: 323–35; doi: https://doi.org/10.1108/10650740610714080.

Zoom Video Communications (2021) Lighting concepts. Available at: https://support.zoom.us/hc/en-us/articles/360028862512-Lighting-Concepts.

The Trainee in Difficulty: Where Are We Now?

Sarah Huline-Dickens

Introduction

In the guide written by Harden and Crosby (2000) for the Association for Medical Education in Europe (AMEE) called *The Good Teacher Is More Than a Lecturer*, the shift from traditional models of learning to a more learner-led one is emphasized and reflects the altered roles and expectations of teachers. Rather than dispensing information the teacher is seen more as a facilitator of learning and providing a supportive relationship for that learning to happen.

Supportive relationships are crucial to the success of training in busy clinical environments. Yet providing support and supportive relationships is still problematic in the health service. In 2019 alone, there were three published reports all highlighting problems and making suggestions for change; one from Health Education England (HEE); one from a National Institute of Health Research (NIHR) funded study undertaken by a team based at the University of Exeter Medical School; and one from the General Medical Council (GMC). It is worth looking at these briefly in turn.

First, as part of the National Health Service (NHS) Staff and Learners' Mental Wellbeing Commission (HEE 2019a) into *all* learners (including non-medical), HEE recommended that:

- there should be an NHS Workforce Wellbeing Guardian in a board-level role in every NHS organization (recommendation 1);
- training in self-awareness, support and suicide risk awareness should be incorporated into every healthcare undergraduate and postgraduate curriculum (recommendation 7);
- when capital allocation is considered, space for staff and learners should be enhanced or created (recommendation 12);
- educational and clinical supervisors should be able to give guidance on support for learners with mental distress (recommendation 14);
- there should be rapid access to help for NHS learners and employees (recommendations 16 and 32);
- there is careful consideration of the way complaints are handled (recommendation 23);
- there are clear organization protocols for responses to death by suicide (recommendation 28);
- all staff should have access to a practitioner psychological treatment service (recommendation 31); and
- there should be the promotion of a positive culture and adoption of tools and resources to tackle bullying and undermining (recommendation 33).

Second, as part of a robust realist review of interventions which have been used to help the mental ill-health of doctors and the subsequent impact on workforce and patient care, the *Care Under Pressure* project, summarized by Carrieri et al. (2020), found that:

- doctors experience mental ill-health when they feel isolated, unable to do the job they were trained for and when they fear consequences of seeking help or support;
- interventions that emphasize relationships and belonging promote wellbeing and improve workplace cultures;
- interventions that create a people-focussed working culture are beneficial; and
- doctors need to have confidence in an intervention and those delivering it, for it to be effective, and trust is easily lost.

The authors added that improving and evaluating existing interventions is likely to be more useful than creating new ones; that complex problems are likely to require complex solutions; and that there need to be clear lines of responsibility across organizations. It is not at all clear, given the current arrangements, that this is the case (see below).

Finally, in *Caring for Doctors Caring for Patients* (West and Coia 2019), a report commissioned by the GMC to investigate and make recommendations about doctors' wellbeing, another set of suggestions were made. This report was co-chaired by the prominent Scottish psychiatrist Dame Denise Coia, and the following were highlighted:

- workplace stress directly affects the quality of care for patients as well as doctors' own health;
- to ensure motivation and wellbeing at work, all three of an ABC of needs (autonomy, belonging and competence, i.e., delivering valued outcomes) must be met;
- the importance of compassionate leadership; and
- the importance of supervision in job plans.

An urgent plea was made to take immediate action in a number of areas to improve the workplace culture and the working environments for doctors. Several examples are cited from around the UK.

It can be seen from these examples, and the fact that there is now in the UK a national conference annually on the doctor in difficulty, that not only do we recognize there is a problem but that we already have many suggestions to deal with the challenges or workplace stress.

In this chapter, the ordinary course of action for doctors with physical health problems will not be discussed. These are rarely controversial in management. Rather, certain individual factors will be considered, including aspects of the culture of medical training, and then the wider training environment that impinge on psychological and mental health. Burnout and differential attainment are discussed; then some practical tools and strategies that may be helpful for trainers; managing difficult conversations and managing performance; and finally there will be some reflections on resilience.

Most of this chapter will assume that trainee problems are related to health or workplace stress. However, under the section on managing performance, attitudinal factors are considered. Conduct may be a feature in cases where referral to the GMC occurs.

Individual Factors

Many would argue that the selection of medical trainees is such that hard-working and conscientious candidates are the very individuals that would find the training environments they are subjected to highly stressful. Medical trainees are widely cited to have perfectionism traits; to be driven to succeed; and to consider help seeking for themselves stigmatizing in some way (Garada 2021). This is why the culture of medical training also needs to be carefully taken into account.

In her opening chapter of *Beneath the White Coat*, Garada (2021) describes the development of her own medical identity: a lengthy process which began in having a general practitioner as a father. She observes that respect and prestige is conferred upon doctors who need to have good grades in order to gain a place at medical school, and training reinforces the sense of specialness. The defence mechanisms which are developed during this training can be helpful and protective in work which is emotionally and physically demanding, but they can also be limiting and lead to institutionalization and enmeshment with work.

When unwell, doctors can often experience feelings of emptiness, self blame, exclusion and stigmatization, and often a crisis occurs before they seek help.

Mental Disorders

Within the category of individual factors lie of course individual mental health disorders. A complete list is not provided here as doctors with psychiatric disorders do not display symptoms that are different to anyone else in the population in so far as they can experience depression, anxiety, post-traumatic stress disorder, eating disorders and personality disorders.

Dyslexia is interesting for falling between the categories of being an educational problem and a medical disorder. As more students and trainee doctors disclose it, it will be increasingly recognized as something individuals need help for, as it is the most common specific learning difficulty, affecting about 6% of the general UK population. It is thought to affect 2% of UK medical students. It requires reasonable adjustments by the employer, but as Newlands et al. (2014) find, it can affect all forms of communication, time management and anxiety.

Less has been written on neurodevelopmental disorders such as attention deficit hyperactivity disorder (ADHD) and autism spectrum disorder (ASD), which are almost certainly under-recognized and often present as disorganization or professionalism difficulties during postgraduate training; or could be the underlying reason for alcohol or drug use. Occasionally, these disorders only become recognized by the trainee during clinical attachments such as child psychiatry. At the time of going to press a national group within HEE has convened to consider the needs of these trainees further.

The Wider Training Environment

Burnout

Although attributed to the psychologist Freudenberger in the 1970s, the editorial by Samra (2018) draws our attention to the fact that this was a phenomenon originally recognized in aviation. US air traffic controllers apparently described feeling exhaustion, with a decline in the quality and quantity of their work, in a context of increasing automation, poor training environments, fatigue and inadequate equipment, among other variables. Links with increased complexity were more salient than emotional demands. Samra concludes: 'Medical workloads need to be reconfigured or redesigned in line with human cognitive, emotional, and physical limitations, with accompanying organisation-wide training and management support' (Samra 2018: p. 2).

Burnout then, an occupational phenomenon according to Montgomery et al. (2019), should not be seen as an individual problem but rather a systemic one. These authors consider that 'the current focus on narrow definitions of burnout as a medical diagnosis and inadequate measurement approaches have hampered progress' (Montgomery et al. 2019: p. 1). And of course they are right, as burnout has not been classed as a psychiatric or medical diagnosis, but rather an occupational condition in eleventh revision of the International Classification of Diseases (ICD 11). For Garada (2020), burnout was a state of physical, emotional and mental and exhaustion caused by a long-term involvement in demanding situations. Not the same as but linked to depression (with an overlap of hopelessness, poor self-esteem and sleep disturbance) she considers it very prevalent and possibly less stigmatizing – calling oneself burnt out may be seen as more acceptable than being described as depressed.

Differential Attainment

This is the term used to describe variations in attainment in average group performance between different groups of doctors. For the purpose of this chapter, we are referring to differentials connected to ethnicity. Doctors who have completed their primary medical qualification overseas are known as international medical graduates and, unfortunately, although their specific needs have been known about for a long time, they still find many obstacles to smooth training in the UK. Doctors who are from ethnic minority groups who trained in the UK (therefore not international medical graduates) are also discussed within this section.

International Medical Graduates

Humphrey et al. (2011) found that inquiries to the GMC concerning doctors qualified outside the UK are more likely to be associated with higher impact decisions at each stage of the fitness to practice process (Humphrey et al. 2011). Why might this be? In the accompanying editorial (Nunez-Smith 2011) the reasons for this are explored and they might include: foreign doctors being viewed as less competent or trustworthy than native doctors by patients; racial and ethnic discrimination; a workplace climate that is hostile and could influence performance; work in specialties that are more likely to be in shortage or in less prestigious areas. These doctors are under-represented in treatment services and over-represented in disciplinary processes (Garada 2021).

It should be pointed out that the GMC have reviewed their fitness to practice practices since then and provided guidance in this area (GMC 2016).

As well as struggling with the demands of moving country and isolation these doctors may face multiple hurdles in language tests, complex visa and registration requirements and financial insecurity. A number of doctors are sending home regular amounts of money to support family in their country of origin. It is much more likely that they are seen as not fitting in or as having inferior qualifications in some way to the established group of senior staff. Discrimination from patients is also understood to be common (see Box 22.1).

Doctors from Ethnic Minorities

However, the findings of Woolf's rigorous meta-analysis study in the same year (Woolf et al. 2011) showed that it was not only international medical graduates who struggled: the ethnic

---

Box 22.1 Case example 1

Zinha referred himself to the professional support team of the deanery. He was an international medical graduate and had been placed in a remote and rural part of the UK in a very different environment to that he was used to in South Asia. He had trouble passing the core training exam in spite of four attempts and sought help at this stage as he had only one remaining chance left.

All of his family except his spouse were abroad; he was helping his own parents financially; and his wife was sick with a second pregnancy. He did not know where to turn or who was going to look after his child.

He was not dyslexic on screening and was given some coaching on exam preparation, a written study guide and general advice about sick leave and carer leave. At follow-up, things were much improved.

After some exam coaching he managed to pass the exam; his wife was better and he was very thankful for the support. 'It is a great relief to know that you care for the trainees', he said.

---

origin of *UK-trained* doctors and medical students was related to their academic performance in both undergraduate and graduate medicine too; and, moreover, this occurred even when tests were written and marked by machine. This was compelling evidence that makes for uncomfortable reading. The outcomes (assessments; exam results; annual progression) for black and minority ethnic doctors differ at all levels from those for white British doctors and show that this is a problem that needs to be acknowledged and tackled.

This effect is now well recognized by the Medical Royal Colleges and GMC. In its 2020 report (GMC 2020), the GMC has made a number of recommendations; on a local level, interventions such as getting to know trainees, providing senior mentoring support and promoting positive relationships; facilitating mixed peer support; addressing biases in recruitment; undertaking learning needs analyses; speaking out about discrimination and racism are all important.

Crucial to the wider training environment for all trainees are matters concerning the higher-level structures of training (at deanery level) and those concerning the immediate environment of the trainee in the clinical environment (supervision).

What Can Help?

Trainers as line managers have a powerful influence: saying thank you can be important. A compassionate conversation, sharing experiences with others and timely access to help are also good ideas. It may be helpful for trainers to be aware of the several useful policy documents about support and wellbeing mentioned earlier, which can be used to make the case for resources in individual NHS trusts.

The Deanery

In England now, HEE has taken over the tasks previously assigned to the postgraduate deaneries and has its own structure of organization and hierarchy of senior staff who manage the process of postgraduate medical and dental education. For example, training programme directors (TPDs) are accountable to the head of school for each specialty, and both are HEE (deanery) appointments, and so accountable in turn to the postgraduate dean. In the NHS trusts, educational supervisors and directors of medical education (DMEs), who are usually consultants appointed to NHS boards, are NHS appointments. In addition, college tutors are the Royal College representative in NHS trusts and these individuals uphold standards in education.

As can be imagined, the complexity of this network brings problems of responsibility and questions of who needs to act when a trainee presents with difficulties. Some of the presenting problems of trainees in difficulty are illustrated in Figure 22.1: a breakdown, according to problem area, of more than 200 cases of trainees open at a given time to one professional support unit of an English deanery region.

On a simple level, a number of problems can be managed with basic advice. For example, failure to pass examinations, or lack of confidence, could be helped with interventions such as the provision of study skills advice, screening for dyslexia, counselling, mentoring or coaching and/or careers advice. These can provide helpful strategies for trainees of any specialty. Very often, such advice is available at deanery level through a professional support unit (PSU) or professional support and wellbeing (PSW) team (see Boxes 22.2 to 22.4). In England, all 10 regions of HEE have such a unit, running along somewhat different lines, in that some employ non-medical coaches; some, medical associate deans; and others have mixed models). The Scottish and Welsh deaneries have similar arrangements. Details can be found at on the HEE website (HEE 2022a).

It is often helpful if a trainee can obtain support from individuals who are outside their usual working environment. Deaneries will often have expert panel meetings so that complex trainees can be discussed and best practice followed, and links established to GMC liaison officers for trainees who have been referred to the regulator.

Helping a Trainee in Difficulty

The following are important to consider when helping a trainee in difficulty:

- early identification;
- keeping an open mind, establishing the facts and circumstances as objectively as possible;

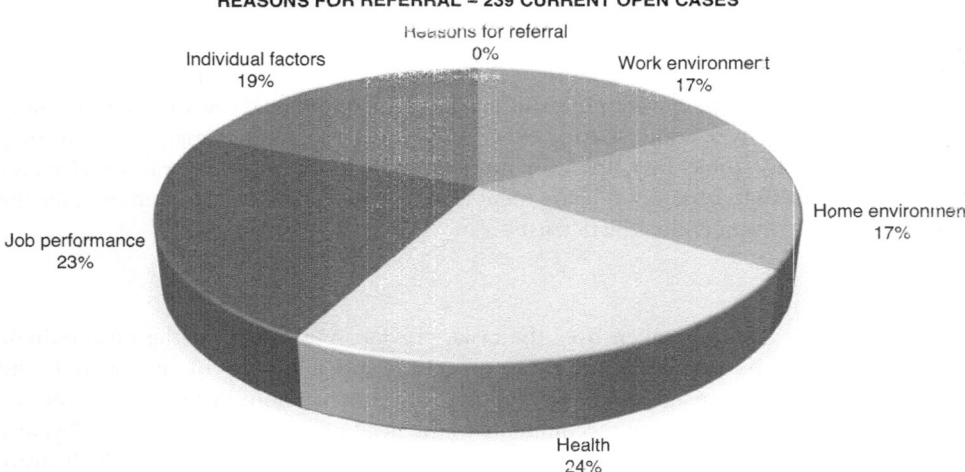

REASONS FOR REFERRAL – 239 CURRENT OPEN CASES

Reasons for referral

Individual factors 19%

0%

Work environment 17%

Home environment 17%

Job performance 23%

Health 24%

Fig. 22.1 Reasons for trainee referral to a professional support unit for help in 2020, from 239 open cases.

Box 22.2 WARD: a trainee-doctor-led initiative

WARD (Well and Resilient Doctors) is a trainee-doctor-led initiative that was established by trainees in the Severn Deanery in the southwest of England. The aim is to provide peer support, sign-posting and education on wellbeing and support for fellow trainee doctors. It is a complimentary support initiative that runs alongside and works together with the systems that are already set up by local and deanery-wide support teams. It is run by trainee doctors for trainee doctors on a voluntary basis and has some funding from the Deanery. It has set up its own website: www.welldoctors.org.

The benefits of the WARD project are numerous for those seeking confidential peer support which becomes continuous throughout the Deanery (as each hospital has a team). It is also beneficial for the doctors involved in running the WARD team as they are engaging in meaningful wellbeing work, being trained in coaching and mentorship and taking part in related quality-improvement projects.

Box 22.3 Case example 2

After some taster days in three specialties Sophia, who was unhappy in her anaesthetics post, applied for a trust grade role in psychiatry in spite of having no previous experience. She moved to Doncaster and is learning on the job but said the team was wonderful, the work environment good and she was happy with the risk she took. In thanking the PSW team for its help, she said 'being able to get some guidance and advice from someone with a clear and objective take on her situation was really helpful and encouraging'.

Box 22.4 Case example 3

After four attempts at her part one exam, Odessa, whose first language was not English, referred herself for advice as she was developing exam anxiety. After a session of understanding her problems and then going through study skills, developing a realistic revision table, emphasizing active recall and professionalizing her learning, she was referred for some coaching sessions. This helped her manage her anxiety and she passed her exam at the next attempt.

- drawing on multiple sources if relevant;
- confidentiality: be wary of inappropriate corridor conversations, emails etc.;
- documentation of the process is crucial;
- solutions will be individual;
- patient safety must be the prime concern; and
- also consider safety of the trainee.

The Supervisor

It is beyond the scope of this chapter to describe all the processes essential to good supervision and the reader is referred to Chapter 14 by Cottrell in this volume. Among these processes are of course induction and a learning agreement, which needs to cover how feedback is given and what needs to happen if things go wrong, including the need for documentation. The agreement also needs to cover who the trainee can approach if they don't get on with the supervisor; and trainers need to be able to recognize a trainee in difficulty and know what to do.

The last five years have led to a professionalization of supervision and a recognition of its fundamental importance in supporting the trainee in difficulty. Chief among the developments is the GMC accreditation process (GMC 2012), which means that doctors are formally recognized on the GMC register as having met certain standards in becoming a clinical or educational supervisor. For England, the HEE framework and its document *Enhancing Supervision for Postgraduate Doctors in Training* (HEE 2019b) describes four types of supervision:

(1) the educational supervisor who is consistent throughout the year;
(2) the named clinical supervisor;
(3) the workplace supervisor who can be anyone in the multi-professional team; and
(4) the clinical supervisor who is the person with overall clinical responsibility for a particular shift.

Managing Coaching Conversations

As outlined the next chapter, the basic skills of having coaching conversations include attentive and reflective listening. These can all be considered advanced communication skills common to both coaching and mentoring and are also skills which psychiatrists have in abundance.

Questioning is a key skill that many psychiatrists have great ability in, and some useful questions are:

• What advice would you give to a friend in your situation?
• What would be most interesting to talk about first?
• What will success look like?

Chapter 23 also describes the GROW model:

• Goal: the proposed outcome of your meeting;
• Reality: an exploration of what is happening right now;
• Options: what is currently under consideration; and
• Will: a sense of motivation to proceed.

There is now work on the importance of coaching and mentoring interventions in the support of marginalized groups such as international medical graduates in the context of differential attainment. Indeed, a useful toolkit is now available on the website of the London and South East Deanery devised by Mendel and MacDonald-Davis (2019) to help trainers train faculty in supporting and supervising trainees from diverse cultural backgrounds using coaching and mentoring approaches. One link to this toolkit can be found on the HEE website (HEE 2022b).

Managing Difficult Conversations

Courses for supervisors can be helpful in reminding or equipping trainers with strategies or structured approaches to this issue. A *stepped approach* is often useful, with time allocated to *preparation*; careful attention to *listening*; and remaining *calm and professional*. It is often helpful to recognize that *avoidance of difficult conversations is often based on fears* about their wellbeing, their reactions, your reputation and your relationship. Some rehearsal with a colleague is often helpful, undertaken as a visualization exercise.

One helpful question when preparing for the conversation is to think through, from your perspective, how you would like your manager to handle the conversation if they needed to speak with you. What skills or qualities would they need to demonstrate to get the best response from you?

Another very helpful tool is to differentiate *facts*, *feedback* and *opinion*. A sickness absence record of 7 days in a month is a fact; the observation of a trainee managing an angry patient is feedback; and someone talking about a trainee having a drink problem is an opinion.

A suggested structure might be:

- Clarify the purpose: 'The reason I wanted to talk with you today is . . . '
- Create a positive context by expressing appreciation of the person and highlight the end goal of your conversation for the other person.
- Clarify the ideal and current position. Be concise, constructive and non-accusatory in tone. Emphasize facts and feedback, and avoid opinions that might inflame the situation.
- Allow the other person to express his/her perceptions: 'Tell me your thoughts about what is happening . . . '. Use open questions, listen and remain receptive
- Move into a problem-solving mode: 'So how do we best move things forward from here?' Ensure the conversation stays focused on the stated purpose/desired outcome
- Clarify your contribution: how you will contribute to success and agree the forms your support will take.
- Summarize, check and close, reflecting again on the agreed plan, the timelines and nature of you support.

Managing Performance

Much of this chapter so far has been centrally concerned with trainees under stress or some kind of crisis at work beyond their control. However, occasionally trainees may present with attitudinal problems, which are more difficult to deal with (see Box 22.5). A difficult trainee from this perspective may:

- display a lack of responsibility for their own learning;
- attract patient complaints early in their attachment;
- demonstrate improved performance only near target times (before ARCP panel) but this is never sustained; or
- have little insight into their poor performance, often blaming others or circumstances for their failure.

Box 22.5 Case example 4

Hatep was a foundation doctor, whose not very well-off family had made great sacrifices for him to attend an international medical school. In his first year of medical training he was found to relay incorrect information about patients at ward rounds, did not respond to attempts to contact him in a timely way. He was not maintaining his portfolio and said that his first job was so relaxed he did not think he needed to try very hard when it came to the second. He also indicated that he could not talk to his family about his problems.

Box 22.6 What do people need from performance management? Adapted from Lewis (2012)

- Acknowledgement that their concerns are valid (if they are)
- A sense that they are being listened to and their fears heard
- A clear rationale and evidence for action
- A clear personal route to improvement and behaviour change
- A clear sense that you want them to succeed with the change
- Practical means of support

Motivation to do medicine and family pressure may be key here: and careers advice and/or coaching in order to help the trainee realize their situation, and that a change of career is needed, may be the preferable route.

Courses exist for supervisors on this topic and it is useful to appreciate the boundary between training matters and employment matters. There is a continuum of process from the least to the most formal, and consistency of approach is desirable. Evidence is also crucial at each step and it is important to keep notes from the beginning of any supervisory encounter. The context of performance management, as with other matters in training, needs to be established with good induction and a learning agreement or contract so that it is clear how feedback will be given.

How such feedback is given is a key issue in performance management and identification of the three (say) most important aspects of behaviour that need to be modified is usually a much better idea than a long list of things that need correction, as this can be demotivating, overwhelming for a trainee who is struggling and can lead to grievances being lodged. If there are concerns about the trainee doing their job, there exists a *capability framework* so that performance can be managed within this scheme.

All employing organizations will have a capability policy and procedure, and it is important to work alongside medical staffing colleagues if this framework is used.

There are only five reasons for dismissing an employee: conduct, capability, redundancy, statutory limitation or 'some other substantial reason'. The two main reasons for dismissing an individual on the grounds of capability are health and performance/competence. Objective setting using SMART (specific, measureable, achievable, realistic, time limited) criteria can be helpful and reviewing these regularly to ensure objectives are being met is useful. Early recognition and management of underperformance using the 'managing difficult conversations paradigm' can be helpful (see above).

A summary of the key factors that trainees need from performance management is given in Box 22.6.

Investigating Concerns: Understanding the Regulatory Environment

It is not the aim of this chapter to describe in detail the operations of the GMC. However, it is important that some basics are covered within the context of the trainee in difficulty. Colleagues can refer to Garada (2021), who describes in three chapters the different stages of the investigatory process of how a complaint is formally handled; suspension and erasure; and how to make the best of situations when things go wrong.

According to Wakeford (2011) the main reason for disciplinary action when the GMC was founded more than a century ago was adultery. In a much later study that he undertook (up to 2011), among the findings were:

- men were four times as likely to be erased as women;
- hospital specialists were erased or suspended at half the rate of general practitioners;
- doctors were more likely to be erased or suspended later in life; and
- non-UK graduates were more than twice as likely to be erased or suspended than those with UK qualifications.

Owing to 28 doctors taking their own lives between 2005 and 2013 whilst undergoing investigation, and the resulting review by Louis Appleby, the number of full investigations was reduced in 2016 and where mental health was a feature of the case, early treatment was recommended instead of investigation wherever possible. (Editorial BMJ 2016)

The GMC referral process is very briefly defined in the report *Fitness to Practise Statistics 2019* (GMC 2019), from initial enquiry, through triage, provisional enquiry, case examiners review, action by assistant registrars (if necessary), the hearing by an investigation committee, an interim orders tribunal and, finally, the medical practitioners' tribunal, which hears the most serious cases.

It is important to note, however, that most complaints to the GMC do not pass through the initial triage process; and less than 2% of doctors who have a case opened with the GMC end in a serious sanction such as erasure or conditions. The two important variables here are the nature of the complaint and the level of engagement of the doctor.

It is also important for trainees and trainers to know that although criminal sanctions against doctors are rare, more than 50% of crimes are due to vehicle offences; and it is likely that many of these are related to drink and drugs. Less often, offences involve forgery, fraud, sexual offences.

Of complaints made against doctors, transgressions often feature involving prescribing for friends or family, inappropriate prescribing (for example of controlled drugs) or dishonesty at work. These might include dishonesty about having undertaken training (when they have not); dishonesty about references or lying about a curriculum vitae; dishonesty in claiming sick pay or submitting time sheets; boundary violations involving the pursuit of sexual or improper emotional relationships and failure to disclose drink driving offences.

The main instances in which a concern should be investigated are summarized in Box 22.7.

Box 22.7 When to investigate a concern (from GMC 2021)

- Misconduct (for example breaches of confidentiality, discrimination, fraud or dishonesty)
- Poor performance (for example serious repeated mistakes of medical treatment)
- A criminal conviction or caution (for example sexual assault, driving offences)
- Physical or mental ill-health that may impact the doctor's ability to practise medicine
- A determination by another regulatory body
- Insufficient knowledge of English

Conclusion

In the last decade, there have been trends to broaden participation in medical training from diverse groups through widening access schemes. The hope is that this more diverse student body will become the trainee doctors in the next few years, whether they are from non professional socio-economic classes or from culturally or ethnically diverse groups. This reflects the recognition that the clinical working and training environment needed to change to be more welcoming and supportive to everyone in the course of their training.

As can be seen from the reports outlined at the start of this chapter, developing resilience is only a small part of the solution. 'No amount of training, yoga, deep breathing or reflection can compensate for a dangerous and flawed system' (Garada 2021: p. 51). An emphasis on acquiring resilience has unfortunately tended to locate system-wide problems in individuals.

This is not to dismiss the need for resilience entirely. In a probably not very well-known work (Cyrulnik 2009) considers the key components of this are the ability to dream and the ability to intellectualize. Those with resilience are able to knit together a feeling of selfhood; an ability to retreat into the inner world when necessary; an ability to conceptualize; and the use of certain defence mechanisms such as sublimation (channelling energy into artistic, intellectual or ethical activities); emotional self control; altruism; and humour. Others would add (e.g., Howe et al. 2012) the ability to engage with help, learning from difficulties and persistence in spite of blocks to progress. Instead of becoming anxious or denying the problem the resilient person uses coping strategies and problem solving to reframe the event.

What does this mean for training schemes and are we selecting the right people to do the work? Fostering *professional resilience* is clearly a good idea and enables a range of training approaches to be taken such as graded exposure to uncertainty; stretching assignments with coaching; use of positive role models; unobtrusive monitoring of wellbeing; and so on. The development of leadership and other professional skills as suggested in the GMC framework will help.

Does this influence the advice we may give to our students or trainees?

Sir Robert Hutchinson (1871–1960) is understood to have given an address to graduating doctors in 1938 at the London Hospital Medical College whilst bestowing them with seven gifts: good health, luckiness, brains, equanimity, a sense of justice, a sense of beauty and a sense of humour (Hutchinson 1938). Kelly and Feeney have elaborated on this in their paper *What every psychiatrist should know* about these principles (Kelly and Feeney 2006), emphasizing the enduring quality of the advice he gave and the importance of a sense of humour in managing the complex demands of medical life.

We should all be wary of thinking that we need to know everything; and mindful that uncertainty and the imposter syndrome (or having fear and doubt) are normal. What is fundamental is the importance of education and learning.

References

BMJ Editorial (2016) GMC adopts more lenient approach. *BMJ*, 353: i2071.

Carrieri D, Pearson M, Mattick K, et al. (2020) Interventions to minimise doctors' mental ill-health and its impacts on the workforce and patient care: the Care Under Pressure realist review. *Health and Social Care Delivery Research* 8: 19.

Cyrulnik B (2009) *Resilience: How Your Inner Strength Can Set You Free from the Past* (translated by David Macey). Penguin Books

Garada C (2020) Understanding burnout. *BMJ*, **369**: m1595; doi: https://doi.org/10.1136/bmj.m1595.

Garada C (2021) *Beneath the White Coat: Doctors, Their Minds and Mental Health.* Routledge.

GMC (2012) Recognising and approving trainers: the implementation plan. Available at: www.gmc-uk.org/-/media/documents/approving-trainers-implementation-plan-aug-12-v2_pdf-66144233.pdf.

GMC (2016) Professional behaviour and fitness to practice. Available at: www.gmc-uk.org/education/standards-guidance-and-curricula/guidance/student-professionalism-and-ftp/professional-behaviour-and-fitness-to-practise.

GMC (2019) Fitness to practise statistics 2019. Available at: www.gmc-uk.org/-/media/documents/fitness-to-practise-statistics-report-2019_pdf-84848269.pdf.

GMC (2020) How to support successful training for black and minority ethnic doctors: actions and case studies for medical Royal Colleges and faculties. Available at: www.gmc-uk.org/-/media/documents/How_to_support_successful_training_for_BME_doctors_20201127.pdf_84687265.pdf.

GMC (2021) Deciding to investigate a concern. Available at: www.gmc-uk.org/concerns/information-for-doctors-under-investigation/how-we-investigate-concerns/deciding-to-investigate-a-complaint-or-concern.

Harden RM, Crosby J (2000) AMEE Guide No 20: The good teacher is more than a lecturer – the twelve roles of the teacher. *Medical Teacher*, **22**: 334–47.

HEE (2019a) NHS Staff and Learners' Mental Wellbeing Commission. Available at: www.hee.nhs.uk/sites/default/files/documents/NHS%20%28HEE%29%20-%20Mental%20Wellbeing%20Commission%20Report.pdf.

HEE (2019b) *Enhancing Supervision for Postgraduate Doctors in Training.* Health Education England. Available at: www.hee.nhs.uk/sites/default/files/documents/SupervisionReport_%20FINAL1.pdf.

HEE (2022a) Professional support for postgraduate medical and dental trainees. Available at: www.hee.nhs.uk/our-work/professional-support-postgraduate-medical-dental-trainees.

HEE (2022b) Differential attainment toolkit. Available at: https://london.hee.nhs.uk/professional-development/differential-attainment/differential-attainment-toolkit (accessed July 2022).

Howe, A. Smajdor A, Stöckl A (2012) Towards an understanding of resilience and its relevance to medical training. *Medical Education*, **46**: 349–56.

Humphrey C, Hickman S, Gulliford MC (2011) Place of medical qualification and outcomes of UK General Medical Council 'fitness to practice' process: cohort study. *BMJ*, **342**: d1817.

Hutchinson R (1938) Seven gifts. *Lancet*, **ii**, 61–2.

Kelly B, Feeney L (2006) What every psychiatrist should know. *Advances in Psychiatric Treatment*, **12**: 462–8.

Lewis C (2012) *Performance Management.* Globis Mediation Group.

Mendel D, MacDonald-Davis J (2019) Differential attainment toolkit. Available at: https://london.hee.nhs.uk/multiprofessional-faculty-development/differential-attainment.

Montgomery A, Panagopoulou E, Esmail A, Richards T, Maslach C (2019) Burnout in healthcare: the case for organisational change. *BMJ*, **366**: l4774; doi: https://doi.org/10.1136/bmj.l4774.

Newlands F, Shrewsbury D, Robson J (2014) Foundation doctors and dyslexia: a qualitative study of their experience and coping strategies. *Postgraduate Medical Journal*, **91**: 121–6.

Nunez-Smith (2011) Migration of doctors and the 'fitness to practice' process. *BMJ*, **342**: 835–6.

Samra R (2018) Brief history of burnout. *BMJ*, **363**: k5268.

Wakeford R (2011) Who gets struck off? *BMJ*, **343**: 1325–7.

West M, Coia D (2019) *Caring for Doctors Caring for Patients: How to Transform UK Healthcare Environments to Support Doctors and Medical Students to Care for Patients.* General Medical Council.

Wolf K, Potts HWW, McManus IC (2011) Ethnicity and academic performance in UK trained doctors and medical students: systematic review and meta-analysis. *BMJ*, **342**: d901.

Chapter 23

Coaching and Mentoring: An Overview for Trainers in Psychiatry

Sarah Huline-Dickens

Introduction

Atul Gawande, a surgeon and professor of public health, delivered a TED talk in April 2017 called 'Want to get great at something? Get a coach' (Gawande 2017). He begins his talk by describing an innovation in coaching by training nurses to observe other nurses acting as birth attendants in rural India. The way the local birth attendants were handling infected material was leading to significant mortality. The coaching intervention completely reversed this trend and the approach of the coaches was found to be just right in facilitating change rather than imposing change from outside. This was transformative in delivering better care.

What has this got to do with the professional development of psychiatrists? The connection is, of course, coaching (or mentoring), but it also symbolizes the way psychiatrists often naturally seek to influence beneficial change in indirect ways.

In the UK in 2003, Dean wrote a brief editorial for *Advances in Psychiatric Treatment* about the importance of having a mentor for newly appointed consultants (Dean 2003). This will be the main context of thinking about coaching and mentoring for many psychiatrists. In the sister journal *Psychiatric Bulletin*, Roberts et al. (2002) had written about mentoring for new consultants in order to mitigate against isolation and the erosion of professionalism; and later Dutta et al. (2010) wrote on how mentoring can have an important effect on personal development, career guidance and research productivity for female academics, who are not well represented in medicine or psychiatry.

Otherwise, very little has been published on the scope of coaching and mentoring within psychiatry in the UK. Coaching and mentoring are, however, approaches that are widely used in the private sector, such as in business (Whitmore 2017).

An English-language literature search between the years 2009 and 2019 using PsycINFO yielded about 30 papers, of which several are relevant to this chapter: and these reveal a much keener interest in the field in the USA and Australia. Teshima et al. (2019), for example, describe the consecutive challenges faced during the course of an academic career and how mentoring has a role at each stage to develop clinical and academic identity, leadership and changes in roles and power. Ahn and Ziedonis (2019) highlight the usefulness of coaches in supporting psychiatrists so that mentors can concentrate giving their guidance on content expertise. Szabo et al. (2019) describe a mentoring programme established in Australia to reduce stress and burnout among first-year trainees; and Rao et al. take the view in their paper that purposeful efforts are needed to 'recruit, mentor, and retain underrepresented students, residents, and faculty within the field of psychiatry to improve the quality of mental health care' (Rao et al. 2018: p. 143). The benefits of mentoring to psychiatric recruitment are extolled by Harper and Roman (2017); and finally Guerrero and Brenner (2016), in an editorial, emphasize how key mentorship is in ensuring creativity and innovation, in order to prepare the workforce in an ever-changing and demanding environment; to grow the workforce in research, education and administration; to diversify the workforce; and to retain it.

In spite of the apparent lack of UK writing on these topics, Viney and Harris (2013) have written on coaching and mentoring as a chapter in *Leadership in Psychiatry* (Bhugra et al. 2013), and there are useful guides published by NHS England (2014) and the London Leadership Academy (2014). The Royal College of Psychiatrists too has established a mentoring champion, with information on mentoring on its website (www .rcpsych.ac.uk/members/supporting-you/mentoring-and-coaching). This article is divided into two sections: the first section provides some background and definitions, describes basic skills, the features of emotional intelligence, the process of contracting, and some coaching questions and models including coaching supervision and evaluation; and the second section discusses organizational context and challenges to implementing change, and summarizes applications. It is hoped that this information will provide psychiatric trainers with an overview of the topic in order to plan their own professional development and to have coaching and mentoring conversations with trainees.

What Do We Mean by Coaching and Mentoring?

The context in which coaching and mentoring developed as a more individualized approach to organizational development in Britain arose in the 1990s. This coincided with an emphasis away from collective life to a more individualistic society. Sport has had a strong influence on the development of coaching and mentoring approaches and there has been an increasing interest in organizational psychology and employee motivation. One notable influence was the *Inner Game of Tennis* by Gallwey (1974), which was a very popular work cited by many opinion leaders in the coaching field, and it emphasized the role of enhancing concentration, confidence and will power. As described in Downey's book (Downey 2014), interference gets in the way between potential and performance, and this is usually rooted in fear and doubt. Another important milestone in the development of coaching and mentoring has been the publication of a number of books by Whitmore, who brought his experience of sporting success to bear on his formulation of the GROW (goal, reality, options, will) model, which he co-created and described in the first edition of *Coaching for Performance* (1992), which is now in its fifth edition (Whitmore 2017). This model is described below.

Coaching and mentoring can be seen to be on a spectrum, but it is useful to see how each of these words is separately defined. It is widely understood that in coaching coaches need not have first-hand experience of the coachee's line of work but in mentoring there is usually a pairing of a more skilled or experienced person with a less experienced person.

Coaching is 'the art of facilitating the performance, learning and development of another' (Downey 2014: p. 39). There are a number of definitions, but the generally accepted view is: that it is a non-directive form of development; that it focuses on improving performance and developing individual skills; that coaching activities have both organizational and individual goals; that it provides people with feedback on both strengths and weaknesses; and that, usually, it is for the short term.

It should be pointed out here that the lack of a precise definition of coaching is a source of confusion, and it is accepted that there is a degree of overlap between coaching and mentoring (see below).

The focus of the coach is therefore to facilitate learning and development through the conversation with the coachee. The role of the coach is to be an equal and not to give advice and the coach will not be a subject specialist. The process of coaching will often be a focus on a short-term goal or goals. The coach is an independent individual, separate from the organization. Within coaching different categories are described, such as business coaching, life coaching and executive coaching.

Mentoring is 'sharing expertise and some guidance' (Whitmore 2017: p. 249). It involves a more experienced person using their greater knowledge and understanding of the work, or of the workplace, to support the development of a less experienced employee. The term mentor appears to derive from a work in the seventeenth century that drew attention to the role of Mentor in the play *Odysseus* by Homer. Mentor is an older friend of Odysseus, who acted in a way that demonstrated wisdom and guidance.

Mentoring involves the long-term development of an individual. It is an essentially supportive form of development; it focuses on helping an individual manage their career and improve their skills; enables them to discuss some personal problems; and can have both organizational and individual goals.

The focus of the mentor is the growth and longer-term development of the mentee, who is often less experienced than the mentor. This contrasts with the focus of the coach, which is facilitating learning and development through the conversation with the coachee, and which may not concern longer-term development.

The role of the mentor may include the giving of advice and the mentor will often be more experienced in the subject than the mentee (in contrast to the role of the coach, who has a more equal relationship with the coachee, will not give advice and is not a subject specialist).

The mentor is often an individual who is part of the organization that employs the mentee. This contrasts with the coach, who, as mentioned above, is an independent individual, separate from the organization.

These differences are summarized in Table 23.1.

In the *Coaching and Mentoring Handbook* (London Leadership Academy 2014), coaching and mentoring are described as ways of giving people time to think, and they are essentially both helping activities. They are not the same as training, although training may involve both or either of them. Neither are they the same as appraisal, educational supervision, teaching, counselling or therapy. The basic skills, the development of the relationships and the basic helping styles are common to both coaching and mentoring, and these will be dealt with consecutively below, after considering the coaching spectrum.

As pointed out in many texts there is a coaching spectrum, attributed to Downey (2003), represented by a sliding scale of interventions, from helping a person find their own solutions in coaching to offering guidance in mentoring.

According to Clutterbuck (2014), the ideal characteristics of a good mentor describe someone who:

- already has a good record for developing other people;
- has a genuine interest in seeing younger people advance and can relate to their problems;
- has a wide range of current skills to pass on;

Table 23.1 Differences between mentoring and coaching

Mentoring	Coaching
On-going relationship that might last for a long time	Relationship generally has a set duration
Can be more informal and meetings can take place as and when the mentee needs advice, guidance or support	Generally more structured in nature and meetings are scheduled regularly
The mentor will share ideas and what they have done	The coach will help the coachee to identify their own solutions
More long term and takes a broader view of the mentee	Short term and focused on specific development areas/problems
The mentor is usually more experienced and qualified than the mentee, and is often a senior person in the organization, who can pass on knowledge, experience and can open doors to otherwise out-of-reach opportunities	Coaching is a more equal relationship and generally not determined by the level of experience the coach has of the coachee's formal occupational role – rather, this professional distance can help to provide a thinking partnership with a different level of challenge and support

Source: London Leadership Academy (2014).

- has a good understanding of the organization, how it works and where it is going;
- can combine patience with good interpersonal skills and an ability to work in an unstructured programme;
- has sufficient time to devote to a relationship;
- can command a mentee's respect;
- has their own network of contacts and influence; and
- is still keen to learn.

Basic Skills

Basic skills include active listening, listening orientation, the technique of reflection and using reflective listening. These can all be considered advanced communication skills common to both coaching and mentoring and are also skills that psychiatrists should have in abundance.

These basic skills and qualities of communication are also reflected in the coaching and mentoring frameworks adhered to by organizations that train coaches. For example, the European Mentoring and Coaching Council (2020) describes a competence framework which is the result of extensive and collaborative research to identify the core competences of a professional coach and mentor. It lists eight competence categories across four levels. These eight core areas comprise:

- understanding self;
- commitment to self-development;
- managing the contract;

- building the relationship;
- enabling insight and learning;
- outcome and action orientation;
- use of models and techniques; and
- evaluation.

Starr (2008) gives more detail on the communication strategies required for being a skilled coach or mentor. These include building rapport, different levels of listening, using intuition, asking questions and giving supportive feedback. She also lists things that should not be done (Starr 2008: p. 324), such as talking too much, seeking to dominate the conversation, trying to solve problems for the coachee, assuming the coach's or mentor's experience is relevant and focusing on what not to do.

Emotional Intelligence

No discussion of coaching and mentoring should avoid mentioning emotional intelligence, even though for the psychiatrist this may be fairly obvious. The term emotional intelligence was first popularized in Goleman's book of the same name in 1995, which makes the point that high emotional intelligence was supposed to confer a significant performance advantage on leaders (Goleman 1995).

Emotional intelligence has become a term used (somewhat vaguely) to describe personal and social skills. However, a more helpful approach is provided by Whitmore (2017), who explains how the competencies of emotional intelligence can be grouped into four domains: self-awareness, self-management, awareness of others and relationship management. Starr (2008) prefers the term emotional maturity and uses this to describe our capacity to deal with our emotions.

Some useful definitions are provided in Box 23.1.

Contracting

Contracting is the process of making an agreement between coach and coachee (or mentor and mentee) on the basis of the relationship: the terms of engagement or ground rules. In any relationship, participants can make implicit assumptions about the purpose, the roles and the responsibilities of the other person involved. An explicit contract can set out the framework of the working relationship, can ensure that best use is made of the time available (that sessions do not degenerate into chat) and that the topics are covered that need to be covered.

Box 23.1 Some useful definitions in relation to emotional intelligence

- **Self-awareness:** The ability to understand and recognize our moods, emotions and drives
- **Self-management:** The ability to choose our responses and behaviour; how we handle change, stress and conflict
- **Awareness of others:** Our ability to understand others' emotional states: an ability closely linked to our ability to empathize
- **Relationship management:** The ability to manage meaningful relationships (communicate clearly, collaborate, negotiate, deal with conflict, motivate and manage others)

The three major functions of the contract therefore are that it:

- ensures alignment: establishing focus, agreement on results, understanding and adjustment to individual needs, clarity of roles and responsibilities and a common language;
- establishes procedures: the coaching methods employed, time frames, boundaries and ground rules and some measurement of progress; and
- models the partnership: serves as an orientation to the partnership and forms the basis for disclosure, enquiry and commitment to the success of the relationship.

The contract might cover the coach as a practitioner and also the process of the coaching. It might include style (usually asking questions), parameters (e.g., the content of the conversations and how they may not be on specialist areas), tools, confidentiality (with a caveat that some things may be challenged, or even shared with others if there were certain concerns; and whether or not there may be supervision with a supervisor), session times, follow-up and feedback (from the coachee to the coach).

Box 23.2 introduces a fictitious coach describing aspects of the coaching role, starting with contracting.

Although the process of contracting is a major consideration in any formal course on coaching and mentoring, within the trainer/trainee relationship this would normally be part of the usual learning or educational agreement established between the two parties at the start of the supervision relationship. Such a learning agreement should cover learning objectives and opportunities; how supervision should occur; a framework for giving feedback; and how strengths and weaknesses will be acknowledged.

Questions and Models

Questioning is a key skill that many psychiatrists have great ability in, but the skill of asking powerful questions can always be enhanced. A survey of useful questions that can be used

---

Box 23.2 Case example: contracting

I phoned the coachee as arranged and went over the practical arrangements about using a colleague's office and that we would aim to meet for four sessions in total (but that this could be reviewed).

We had already established by email that Thursday afternoons are best.

I said that I would bring a contract to the first meeting.

I checked that it would be alright with him to give him feedback as we went along.

I briefly mentioned that there were models that it might be helpful to use, and that I would be quite active in the sessions in reminding him of the goals he had set.

I explained that I would be making notes that I would share with him but that our sessions would of course be confidential except for the ordinary professional obligations that we all have concerning patient harm.

I would, however, be discussing some aspects of our sessions in supervision of my coaching and explained what this might look like.

Finally, I would be asking for feedback from him at the end.

He thought this was all rather formal but was happy to agree.

when mentoring and coaching is beyond the scope of this chapter but many examples are given in Whitmore (2017). He lists some of his favourites as:

- What advice would you give to a friend in your situation?
- What would be most interesting to talk about first?
- What will success look like?

Other questions that I have found useful include:

- What do you sense your colleague needs from you?
- What has been different about the way you have been working with your colleague?
- What would you do if you were in charge?
- What support do you need to do that?

Avoiding 'why?' questions, questions with multiple layers and leading questions is advised in many texts. Questions that are open and questions that encourage the individual to choose the next step and to think about what support they will need to take that step are often fruitful.

The models used in coaching and mentoring are useful for structuring these conversations. The GROW model, probably the best known, was originally published by Whitmore in 1992 and appears in his more recent titles (Whitmore 2017). The acronym stands for:

- **Goal**: the proposed outcome of your meeting;
- **Reality**: an exploration of what is happening right now;
- **Options**: what is currently under consideration; and
- **Will**: a sense of motivation to proceed.

The following are examples of questions that might be used when applying the GROW model, from Whitmore (2017):

Goal questions:

- What would you like to achieve in this conversation?
- If you had a magic wand, where would you like to be at the end of this?
- It sounds like you have two goals, which would you like to focus on first?

Reality questions:

- What is happening at the moment?
- What impact is this having on you?
- Who else is involved?

Options questions:

- What could you do?
- Who could help you with this?
- What else could work here?

Will questions:

- When precisely are you going to start?
- What will you do to make sure that happens?
- What is your commitment to taking that action, on a scale of 1–10?

Many of these questions will be familiar to psychiatrists from therapeutic work with patients, for example, using the magic wand (miracle) question in solution-focused therapy; scaling questions to monitor, say, levels of confidence; and posing questions to connect progress to tangible changes in behaviour or emotional management.

Considering other tools that might be used in coaching and mentoring, notwithstanding the lack of evidence, Starr (2008) highlights that personality profiling is used in coaching to increase the coach's understanding of an individual. One advantage this might have is that it allows the coachee to discuss themselves in a less self-conscious way. It might help the coach to understand what the coachee is good at, what they value and what they want to improve. Some useful objective material to work on in a coaching or mentoring relationship can be gleaned by means of 360-degree (or 360) feedback.

Coaching involves learning, and many tools have been developed to try to elicit learning styles or communication preferences. Although there is little evidence to support the questionnaire devised by Honey and Mumford (1982) as a valid instrument in assessing learning styles, a more recent system of learning preferences developed by Fleming in 1992 known as VARK, using the **V**isual (e.g., watching a video), **A**uditory (e.g., engaging in discussion), **R**eading/writing (e.g., making a written summary) and **K**inaesthetic (e.g., participating in role-play) methods of learning, has been proposed (see Fleming 2001). It is now thought, somewhat more realistically, that a learning approach is student and task specific, that is to say that an individual will adopt one approach for one task and a different one for another (Bandaranayake 2001).

Box 23.3 continues our case example with an extract from the coach's questioning of her coachee.

Coaching Supervision

The supervision in coaching and mentoring provides for continuous development of coaches and mentors. Supervision is typically provided by an experienced person and accreditation bodies require that coaches are supervised, rather as in other fields of therapy practice.

Box 23.3 Case example: some coaching questions

I began the session with an open question: How has your week been?

He said it had been difficult, especially as the Care Quality Commission had sprung a visit on the unit.

After he had said enough about this to satisfy himself, I asked how had he got on with the goals he set himself last time: in particular, chairing the team meeting with B present.
I reminded him that we had discussed this last time and he was anticipating some challenge from her.

He said that it had gone much better than he had expected. Although she did not like the plan, she appeared more thoughtful than she had been and seemed less angry.

I said that sounded encouraging. What had he done differently?

He said he had tried to talk to her in advance of the meeting and had also been speaking to her colleagues, who had told him that she was having some personal difficulty.

Rehearsing the conversation with a housemate had also helped.

I asked: 'And so what impact did this change have on you?'

He said it had made him realize that some planning had made quite a lot of difference to the meeting, and the rehearsing especially.

I asked whether that was a technique that could be useful in the future.

Who else would it be helpful to involve? So to summarize . . .

There are different models for coaching supervision, such as the double-matrix model by Hawkins and Shohet, first developed in 1989 (Hawkins and Shohet 2006). It has (rather unfortunately, in my view) become known subsequently by the term 'seven-eyed' by other writers in the field.

This model has seven domains or areas of focus:

- the coachee and how they present;
- the strategies and interventions used by the coach;
- the relationship between the coachee and the coach;
- the coach;
- the supervisory relationship;
- the supervisor's own process; and
- the wider organizational context.

The justification for such a model is that all aspects of the encounter that have relevance are considered. It also supports safe, ethical practice and accountability. This improves the quality of the work, can help transform the relationship with the coachee and provides a space for reflection. It allows the coach to become aware of their own responses to the coachee and to be able to question these and to avoid becoming ensnared by, shall we say, less than conscious material that could be problematical if not recognized. There is also a justification for this model on the grounds that it may prevent burnout and may encourage giving constructive feedback and support for ongoing professional development.

Clearly, however, one disadvantage is the cost in terms of time and resources needed.

In Box 23.4, our coach describes an interaction with her coaching supervisor.

Box 23.4 Case example: an interaction from coaching supervision

I presented to my supervisor an extract of another coaching session.

He said 'The goals as you describe them seem very broad. Is there any way of focusing one or two? Does one influence any of the others?'

I said 'Yes, it does seem difficult to pursue just one or two as the lists he sets himself are long. Maybe this is about his anxiety.'

He asked 'What do you need to do to help him focus on one at a time?'

I thought for a moment and said 'I think I will need to come back to this in the next session. The other problem I am finding is that he seems to expect me to tell him how to be a leader.'

He replied 'Well, of course that may be a reflection of the positive relationship you have developed. However, that is not your role, which is rather to facilitate understanding and facilitate change.'

I remembered 'He is thinking of doing a course in leadership as well.'

He said 'It is possible then that this course fulfils the other goals in helping him learn about leadership?'

I replied 'Yes – that's helpful. We can certainly discuss that.'

He summarized 'Well, it sounds as if it is going well. What do you think are the best ways of keeping him focused on the priorities?'

Evaluation

The kinds of methods and sources of data capture to evaluate coaching and mentoring include hard data, which might be easier to measure and quantify, can be more easily translated into resources, can give common measures of performance and can be more credible with management if a business case is needed. Soft data may be less credible as a performance measure, but often are more interesting on a human level. Evaluation could include:

- 360 feedback;
- surveys, interviews and structured questioning;
- observed performance;
- records of objectives or achievements;
- number of coaches or mentees seen; and
- feedback from other staff.

It is relevant to recognize that research on coaching and mentoring in all fields is still in its infancy, has many challenges and can be likened to complex health services research, in that there are many variables. Much of the research to date concerns case studies, but mixed-methods studies, drawing on triangulation between qualitative and quantitative methods, are likely to be most useful.

Indeed, Carter (2006) in her work *Practical Methods for Evaluating Coaching*, published by the Institute for Employment Studies, concludes that there should be more evaluation in order for coaching to gain credibility and that there has been a lack of neutrality and objectivity in evaluations generally.

At an individual level, evaluation could encapsulate any of the following:

- an improved sense of support;
- improvements of knowledge, skills and experience;
- innovations;
- enhanced performance (as measured by completed work, attendance, sickness absence, career progression);
- evidence of reflective practice (e.g., in reflective logs);
- developments in leadership expertise;
- enhanced networks;
- evidence of independence, autonomy and self-development;
- more effective prioritization;
- achieving balance between work and personal life; and
- an improved sense of connection with the workplace.

At an organizational level, an appealing and diagrammatic scheme can be found in O'Neill (2016).

Organizational Context

The UK's National Health Service (NHS) (and organizations related to it, such as Health Education England) are learning organizations and have been founded on principles of teaching and learning since their inception. Maintaining a culture in which learning is entwined with day-to-day work needs not only the involvement of everyone in the organization but also, crucially, the involvement of the executive team.

For coaching and mentoring to be established in organizations, there needs to be emphasis on support and continuous learning, so that the following can apply:

- coaching and mentoring are seen as essential skills at all levels and as a fundamental element of leadership;
- learning is a priority and supported by top management;
- people are encouraged to find ways of improving skills and knowledge alongside more general personal development;
- people are not afraid to ask for help;
- communication is open and information is shared freely;
- continuous improvement is emphasized;
- reflective practice is understood; and
- learning experiences are widely available.

The context of the coaching and mentoring and the relationships between the coach/mentor and the coachee/mentee will clearly be influenced by these wider considerations.

Organizational Challenges for Doctors Undertaking Coaching and Mentoring

There are challenges in establishing coaching and mentoring in organizations such as the NHS. Some of these are structural and some ideational. Hawkins (2012) has described the creation of a coaching culture and some of the barriers to this.

The first perhaps is the organizational support and the resources – financial and meeting space, for example – that are needed. The second challenge is the consultant job plan. To include time for being a mentor or coach within an already full clinical timetable, including other already existing training responsibilities, would be a challenge in many clinical services. And this relates the third point, which concerns roles. According to Clutterbuck (2014), failure to distinguish between the roles of line manager and mentor can lead to confusion and even conflict. This is especially so when a line manager undertakes appraisals as well.

Finally, in the chapter entitled 'Problems of Mentoring Programmes and Relationships' (Clutterbuck 2014: pp. 109–118), there is a description of personal and organizational factors that can go wrong in mentorship programmes, such as lack of clarity about role, too little or too much formality, power alignments, being mentored by one's line manager, failure to establish rapport in the relationship, perpetuation of narrow ways of thinking, differences in maturity and difficulties that can arise with mixed-sex mentoring relationships. This is why coaching (and mentoring) supervision can be important.

Opportunities for More Coaching and Mentoring

As the pressure on services grows, so the pressure on doctors and other NHS colleagues grows too. Fortunately, the calls to support staff are growing louder, and in the past year alone there have been several major documents from the General Medical Council (GMC) and Health Education England about doctors' (and other health service colleagues') well-being. The NHS Staff and Learners' Mental Wellbeing Commission (Health Education England 2019) has recommended an NHS Workforce Wellbeing Guardian, a board-level role, in every NHS organization; and the GMC document *Caring for Doctors Caring for*

Patients (West and Coia 2019) was based on a review co-chaired by a psychiatrist. There are eight references to coaching within it and nine references to mentoring, with a call to action that the culture of the NHS must change and for the leadership to become more compassionate. There is now work on the importance of coaching and mentoring interventions in the support of marginalized groups such as women in academic roles or international medical graduates in the context of differential attainment (a concept written about extensively by Woolf et al. (2011)). Indeed, a useful toolkit is now available on the website of Health Education England's London and South East Deanery devised by Mendel and MacDonald-Davis (2019) to help trainers train faculty in supporting and supervising trainees from diverse cultural backgrounds using coaching and mentoring approaches. Coaching and mentoring have important roles to play not only in mitigating against the risks of burnout, but also in offering support and professional development opportunities to doctors who wish to enter leadership roles and for those who may otherwise need additional support.

Conclusion

Although there are obstacles in current clinical practice to undertaking coaching and mentoring, there are persuasive arguments for the use of both types of support beyond the well-recognized application of mentoring for the newly appointed consultant. Coaching and mentoring can be useful at other times of role change in professional life when leadership skills need developing, but a wider availability of coaching and mentoring might also contribute to the retention of senior workforce and to the reduction of workplace exhaustion. It could contribute to the greater attractiveness of psychiatry in improving a sense of personal development, engagement and a sense of belonging.

Coaching and mentoring conversations with trainees can facilitate learning and be used to give meaningful feedback. As clinical and educational supervisors are increasingly being called on to support trainees from international backgrounds and to mitigate the effects of differential attainment, it is perhaps time to consider the adoption of these approaches more widely in psychiatric training culture and time for coaching and mentoring to become professionalized in psychiatry.

References

Ahn M, Ziedonis D (2019) Coaching health care leaders and teams in psychiatry. *Psychiatric Clinics of North America*, **42**: 401–12.

Bandaranayake R (2001) Study skills. In Dent J, Harden R (eds.), *A Practical Guide for Medical Teachers*. Churchill Livingstone, ch. 37.

Bhugra D, Ruiz P, Gupta S, et al. (2013) *Leadership in Psychiatry*. John Wiley & Sons, Inc.

Carter A (2006) *Practical Methods for Evaluating Coaching* (IES Report 430). Institute for Employment Studies.

Clutterbuck D (2014) *Everyone Needs a Mentor*. Kogan Page.

Dean A (2003) Mentors for newly appointed consultants. *Advances in Psychiatric Treatment*, **9**: 164–5.

Downey M (2003) *Effective Coaching: Lessons from the Coach's Coach*. Texere Publishing.

Downey M (2014) *Effective Modern Coaching: The Principles and Art of Modern Business Coaching*. LID Publishing.

Dutta R, Hawkes SL, Iversen AC, et al. (2010) Women in academic psychiatry. *Psychiatrist*, **34**: 313–17.

European Mentoring and Coaching Council (2020) Competence framework. Available at:

https://emccuk.org/Public/Accreditation/Competence_Framework.aspx.

Fleming N (2001) VARK: a guide to learning styles. Available at: https://vark-learn.com.

Gallwey WT (1974) *Inner Game of Tennis: The Ultimate Guide to the Mental Side of Peak Performance*. Random House.

Gawande A (2017) Want to get great at something? Get a coach. Available at: www.ted.com/talks/atul_gawande_want_to_get_great_at_something_get_a_coach.

Goleman D (1995) *Emotional Intelligence*. Bantam Books.

Guerrero A, Brenner A (2016) Mentorship: a return to basics. *Academic Psychiatry*, **40**: 422–3.

Harper BL, Roman BJB (2017) The changing landscape of recruitment in psychiatry. *Academic Psychiatry*, **41**: 221–5.

Hawkins P, Shohet R (2006) *Supervision in the Helping Professions*, 3rd ed. Open University Press.

Hawkins P (2012) *Creating a Coaching Culture*. Oxford University Press.

Health Education England (2019) *NHS Staff and Learners' Mental Wellbeing Commission*. Health Education England.

Honey P, Mumford A (1982) *Manual of Learning Styles*. Peter Honey Publications.

London Leadership Academy (2014) *Coaching and Mentoring Handbook*. Health Education England.

Mendel D, MacDonald-Davis J (2019) Differential attainment toolkit. Available at https://london.hee.nhs.uk/multiprofessional-faculty-development/differential-attainment/differential-attainmenttoolkit.

NHS England (2014) *A Guide to Mentoring*. NHS England.

O'Neill P (2016) The Leadership Development Evaluation Framework: developing evidence based interventions and creating a learning culture. Available at: www.hee.nhs.uk/sites/default/files/documents/Evaluation%20Framework%20vF1.2.pdf.

Rao S, How P, Ton H (2018) Education, training, and recruitment of a diverse workforce in psychiatry. *Psychiatric Annals*, **48**: 143–8.

Roberts G, Moore B, Coles C (2002) Mentoring for newly appointed consultant psychiatrists. *Psychiatric Bulletin*, **26**: 106–9.

Starr J (2008) *The Coaching Manual: The Definitive Guide to the Process, Principles and Skills of Personal Coaching*, 2nd ed. Pearson Education.

Szabo S, Lloyd B, McKellar D, et al. (2019) 'Having a mentor helped me with difficult times': a trainee-run mentoring project. *Australasian Psychiatry*, **27**: 230–3.

Teshima J, McKean AJS, Myint MT, et al. (2019) Developmental approaches to faculty development. *Psychiatric Clinics of North America*, **42**: 375–87.

Viney R, Harris D (2013) Coaching and mentoring. In Bhugra D, Ruiz P, Gupta S (eds.), *Leadership in Psychiatry*. Wiley-Blackwell, pp. 126–36.

West M, Coia D (2019) *Caring for Doctors Caring for Patients: How to Transform UK Healthcare Environments to Support Doctors and Medical Students to Care for Patients*. General Medical Council.

Whitmore J (2017) *Coaching for Performance: The Principles and Practice of Coaching and Leadership*, 5th ed. Nicholas Brealey Publishing.

Woolf K, Potts HWW, McManus IC (2011) Ethnicity and academic performance in UK trained doctors and medical students: systematic review and meta-analysis. *BMJ*, **342**: d901.

Index

Note: Locators in **bold** indicate tables; locators in *Italics* indicate figures.